"The systemic perspective on family dynamics adds fresh insight to existing approaches to parent education. Dr Roberts proposes that second order parenting can enhance the education process by focusing on parental attitudes and behaviors as well as techniques to alter children's behavior. Parent–child interaction is viewed from a wide-angle systemic perspective. Transformational change in the affective climate of the family can arise from unconscious and implicit processes happening within family relationships. I am impressed with the extensive research presented in Dr Roberts's work. Readers from the fields of psychology, child development, family relations, and parent education will appreciate the thorough documentation supporting his recommendations."

—Del Hayden, Professor of Counseling (Emeritus),
Western Kentucky University

"Consistent with the tradition of Carl Whitaker's Symbolic Experiential Psychotherapy model, Dr. Thomas Roberts has written a very controversial book on second order parenting that veers away from typical parenting models in that it focuses on both explicit parenting interventions (first order change/parenting) and implicit parenting interventions (second order change/parenting) where the unconscious and emotional process of learning is emphasized. Using his understanding and knowledge of up-to-date neuroscience research and attachment theory, Dr. Roberts has written a cutting-edge and much-needed parenting book that will resonate with many parents with who want to connect creatively with their children."

—Michael Chafin, Psychotherapist and Former President of the American Association for Marriage and Family Therapy (AAMFT)

INDIRECT PARENTING INTERVENTIONS, NEUROSCIENCE AND THE PARENT-CHILD RELATIONSHIP

This volume explores indirect parenting behavior that changes the structure of the parent–child relationship, examining the ecological dimension of parenting in addition to nurturance and control.

Drawing on neuroscientific research in parenting, it provides a model for how children learn implicitly and how parents can relate to children through indirect means. Thomas W. Roberts argues that first-order parenting techniques, teaching specific behaviors to reduce unwanted child behaviors, are overused. He examines and offers guidance on how indirect interventions that place emphasis on the interactional components of the parent–child relationship, such as modeling, storytelling, reframing, humor, and paradox, referred to as second order parenting, can support parents and children in developing positive relationships.

- Addresses the latest brain research and its application to parent–child interactions
- Introduces the student to aspects of the parent–child relationship that are not covered in most courses
- Useful to clinicians who work directly with parents
- Offers a perspective on parenting that differs from most parenting models
- Facilitates awareness of how unconscious and nonverbal communication affects parenting
- Serves to deepen the relationship with the child and curb unwanted behavior

Indirect Parenting Interventions, Neuroscience and the Parent-Child Relationship will be thought-provoking reading for students and scholars of parenting and family systems, as well as clinicians who work directly with parents, giving them a broader perspective in dealing with parent–child interactions.

Thomas W. Roberts received his Ph.D. degree from the University of Georgia in Child and Family Development. He came to San Diego State University in 1999 as Chair of the Department of Child and Family Development and was chair for nine years. He taught courses in family relationships and public policy and ethics. His research interests include divorce and remarriage, parenting, and applying neuroscience to family relationships. His current projects include how the unconscious plays the pivotal role in intimate family relationships. He has written grants on single-parenting, childhood obesity, early literacy, professional development for early childhood educators, and childhood safety.

INDIRECT PARENTING INTERVENTIONS, NEUROSCIENCE AND THE PARENT-CHILD RELATIONSHIP

Second-Order Parenting

Thomas W. Roberts

Routledge
Taylor & Francis Group
NEW YORK AND LONDON

Designed cover image: Choreograph via Getty Images

First published 2025
by Routledge
605 Third Avenue, New York, NY 10158

and by Routledge
4 Park Square, Milton Park, Abingdon, Oxon, OX14 4RN

Routledge is an imprint of the Taylor & Francis Group, an informa business

Library of Congress Cataloging-in-Publication Data
Names: Roberts, Thomas W., author.
Title: Indirect parenting interventions, neuroscience and the parent-child relationship : second-order parenting / Thomas W. Roberts.
Description: New York, NY : Routledge, 2025. | Includes bibliographical references and index.
Identifiers: LCCN 2024031035 (print) | LCCN 2024031036 (ebook) | ISBN 9781003381679 (hardback) | ISBN 9781032464336 (paperback) | ISBN 9781003381679 (ebook)
Subjects: LCSH: Parent and child—Psychological aspects. | Parenting—Psychological aspects. | Neurosciences.
Classification: LCC BF723.P25 R623 2024 (print) | LCC BF723.P25 (ebook) | DDC 155.9/24—dc23/eng/20240717
LC record available at https://lccn.loc.gov/2024031035
LC ebook record available at https://lccn.loc.gov/2024031036

ISBN: 978-1-032-46428-2 (hbk)
ISBN: 978-1-032-46433-6 (pbk)
ISBN: 978-1-003-38167-9 (ebk)

DOI: 10.4324/9781003381679

Typeset in Times New Roman
by Apex CoVantage, LLC

This book is dedicated to my grandsons: Thomas Judah Roberts and Jesse Solomon Roberts.

CONTENTS

PREFACE

The idea for this book is at least 30 years old and emerged while I was writing *A System's Perspective of Parenting: The Individual, the Family, and the Social Network*. It was in this book where I coined the term *second order parenting* to describe indirect and implicit methods of parenting. I had intended to write this book as a sequel but, as the years passed and I was involved in other academic efforts, it stayed on the back burner. While the term originally referred to indirect interventions, such as storytelling, in the intervening years and with the advent of neuroscience and new research on emotion, the unconscious, and learning, the concept of second order parenting took on a broader meaning. Neuroscience has taught us much about how the unconscious is involved in the conscious and is the major factor in solving problems and learning new information. According to current research, the conscious mind has gotten credit for rational decision making when, in fact, the decision is made in the unconscious before it becomes conscious.

Many of our theories of learning are still based on the view that the conscious mind has an executive function and is in control of what we think and how we act. Subject matter for learning, for the most part, is expected to engage the rational centers of the brain. Effort is made to limit emotional, humorous, and confusing content to a minimum and present material in a logical, rational way. New research has demonstrated that learning does not take place without emotions and that humor and confusion increase learning instead of blocking it. Second order parenting incorporates this research to allow for outside-the-box thinking in parenting, in terms of both the content and the methods of parent training and parental parenting.

The book draws from other disciplines, especially from systemic psychotherapy, because of the focus on paradoxical, indirect, and dialectical thinking. The work of a few therapists, including Milton Erickson, provides invaluable insight into defining how transformational change occurs. This book is an attempt to apply those insights to parenting.

While I have been influenced by many great minds in the parenting literature, as a parent I deviated from the expected ways of parenting. I found myself often using humor, confusion, paradox, storytelling, observation, and mutual relationship-building with my children. These parenting behaviors arose spontaneously and naturally rather than attempting to implement specific interventions.

Writing this book was not meant to provide answers and, in fact, it may raise more questions than it answers. It may be controversial and even considered "wrong" to some readers. What I would ask is that it be taken with an open mind. The purpose is not to undermine current methods of parenting and parent education, but to supplement them with methods that have been underdeveloped in the literature. With progress and research advancements, humanity often learns it does not know what it thinks it knew. Understanding is not a static state we come to, but a constantly revolving door of *aha* moments. My hope is that this book and the contents therein will spark insight in others, lighting the path toward greater awareness of human development.

ACKNOWLEDGMENT

I wish to thank my editor, Molly Selby, and her staff at Routledge for their assistance of this publication. Additionally, I am grateful to Michael Chafin, former President of the American Association for Marriage and Family Therapy, and Delbert Hayden, Emeritus Professor in the Department of Counseling at Western Kentucky University, both of whom read chapters and offered feedback. I am indebted to my daughter, Kara Roberts, who copyedited the chapters and made valuable suggestions on chapter content, figures, and tables, and without whose help this book would not have been completed. I thank my wife, Karen, for her patience and support during the writing of this book.

PART I

The Basics of Parenting and Family Development

1

INTRODUCTION TO PARENTING MODELS

Evolution of Parenting

The primary role of parents in their offsprings' lives is to ensure that the children grow up and become functioning adults. This role has been noted in ancient literature, such as in the Greek writings of Plato and in the words of the Christian Bible, "Train up a child in the way he should go and when he is old, he will not depart from it" (*King James Bible*, 2008). Parenting today differs greatly from parenting in times past (Buchanan & Glatz, 2022). There are less definable paths into adulthood in modern society and assuming an adult role belies the unencumbered transition from childhood to adulthood of our ancient ancestors. Far from being natural in the 21st century, parenting is an endeavor that requires parents who possess healthy habits and social behaviors, and who also have knowledge of child development.

Advances in technology and social media over the past half century have affected both the types of interaction and the quality of those interactions of parents and their children. Social media, the availability of cell phones, video games, and other forms of technology have decreased the contact between parents and their children. The main consequence of the increase of social media on the parent–child relationship is less face-to-face interaction and a higher risk for attachment disorder (Ante-Contreras, 2016).

Coupled with the advances in technology and social media, cultural and historical changes have made a mark on the frequency and quality of the parent–child relationship. For example, as late as the 1940s and 1950s, *extended families* lived near the *nuclear family* to provide physical and mental support. The transformation from a mainly agrarian to an urban society that took place beginning in the 1950s led to greater mobility within families. Adult children followed job opportunities, which resulted in being more distant from their family of origin. Thus, the familial

DOI: 10.4324/9781003381679-2

support system was no longer possible in the fast-paced and mobile societal structure (Atkinson, 2022).

The changes within the American society over the past four decades have increased the stress of parenting (Walper & Kreyenfeld, 2022), which appears exacerbated by certain factors such as the presence of *poverty* (Beasley et al., 2022). Forty percent of children today are being raised in low-income families, which are beset with economic, social, educational, and occupational deficits. Substance abuse, mental illness, childhood diseases, and developmental delays are significantly higher in poverty and low-income families and create a condition of chronic stress (Chen, 2022). While all families were impacted by COVID-19, parenting within low-income families tended to be more affected (Czeisler et al., 2020).

Other factors related to stress in parenting in the 21st century include extending the period of *adolescence*, which has resulted in children residing in their parents' home until their mid- or late-20s and, in some cases, returning home after being on their own. In general, adult children living at home feel greater stress, especially if there are unresolved issues from childhood with their parents. This interruption in young adults taking on adult roles is related to several emotional and social issues (Fass, 2016). According to Fass, from the earliest times in American history, childhood was characterized by autonomous behavior and independence that transitioned into adulthood in the late teens.

What was considered the end of childhood in 1950 was around 20 years of age, but today childhood extends to 26 or even older with detrimental effects on children. Child development theorists, such as Erik Erikson (1950), believed that adolescence ended at approximately 20 years of age which ushered in adulthood. Young adults were expected to be on their own. This longer reliance on parents today impedes the young adult person from establishing their own independence and self-reliance, and may foster the existence of the overinvolved parent.

All these factors are related to greater *stress in parenting*, which has resulted in a proliferation of parenting education models (Figure 1.1). While parenting was considered natural in times past, today it is generally believed that parents need support and training to be effective parents. In the past 50 years, there has been an inundation of books on parenting. Initially, theories of human behavior guided the development and application of parenting models. Slowly, as research began to paint a picture of effective parenting skills, theoretical applications became less important. Today, evidence-based interventions tend to cross theoretical lines and meld interventions into less identifiable theoretical perspectives. One common theme throughout this transition in parent education models is that parenting is natural behavior only to a point, and knowledge and skill development are needed.

Parent education models developed out of a desire to improve parent–child relationships in families in which children were having behavior problems at home, at school, and with peer relationships. High-risk families were identified and in many of these families, significant dysfunction and instability existed. Interventions for the most part assumed a psychotherapeutic flavor that developed from applying

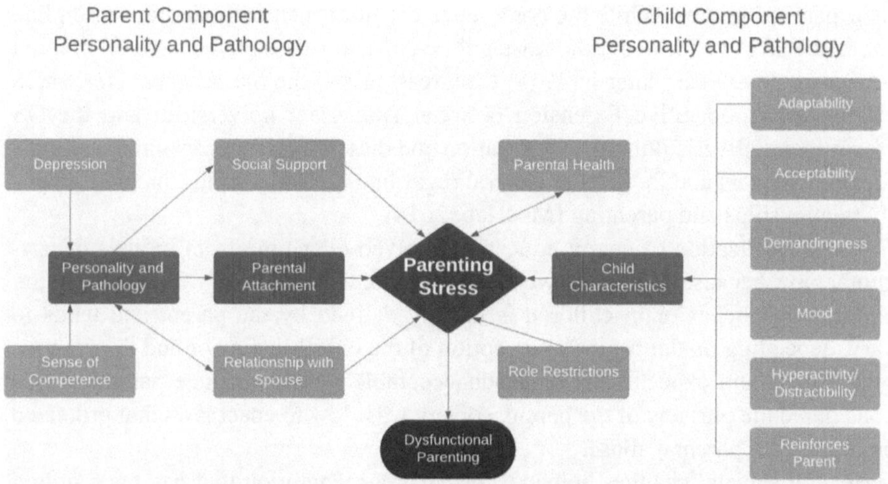

FIGURE 1.1 Parenting stress develops from a combination of many factors from both the parent's personality and pathology, and the child's personality and pathology. (Kim, 2019, CC BY-SA 4.0)

therapy techniques to working with these families. Stopping and preventing child abuse and neglect has remained a major focus of parent education programs.

Generally, early parent education models assumed that parents needed specific skills to effectively counter their children's misbehavior. Parents who were abusive or neglectful had to attend parent education to be reunited with their children. While parent education models have evolved over the past several decades, it is important to understand the basic structure of the early approaches, including the Behavioral model, Parent Effective Training (PET), and Adlerian approach. The next section of this chapter will review parent education models and how models have evolved over the years.

Models of Parenting Education

While concerns about parenting were present in periods before laws exited to protect children and before parent education models formally existed, support for parents with child problems was provided by families and community. Beginning in the early 1800s, concerns about the welfare of children were initiated by mothers who often formed small groups to discuss their concerns (Croake & Glover, 1977). As time passed and the need to address parenting concerns became more apparent, various initiatives were untaken. One change that occurred was the engagement of the government which organized the first *Conference on the Welfare of the Child* in 1909 (Stretch, 1970). President Theodore Roosevelt assigned the conference the responsibility of determining future pathways for children who resided outside their parents' homes. While the conference did not specifically address discipline for misbehaving children, it did raise public consciousness on the state of children in society. Five years later in 1914, Congress passed the *Smith–Lever Act* which established Cooperative Extension between land grant universities and the US Department of Agriculture for the creation and dissemination of resource materials for rural farmers and families in general regarding a host of topics, including family relationships and parenting (MacNab, 2014).

The formalization of parent education evolved over time from models of psychotherapy because therapists were the first contact for help with misbehaving children. Misbehavior in children is usually defined by the parent and tends to vary, depending on the parent's perception of the child's behavior and the parent's own beliefs and expectations about unacceptable behavior. Since parenting was considered the purview of the parent, society was slow to enact laws that protected children from parental abuse.

Several societal changes helped to usher in a recognition that parents required guidance and that parent education was needed (Lantsburg, 2016). One concern was the increase in the number of families below the poverty line and inequity of resources available to these families. This growing concern about the vulnerability of *at-risk families* occurred in the 1960s and was noted by the *Moynihan Report* (1965), an analysis of the Black family which noted specifically the vulnerability of Black children to succeed due to educational and economic disadvantages. Beginning in the 1960s and extending into the present day, an increase in single-parent families began that affected Black families in great numbers. Research on single-parent families began to show problems with parenting, school behavior, and educational achievement in significantly greater numbers than two-parent families (Brennan, 2021). Other factors, such as technological advances in the form of access to social media, drug and alcohol addiction, domestic violence, and child abuse and neglect, had negative effects on families and particularly low income and poverty level families. One way to counteract these negative factors was to intervene at the parenting level to increase parenting effectiveness in these families.

The earliest models of parenting education tended to emphasize different aspects of child misbehavior. For example, the misbehavior of the child and the reinforcing of the misbehavior by the parent was the main concentration of the *Behavioral model* (Patterson, 1982). *Parent Effectiveness Training (PET)* (Gordon, 1975) emphasized communication between the child and parent, while aiding the child in learning responsibility and the consequences of the misbehavior was the focus of the *Adlerian model* (Adler, 1927/2003), as developed by Rudolph Dreikurs (1964). While these first approaches do not appear so much today in their original forms, they heavily influenced the evolution of parent education models and are briefly discussed later.

The Adlerian Model

The Child Guidance Center developed by Adler was aimed at improving social relations among the family and within the community. His method of working with a family while other families watched was seminal for later approaches to family therapy that involved the whole family. Adler's methods were expanded and specifically applied to parenting by Dreikurs.

The Adlerian approach offered a unique perspective by focusing on the child's goals in purposeful behavior that the parent views as misbehavior. To find a secure place within their social environment, children adopt mistaken immediate-level goals, including attention, power, revenge, and inadequacy (Dreikurs, 1964). These goals represent a lineal progression from attention to inadequacy, depending on the parent mishandling the goals.

The approach also views the role of the parent as providing respect and understanding in place of showing power and control over the child. If the parent can understand the motivation for the child's behavior, a strategy of providing a logical consequence for the behavior can be enacted. *Logical consequences* do not follow directly from the children's behavior like a *natural consequence*, but describe the relationship between statements and action, acting as a true consequence of the behavior. It must make sense to the child, or it will not be effective. From this perspective, parents are encouraged not to engage in power struggles or to react in anger at the child's misbehavior. Punitive behavior by the parent only leads to greater defiance by the child. Forming a cooperative alliance with the child in a democratic-style relationship of respect and equality is the ideal parenting stance.

At the heart of parent–child relationship within the family, according to Dreikurs (1955), is a democratic model that undercuts the parents' superiority position and the child's inferiority position. The parents and child must be viewed as equals within the family unit. *Democratic families* are not to be confused with permissive parents who abnegate their responsibility. Allowing for mutual respect and freedom gives the child a framework for learning that choices can have consequences, which result from the behavior itself or logical consequences that the parent imposes because of the child's behavior. The Adlerian parenting education model is based on education and assumes that pathology is not the cause for the child misbehaving (Hoffman, 2020). Parents must foster a family environment that is open to learning new skills and ways to adapt to changing circumstances.

Parent Effectiveness Training (PET)

PET was developed by Thomas Gordon (1975) and has similarities with Adlerian parenting in that it is non-punitive and embraces a democratic posture between parent and child. Contrary to models that use punishment, PET resolves conflicts between parents and children by recognizing the needs of both. PET focuses on developing positive communication patterns that prevent a win–lose dynamic where the parent wins and the child loses (Gordon, 2000). Instead, PET's *no-lose approach* will allow for mutual resolution of conflicts that benefit both parent and child. Based on the belief that children do not misbehave, the goal of parenting intervention is to understand the need the child is attempting to meet by their behavior. While acknowledging that the child's behavior is undesirable, the parent must direct the child in more acceptable ways of behaving. The parent communicating in this fashion reduces the loss of self-esteem and negative self-image that accompanies punitive models.

Understanding that both the parent and the child have needs that should be met leads to negotiating ways to meet those needs (Gordon, 2000). Thus, children are involved in the process of resolving the conflict by offering their thoughts and suggestions. In this way, children are encouraged as participants in the resolution process to solve their own problems. This participation allows children to buy into the solution rather than having it forced on them.

While this approach seems straightforward, it would be difficult for most parents, especially those who are unfamiliar with child development theories. Parents must be good communicators, emotionally stable, and patient. Numerous research studies have provided support for this model which continues to be used today (Cedar & Levant, 1990; Davidson & Wood, 2004). However, some research has been mixed. For example, Haffey and Levant (1984) found that while PET did improve parents' communications skills, it did not improve children's communication skills. Oryan and Gastil (2013), in an exhaustive review of PET and Adlerian models, found that neither were truly democratic and that parents guided the process. The researchers recommended that both models be reconfigured, with the parent as a type of manager that guides the process.

The benefits of the PET model include improving communication skills, teaching children effective ways of negotiating conflict resolutions peacefully which can carry over to their peer relationships, improving self-esteem and *self-efficacy*, creating and maintaining a firm bond with parents, reducing parenting stress, and reducing adversarial relationships within the family. The effectiveness of the PET model weakens, however, when employed by less educated parents or parents who have already established entrenched negative patterns.

Behavioral Model

The Behavioral Model posits that children learn how to behave in social situations through others' reinforcement (Patterson, 1982). Punishment, administered via strict guidelines, can be used by the parent to change behavior. A child's behavior stems from the parents' behavior, mirrors the parental behavior, and is subsequently reinforced or rewarded by the parent. Put simply, the parent changes their rewarding or reinforcing behavior to change the child's behavior. The child's misbehavior is the result of socialization, rather than from a diagnosed mental or emotional disorder. Misbehavior displayed at home is likely to continue in other social settings, such as at school when authority figures try to regulate behavior (Fox et al., 2002). This makes it more critical for the parent to learn specific techniques for adjusting unwanted behavior.

To change behavior, parents are taught new skills to reward behavior they want to see continue and to stop bad behavior. This process is done in a stepwise fashion to shape the new behavior over time. Rewards, consisting of social features, material effects, and privileges are introduced to parents as a means to shape behavior. Social rewards are generally more effective depending on the quality of the overall relationship with the parent. Parents are taught specific techniques for how to give rewards, which generally are done repeatedly until firmly established and then continued intermittently.

When rewards fail to change the undesired behavior, parents are taught other techniques such as various forms of punishment, including timeout. Timeout removes the child from the present situation and is useful for aggressive children. There are specific guidelines for how to use timeout effectively. Timeout and other forms of punishment may be appropriate for aggressive acting out behavior, but less effective for sensitive children and nonacting out behavior. The parent tends to take more control of the situation from a behavioral approach than other parenting approaches (Pinsker & Geoffrey, 1981).

Other researchers have also found limitations to the behavioral parenting approach (Figure 1.2). Cagan (1980) was concerned with the mechanistic features of the approach due to the one-way dynamic of influence, with the parent influencing the child through rewards and reinforcements. The parent–child relationship is a reciprocal two-way interaction in which both influence each other. Fabes et al. (1989) concluded that children may not continue desired behaviors unless parents continue to reward them. The use of rewards does not seem to change underlying attitudes of the child. The Behavioral approach does not consider the child's internal emotional system as important in changing or maintaining behavior (Schwartz, 1986). The behavioral change is guided by external means and the *relationship* between parent and child is of little concern. While the application of the behavioral model has been largely ineffective in a broad general use, researchers have concluded that it is effective with two clinical populations—children with learning disabilities (Gates et al., 2001) and children who engage in high-risk behavior (Stolz et al., 2010).

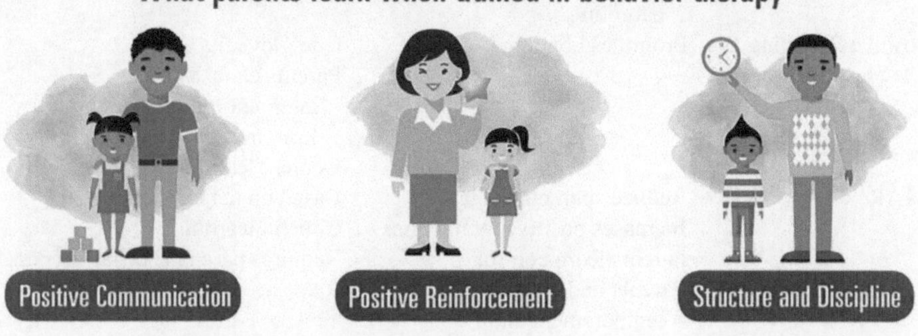

FIGURE 1.2 Behavioral parent training teaches parents how to reinforce and reward behavior (Commons Wikimedia) https://commons.wikimedia.org/wiki/File:What_parents_learn_when_trained_in_behavior_therapy.jpg

Evolution of Parenting Education Models

While the above three parent education models had seminal influence over the parent education field, they spawned a proliferation of new models that attempted to address issues raised by research evaluations. Importantly, it became clear that families are more diverse and culturally different than the above models implied (Fine & Lee, 2001). Furthermore, these models failed to acknowledge the difference in families because of poverty and social disadvantages (see Table 1.1).

Another major concern about all three models is that they failed to include developmental stages. Rather than focusing on children's needs and reasons for

TABLE 1.1 Comparing Models of Parent Education

Model	*Pros*	*Cons*
Adlerian	Improves bonding Improves communication Uses both explicit and implicit methods	Fails to identify development Ineffective with aggression Family culture and background unimportant
Parent Effectiveness Training	Improves communication Improves negotiating skills Improves bonding Creates positive interactions	Geared to educated parents Ineffective with aggression Family background unimportant
Behavioral	Effective with aggression Effective in residential settings	First order change Explicit learning model Overemphasis on rewards Not generalizable Family background unimportant Content learning
STEP	Improves communication skills Promotes bonding Decreases authoritarian parenting	Unreliable research results
Positive Parenting	Promotes bonding	One glove fits all Parents choose online interventions without input from trainers Content learning
STAR	Reduces parental anger Increases positive interactions Parents learn control Parents understand child's temperament and developmental level	Based on deficit model Content learning Requires parental self-awareness Requires educated parents
SFP 10–14	Reciprocal interaction Adapts for culture	Based on deficit model Content learning

misbehavior at different ages, the models implied that "one size fits all," meaning age and developmental level were not addressed. For example, PET and Adlerian models do not distinguish between the cognitive level of the child at different ages but assume that children of all ages are able to participate equally with the parent in negotiating outcomes. Later evolution of parent education models have attempted to address developmental matters. Table 1.1 provides a summary of some of the current parent education models that evolved from these early models.

Systematic Training for Effective Parenting (STEP)

Following in the Adlerian tradition of parenting as developed by Rudolph Dreikurs (1964), Don Dinkmeyer and Gary McKay (1973) developed the STEP parenting education program, which can be used for all ages of children and types of families. The model was developed to help parents of misbehaving children and expectant parents who want to create more harmonious relationships with their children. It has been an effective model when used with parents who are trying to regain custody of their children after the children's removal from the home (Adams, 2001). The goals of the nine-week STEP training program are to improve communication, create mutual respect among family members, improve cooperation among members, and increase children learning the consequences and taking responsibility for their behavior. The nine sessions are approximately of 1.5 hours in a group setting of 6–12 parents. Parents learn good methods of communicating with their children, how to listen and give support, how to facilitate responsibility and understanding consequences of behavior, and the structure and importance of family meetings.

To address developmental matters, the program is offered in four different versions—early childhood for parents of young children; children 6–12; a Spanish version of children 6–12; and a version with parents of teenagers. Since 1976, there has been wide use of STEP, which has generated numerous research evaluations. The STEP program is based on a belief that children have faulty views of their experiences that activate negative emotions and uncooperative behavior. Also, the program is founded on the belief that when parents change their behavior by helping children understand their faulty beliefs and misinterpretations, children concomitantly change their behavior (Brock et al., 1993).

In a review of *evidence-based research* designs and findings, research to evaluate the effectiveness of the STEP program found that studies generally used measures that had high validity and reliability (SAMHSA'S National Registry of Evidence-Based Programs and Practices, no date). Generally, the studies adjusted for sample size and outcomes were measured by participants improving from clinical to healthy functioning. The evaluation also found some major weaknesses in the studies, including not comparing the outcomes of those who dropped out to participants who completed the program, very small sample sizes, inadequate comparison groups, and in some cases changing the research design during applying the program.

Other research studies on STEP have produced more positive results. For example, a study conducted by Larson (2000) on the use of STEP with parents of teens found that there was a decrease in *authoritarian parenting* and an increase in the overall quality of the parent–child relationship. A weakness of the study was that there was no comparison group, and the sample was only English-speaking middle-class White families. Another study by Jonynienė (2013) on the efficacy of STEP found that it was effective in decreasing authoritarian parenting and improving the parent–child relationship. The follow-up reports revealed that the changes were lasting.

To date, STEP is used extensively in various settings in schools, by therapists, and by parent educators who continue to do research on the effectiveness of the program (Kubli, 2022). It is believed to be a promising evidence-based model for parent education.

Recent Application of Behavioral Modification Parenting Education Programs

Behavioral modification parenting programs continue to be used widely for specific child problems that need intensive managing, such as attention-deficit/hyperactivity disorder (ADHD), and research has confirmed the effectiveness of the programs (Chacko et al., 2020). Behavioral parenting when coupled with medication has been found to be very effective in controlling ADHD. Behavioral parenting is based on the belief that parenting children, especially those with management issues, is stressful on parents who need better skill development and knowledge to be effective. Several behavioral parenting training models using similar interventions have been developed in recent years. Below is a brief discussion of some of the most used and researched models.

Positive Parenting Program

Referred to as the Triple P, this model is an integrative parenting approach that pulls from cognitive behavioral theory, social learning theory, and developmental components (Padilla-Walker et al., 2012). Triple P is a skills-oriented program that teaches parents specific interventions to use for specific problems. Research studies over the past three decades have shown how this model has improved parent–child relationships and increased parents' confidence in their ability to effectively deal with their child's misbehavior and prevent problems from arising in the future (Rodrigo et al., 2012). The training is offered in both in-person and online sessions, which allows parents to work through the program at their own pace and time.

Triple P offers specific interventions for temper tantrums, bedtime dawdling, openly defiant behavior, disrespectful behavior toward parents and other authority figures, problems with social relationships, and other problems that parents identify.

The developers of this model integrated behavioral family therapy, child parenting developmental theory, behavioral analysis, and psychotherapy to apply to a broad range of family and child problems. The program has generated a wide range of research support for young children, teens, and adolescents (Turner et al., 2007).

STAR Parenting

STAR parenting is an acronym for S—stop yourself from immediately responding; T—think about emotions; A—ask self about expectations for child's behavior; R—respond in an appropriate developmental way (Fox & Fox, 1992). The underlying theoretical base is cognitive behavioral theory, influenced heavily by the writings of Baumrind (1966) on authoritative parenting.

The goals of STAR parenting are to reduce parental anger and authoritarian interactions with children and, therefore, increase the positive interaction with children. The focus is on how the parents interact with the child. It gives parents a process to repeat for different problems. The process is meant to give parents choices of how to act toward their misbehaving child rather than tell them how to act. While the program is geared toward the parent, the reciprocal nature of parent–child interaction is of primary concern. The child's temperament, developmental level, and long-term goals are necessary for the parent to know to respond in the most effective manner. Research studies typically show a decrease in parental anger and distress and harsh punishment (Collins & Fetsch, 2017).

Strengthening Families Program for Parents and Youths 10–14 (SFP 10–14)

The SFP 10–14 parenting education program is a seven-session parenting program based on combining two approaches that support healthy family development—the biopsychosocial model (DeMarsh & Kumpfer, 1986) and the risk and prevention model (Spoth et al., 2001). SFP 10–14 intends to build adaptive skills for both parents and children, improve family strengths, and improve the overall relationship of parents and their children in a reciprocal interactional loop. Research by Spoth et al. (2013) and Trudeau et al. (2016) confirm the effectiveness of the program in treating and preventing substance abuse in young teens.

SFP is innovative in that it adjusts for cultural considerations and requires at least five families, providing an environment for group dynamics and learning (Hockaday, 2020). Parents and children have concurrent but separate sessions in the first hour, followed by family group sessions. Multiple facilitators lead the sessions, who then provide feedback and input for processing sessions. Each session utilizes several delivery methods, including didactic information from facilitators, media presentations, role-playing, and group activities and ends with participants sharing what they learned.

Current Concerns Addressed in High-Quality Models

The above highlights only a few of the numerous parenting education models and space does not allow for elaboration on all of them. While models vary in specific content and focus, they share common purposes and goals (see Table 1.2). Parent education models predictably emphasize several similar aspects (National Academies of Science, Engineering, and Medicine (NASEM), 2016): Improving communication between parents and children, increasing positive prosocial behavior in children, and decreasing negative behavior, improving the overall quality of family interactions, increasing the emotional well-being and mental health of parents through skill development, increasing self-efficacy of parents in their role as parents.

A major shift in parenting interventions has occurred over the past several decades resulting from the emphasis on evidence-based programs (NASEM, 2016). Evidence-based programs have solid high-quality research that supports the effectiveness of the program. Generally, research evidence supports interventions that improve the overall quality of the family environment (Barth & Liggett-Creel, 2014). Home visitation programs are the most common for families with 0- to 4-year-old children, but a paucity of research exists for this age group.

Evidence-based programs reveal that the involvement of at-risk fathers is a missing link of parenting education programs in the past and increases the possibility of successful outcomes. The *Nurturing Fathers' program* is an example of how fathers can be trained in family strengths and knowledge of child development (Nurturing Fathers' Program, n.d.) The program consists of 2.5-hour sessions for 13 weeks. Fathers are exposed to nurturing interventions which can enhance their ability to communicate more effectively and be a more involved family member. This greater involvement as a parent has positive effects on the marital relationship

TABLE 1.2 Common Elements of Parent Education Programs

Pros	*Cons*
• *Promotes positive communication patterns* • Facilitates interactions that improve nurturing behavior • Increases emotional regulation in children • Reduces parental punishing behavior • Establishes parental consistency in applying discipline • Offers parenting material in a variety of media • Focuses on new skill-building exercises • Reflects evidence-based research • Uses predetermined training material • Improves family relationships	• *Does not allow for individualized interventions* • Does not require all persons involved in parenting to attend • Program evaluation is based on verbal assessment, not on observed behavior

as they learn how to be more vulnerable in their marital relationship (Carlson & Turner, 2010). According to Daire et al. (2007), involvement in the Nurturing Program improved fathers' knowledge of child development, changed their attitude toward corporal punishment, decreased attitudes that are associated with abuse, and increased aptitudes related to empowerment of children.

The *Incredible Years program* is an evidence-based parenting education program that offers individual programs for parents with infants (0–1), toddlers (1–3), preschoolers (3–6), and school-age (6–12) (Incredible Years Program, n.d.). The goals of the program are to improve attachment, reduce harsh and punitive parenting, and prevent disruptive behavior with conduct disorder and ADHD. A long-term goal is to improve academic success by reducing school dropout and reducing acting out behavior.

Intervention parent education programs for fathers in prison has become a new trend in parenting education because the number of fathers in prison has increased and the impact of father absence in these homes can be very stressful for mothers and children (Bushfield, 2004). Bushfield conducted a three-day parent education program with incarcerated fathers. Results indicated that incarcerated fathers changed attitudes of corporal punishment and were more receptive to role reversal.

The *Responsible Fatherhood (RF) program* is a federally funded program that works primarily with fathers who are currently incarcerated or fathers reentering society who have been involved in the criminal justice system (Alamillo et al., 2021). While the RF program does not include children or one-on-one sessions, the group setting produces changes in knowledge, and attitudes toward parenting that show improved changes. The RF program does not address the crucial issues of the quality of the parent–child relationship and the well-being of the child.

Parent education programs have been translated into Spanish to be more fitting for Spanish-speaking parents. Given that there are increasing numbers of Latino families in the United States, many of which speak Spanish in the home with small children, there is an urgent need to provide parent education materials in Spanish and to adapt the programs to fit the Latino culture (Calzada, 2010). Programs adopt concepts and practices that are common in the Latino community, such as *familismo*, stressing the importance of strong family ties and loyalty (Lakes et al., 2011; Montanez et al., 2010). Providing meals and family sharing improve attendance to parent education programs and reduce recidivism.

Future Trends in Parent Education

The purpose in this section of the chapter is to point out what is missing in parent education programs and how to include new ideas that are supported by recent neuroscience research. In a comprehensive review of the parent education literature, Morris et al. (2020) gave several suggestions for further development of parent education models. These suggestions include (1) greater focus and visibility on the earliest years of development because of the vulnerability of this group for abuse and trauma; (2) provide more resources for parents whose children vary from developmental norms; (3) articulate more clearly the programs geared toward minority populations; (4) understand more clearly the needs of parents and children in all types of family structures; (5) develop models that are more conducive to involvement of fathers; (6) develop new ways of disseminating materials so that underrepresented parents are included; (7) increase research efforts; and (8) allow for flexibility in presenting programs.

While Morris et al. (2020) have focused on important issues of future development of parent education models, their suggestions can be considered thinking "inside the box" and focuses on how to change existing content and structure to better deliver information. This is needed and important to do, but this book takes the position that there is also a need to think "outside the box," or what we can learn from other disciplines and research, namely, neuroscience, which can inform new directions in parent education (see Table 1.3).

One issue that needs further illuminating regarding thinking outside the box is the structure of parent education models. While models of parent education differ in specific content, they tend to have similar structure and purpose. The structure is educational in the sense that information is presented to participants in the form of didactic activities, group discussion, role-play, and media, such as videos. The underlying structure assumes that participants are missing specific parenting skills that are needed to have a fully functioning parent–child relationship (Morris et al., 2020). These skills include improving the quality of parent–child communication, helping children learn emotional regulation, helping parents learn effective discipline interventions, problem-solving skills, and reducing stress (Borden et al., 2016). Models further assume that the training materials are sufficient to correct those deficiencies and evaluation of the outcomes will demonstrate that the model mostly achieves the desired purpose.

The basic structure of parent education models can be labeled a **deficit approach** because it views participants as needing to develop new skills. Because of this assumption, participants are viewed as subjects who lack certain skills and who can be taught in ongoing sessions, which vary from model to model. Some critics

TABLE 1.3 Thinking Outside the Box for Future Directions in Parent Education

Change the structure form educational to experiential
Eliminate deficit thinking in program construction
Focus on the parents' strengths
Use positive input and humor
Construct programs based on learning theory and neuroscience
To enhance learning, focus on emotions and how parents feel about the training
Use implicit interventions, such as storytelling and dialectical/implicit methods
Encourage confusion and the resolution of confusion
Provide for periods of distraction to enhance aha experiences

of the deficit model believe that instead of strengthening participants, the long-term effects are detrimental because the deficits of participants can be overemphasized, and the strengths can be minimized (Davidson & Orsini, 2013). The deficit approach, particularly with manualized models that present the same material to all participants, assumes that all participants have similar deficits and need the training that is either general or individualized for participants.

To counteract the deficit model of **skill-building**, the trend in several recent models is to focus on the strengths and skills of the participants and expand on them (Morris et al., 2020). This positive approach is based in the belief that persons have hidden skills and strengths that need to be recognized and broadened. This approach assumes that negative emotions reduce the motivation to change, while positive emotions increase self-efficacy and empowerment (Miller, 2008). The emphasis on positivity reflects the work of Martin Seligman (2007) and operates on conscious control of staying attentive to positive thoughts and emotions. Some have criticized the positive focus because motives and emotions are not controlled by conscious thought (Ryle, 1990; Miller & Buckhout, 1973). It is worth asking if trying to apply conscious control to emotions in relatively short training sessions, like parent education, has desired lasting effects. While we can certainly reflect on thoughts, behaviors, and motivations, the actual progression of doing so reflects unconscious inklings that we are not aware of (Ayan, 2018). How the unconscious guides thoughts, behaviors, attitudes, and other mental processes needs greater emphasis in parent education models and these concerns will be addressed in more detail throughout this book.

Another assumption that is present in models of parent education is that participants learn new skills that are presented in a variety of formats. *How* a person learns a new skill is extremely important. Since learning is the basic way change in behavior will occur, a developed concept of learning should be addressed in parent education models. The model for learning employed by parent education programs is referred to as content learning (Merriam, 2015), placing learning within a particular context. This context includes the participants and the method of presentation. What is implied in parent education models is that learning is the result of explicit and rational presentations. This view of learning as the most efficient way may be limited, and recent neuroscience research raises questions regarding how learning takes place. The underlying focus on using different types of presentations, such as didactic information, group discussion, role-play, and the like, fail to shed light on brain processes that are involved in learning. For example, *observation* is the key to learning by young children (Harris, 2012). Parent education models typically do not emphasize observation as an intervention. A full discussion of neuroscience and how we learn unconsciously will be discussed in greater detail in other chapters.

Human relationships, including parenting, form based on emotional attachments that are mainly outside of conscious thought. *Attachment*, which is so important for later emotional security, forms early in development without rational or conscious awareness. While attachment theory is prominent in some recent models of parent education, the process of *reattachment* as an implicit and nonconscious process is not clearly articulated. Attachment and reattachment are not direct, rational processes. Furthermore, there is evidence that one's attachment style remains relatively consistent throughout the lifespan and forms the basis for adult romantic relationships (Campbell & Stanton, 2019). The neocortex is later in developing and the emotional areas of the brain develop first, including one's attachment style. Learning at this early age is characterized as occurring outside of conscious awareness, and the main avenue for learning arises from play, not a structured learning situation.

The structural paradigm of most parent education models can be labeled *First Order Parenting (FOP)*. First order parenting reflects the concept of first order change in systems theory (Maier, 2008), which is change brought about by direct, conscious efforts to change the system (see Table 1.2). This book suggests that parent education models should include more experiences in which participants can learn implicitly, referred to as *Second Order Parenting (SOP)*. Second order parenting refers to change that occurs unconsciously or implicitly. Chapter 2 will discuss first order and second order parenting at length (see Table 1.4).

In addition to the above concerns, parental love is not a concept generally associated with parent education models, yet it is a fundamental aspect of parenting. To operationalize love is a difficult task because prescribing behaviors viewed to be loving fail to encapsulate its deeper meaning. Much of what we consider as love is implicit, unconscious, and nondescript. While love may have many characteristics like positivity, nurturance, and attachment, it is a unique concept that lacks development in parent education models. Essentially, parents cannot be trained to love their children; love is an instinctual, innate feeling presented externally to others via specific behaviors.

Parent education models tend to focus on the neocortex or rational brain processes in learning while minimizing emotions and emotional processes. Recent brain research makes less distinction between them and indicates that emotional and implicit processes dominate brain activity (Ayan, 2018). What is thought of as

TABLE 1.4 Comparing First Order and Second Order Parenting

First Order Parenting	*Second Order Parenting*
Direct change	Indirect change
Change in an individual	Transformational change in system
Direct interventions	Indirect interventions
Predetermined	Spontaneous
Scripted	Creative
Rational	Paradoxical
Reflects linear thinking	Reflects circular thinking

rational activity engaging the neocortex is in reality the activation of the emotional centers of the brain and not the neocortex. This book will show that emotional processes are paramount, and interventions should be broadened to access emotional centers of the brain.

The following chapters will present a model of parenting and parent education that will emphasize indirect, implicit, unconscious, and creative interventions that hopefully will further advance the evolution of ideas and interventions for parenting and parent education. These suggestions are not meant to replace or undermine parenting and parent education practices already in use. Rather, parenting and parent education models are deemed to be evolving and must reflect the latest research. Neuroscience offers new research, which to date has had little application to parenting and parent education models. This book is an attempt to fill that void.

References

Adams, J. F. (2001). Impact of parent training on family functioning. *Child and Family Behavior Therapy, 23*(1), 29–42.

Adler, A. (2003). *The collected works of Alfred Adler*. The Alfred Adler Institute of Northwestern Washington. (Original work published 1927)

Alamillo, J., Williams, B., & Avellar, S. (2021). *The effects of parenting programs for incarcerated and reentering fathers*. Framing Research: Brief Reports, OPRE Report 2021–140. Office of Planning, Research, and Evaluation, Administration for Children and Families, U.S. Department of Health and Human Services.

Ante-Contreras, D. (2016). Distracted parenting: How social media affects parent-child attachment. *Electronic Theses, Projects, and Dissertations, 292*. https://scholarworks.lib.csusb.edu/etd/292

Atkinson, V. S. (2022). Every picture tells a story: Parenting advice books provide a window on the past. *Social Sciences, 11,* 11. https://doi.org/10.3390/socsci11010011

Ayan, S. (2018). The brain's autopilot mechanism steers consciousness. *Scientific American*. Retrieved November 30, 2022, from https://www.scientificamerican.com/article/the-brains-autopilot-mechanism-steers-consciousness/

Barth, R. P., & Liggett-Creel, K. (2014). Common components of parenting programs for children birth to eight years of age involved with child welfare services. *Children and Youth Services Review, 40,* 6–12. https://doi.org/10.1016/j.childyouth.2014.02.004

Baumrind, D. (1966). Effects of authoritative parental control on child behavior. *Child Development, 37,* 887–907.

Beasley, L. O., Jespersen, J. E., Morris, A. S., Farra, A., & Hays-Grudo, J. (2022). Parenting challenges and opportunities among families living in poverty. *Social Sciences, 11*, 119. https://doi.org/10.3390/socsci11030119

Borden, L. M., Gunty, A., Lu, Z., Mischel, E., Otto, M., & Richmond, A. (2016). *Enhancing child outcomes through high quality parent education programs*. Research Outreach, Center for Research and Outreach (REACH), University of Minnesota.

Brennan, D. (2021). How does single parenting affect a child? *MedicineNet*. Retrieved December 1, 2022, from https://www.medicinenet.com/how_does_single_parenting_affect_a_child/article.htm

Brock, G. W., Oertwein, M., & Coufal, J. D. (1993). Parent education: Theory, research, and practice. In M. Arcus, J. Schvaneveldt, & J. Moss (Eds.), *Handbook of family life education: The practice of family life education* (Vol. 2, pp. 87–114). SAGE.

Buchanan, C. M., & Glatz, T. (2022). Introduction to special issue: Parenting in the 21st century. *Social Science, 11,* 484. https://doi.org/10.3390/socsci11100484

Bushfield, S. (2004). Fathers in prison: Impact on parent education. *Journal of Correctional Education, 55*(2), 104–166.

Cagan, E. (1980, January–February). The positive parent: Raising children the scientific way. *Social Policy, 10*(4), 40–48.

Calzada, E. J. (2010). Bringing culture into parent training with Latinos. *Cognitive and Behavioral Practice, 17,* 167–175.

Campbell, L., & Stanton, S. C. E. (2019). Adult attachment and trust in romantic relationships. *Current Opinions in Psychology, 25*(1), 148–151. https://doi.org/10.1016/j.copsyc.2018.08.004

Carlson, M. J., & Turner, K. J. (2010, April 15–17). *Fathers' involvement and fathers' well-being over children's first five years.* A presentation at the Annual Meeting of the Population Association of America, Dallas, TX.

Cedar, B., & Levant, R. F. (1990). A meta-analysis of the effects of parent effectiveness training. *American Journal of Family Therapy, 18,* 373–384.

Chacko, A., Hopkins, K., Acri, M., Mendelsohn, A., & Dreyer, B. (2020). Expanding attention-deficit/hyperactivity disorder service provision in urban socioeconomically disadvantaged communities: A pilot study. *Clinical Practice in Pediatric Psychology, 8*(2), 189–194. https://doi.org/10.1037/cpp0000321

Chen, J. (2022). *Poverty.* Retrieved October 20, 2022, from https://www.investopedia.com/terms/p/poverty.asp

Collins, C. L., & Fetsch, R. J. (2017). A review and critiques of 16 parent education programs. *Journal of Extension, 50*(4). https://archives.joe.org/joe/2012august/pdf/JOE_v50_4a8.pdf

Commons Wikimedia. (n.d). What parents when trained in behaivor therapy. https://commons.wikimedia.org/wiki/File:What_parents_learn_when_trained_in_behavior_therapy.jpg

Croake, J. W., & Glover, K. E. (1977). A history and evaluation of parent education. *The Family Coordinator, 26*(2), 151–158. https://doi.org/10.2307/583363

Czeisler, M. É., Lane, R. I., Petrosky, E., Wiley, J. F., Christensen, A., Njai, R., Weaver, M. D., Robbins, R., Facer-Childs, E. R., Barger, E. R., Czeisler, C. A., Howard. E., & Rajaratnam, S. M. W. (2020). Mental health, substance use, and suicidal ideation during the COVID-19 pandemic—United States. *Morbidity and Mortality Weekly Report, 69,* 1049–1057.

Daire, A. P., Greenidge, W., & Johnson, N. (2007). *Parental attitudes and behaviors of participants in the nurturing father program* [Unpublished manuscript].

Davidson, J., & Orsini, M. (2013). *Worlds of autism: Across the spectrum of neurological difference.* University of Minnesota Press. https://doi.org/10.5749/minnesota/9780816688883.001.0001

Davidson, J., & Wood, C. (2004). A conflict resolution model. *Theory into Practice, 43*(1), 6–13.

DeMarsh, J., & Kumpfer, K. L. (1986). Family-oriented interventions for the prevention of chemical dependency in children and adolescents. *Prevention, 18,* 117–151.

Dinkmeyer, D., & McKay, G. D. (1973). *Raising a responsible child: Practical steps to successful family relationships.* Simon & Schuster.

Dreikurs, R. (1955). Adlerian analysis of interaction. *Group Psychotherapy, 8*(4), 298–307.

Dreikurs, R. (1964). *Children the challenge.* Hawthorne.

Erikson, E. H. (1950). *Childhood and society.* W.W. Norton.

Fabes, R. A., Fultz, J., Eisenberg, N., May-Plumlee, T., & Christopher, F. S. (1989). Effects of rewards on children's prosocial motivation: A socialization study. *Developmental Psychology, 25,* 509–515.

Fass, P. S. (2016). *The end of American childhood: A history of parenting from life on the frontier to the managed child*. Princeton University Press.

Fine, M. J., & Lee, S. W. (2001). *Handbook of diversity in parent education: The changing faces of parenting and parent education*. Academic Press.

Fox, L., Dunlap, G., & Cushing, L. (2002). Early intervention, positive behavior support, and transition to school. *Journal of Emotional and Behavioral Disorders, 10*(3), 149–157. https://doi.org/10.1177/10634266020100030301

Fox, R. A., & Fox, T. A. (1992). *Leader's guide: STAR parenting program*. STAR Parenting.

Gates, B., Newell, R., & Wray, J. (2001). Behavior modification and gentle teaching workshops: Management of children with learning disabilities exhibiting challenging behavior and implications for learning disability nursing. *Journal of Advanced Nursing, 34*, 86–95. https://doi.org/10.1046/j.1365-2648.2001.3411730.x

Gordon, T. (1975). *P.E.T. parent effectiveness training: The tested new way*. Plume.

Gordon, T. (2000). *Parent effectiveness training: The proven program for raising responsible children*. Three Rivers Press.

Haffey, N., & Levant, R. F. (1984). The differential effectiveness of two models of skills training for working class parents. *Family Relations, 33*, 209–216.

Harris, P. L. (2012). *Trusting what you're told: How children learn from others*. Belknap.

Hockaday, C. (2020). *Strengthening families program: Parents and youth 10–14 (SFP 10–14)*. The California Evidence-Based Clearinghouse for Child Welfare, Information and Resources for Child Welfare Professionals. https://www.cebc4cw.org/program/strengthening-families-program-for-parents-and-youth-10-14-sfp-10-14/

Hoffman, R. (2020). Alfred Adler's theories of individual psychology and Adlerian therapy. *Simply Psychology*. https://www.simplypsychology.org/alfred-adler.html

The incredible years, parents, teachers, and children training series. (n.d.). https://incredibleyears.com/programs/

Jonynienė, J. (2013). *Lifestyle dynamics and efficacy of systematic training for effective parenting (STEP) on parenting style and perception of child behavior* [Doctoral dissertation]. https://gs.elaba.lt/object/elaba:1838942/

Kim, H. (2019). *Parenting stress*. Open Science Framework. https://doi.org/10.17605/osf.io/9cg58

King James Bible. (2008). Oxford University Press. (Original work published 1769)

Kubli, K. (2022). *A review of systematic training for effective parenting (STEP) curriculum*. Everett Christian Counseling. https://everettchristiancounseling.com/a-review-on-systematic-training-for-effective-parenting-step-curriculum/

Lakes, K. D., Vargas, D., Riggs, M., Schmidt, J., & Baird, M. (2011). Parenting intervention to reduce attention and behavior difficulties in preschoolers: A CUIDAR evaluation study. *Journal of Child and Family Studies, 20*, 648–659.

Lantsburg, M. E. (2016). Parenting in today's world: New trends. *Journal of Modern Foreign Psychology, 5*(2), 62–66.

Larson, B. J. (2000). *Systematic training for effective parenting of teens (STEP/teens): Parenting authority, adolescent externalizing behavior and parent-child relationships*. Bell.

MacNab, S. (2014). *100 years of cooperative extension: The Smith-Lever Act of Centennial*. University of California, UC Calfresh Fresno/Medera Counties. https://ucanr.edu/blogs/blogcore/postdetail.cfm?postnum=13261

Maier, H. (2008). First and second order change: Powerful concepts in preparing child care practitioners. *Journal of Children in Contemporary Society*. https://doi.org/10.1300/J274v17n03_04

Merriam, S. B. (2015). Adult learning: A review and an update. *Culture, Biography & Lifelong Learning, 1*(1), 59–71. https://doi.org/10.1016/B978-0-08-044894-7.00003-8

Miller, A. (2008). A critique of positive psychology—or the new science of happiness. *Journal of Philosophy of Education, 42*(3–4), 591–608.

Miller, G. A., & Buckhout, R. (1973). *Psychology: The science of mental life*. Harper and Row.
Montanez, M., Devall, E., & Van Leeuwen, D. M. (2010). Social capital: Strengthening Mexican American families through parenting education. *Journal of Family & Consumer Sciences, 102*(3), 27–33.
Morris, A. S., Jespersen, J. E., Cosgrove, K. T., Ratliff, E. L., & Kerr, K. L. (2020). Parent education: What we know and moving forward for greatest impact. *Family Relations, 69*, 520–542. https://doi.org/10.1111/fare.12442
National Academies of Science, Engineering, and Medicine. (2016). *Parenting matters: Supporting parents of children ages 0–8.* https://www.nap.edu/catalog/21868/
The nurturing father program. (n.d.). https://nurturingfathers.com/
Oryan, S., & Gastil, J. (2013). Democratic parenting: Paradoxical messages in democratic parent education theories. *International Review of Education, 59,* 113–129. https://doi.org/10.1007/s11159-13-9351-7
Padilla-Walker, L. M., Carlo, G., Christensen, K. J., & Yorgason, J. B. (2012). Bidirectional relations between authoritative parenting and adolescents' prosocial behaviors. *Journal of Research on Adolescence, 22*(3), 400–408. https://doi.org/10.1111/j.1532-7795.2012.00807.x
Patterson, G. R. (1982). *A social learning approach to family interventions: Vol. 3. Coercive family process*. Castalia.
Pinsker, R., & Geoffrey, K. (1981). A comparison of parent effectiveness training and behavior modification parent training. *Family Relations, 30,* 61–68.
Rodrigo, M. J., Almeida, A., Spiel, C., & Koops, W. (2012). Introduction: Evidence-based parent education programs to promote positive parenting. *European Journal of Developmental Psychology, 9*(1), 2–10. https://doi.org/10.1080/17405629.2011.631282
Ryle, G. (1990). *The concept of mind*. Penguin.
SAMHSA'S national registry of evidence-based programs and practices. (n.d.). https://www.coastalpreventionresources.org/wordpress/wp-content/uploads/2014/01/STEP.pdf
Schwartz, B. (1986). *The battle for human nature: Science, morality, and modern life*. Norton.
Seligman, M. E. P. (2007). *Authentic happiness*. Free Press.
Spoth, R. L., Redmond, C., & Shin, C. (2001). Randomized trial of brief family interventions for general populations: Adolescent substance use outcomes 4 years following baseline. *Journal of Consulting and Clinical Psychology, 69,* 627–642.
Spoth, R. L., Trudeau, L., Shin, C., Ralston, E., Redmond, C., Greenberg, M., & Feinberg, M. (2013). Longitudinal effects of universal preventive intervention on prescription drug misuse: Three RCTs with late adolescents and young adults. *American Journal of Public Health, 103*(4), 665–672.
Stolz, H., Vargas, L., Clifford, L. M., Gaedt, H., & Garcia, C. F. (2010). Evaluating parent project: A multi-site inquiry. *Family Science Review, 15*(1), 1–15.
Stretch, J. J. (1970). The rights of children emerge: Historical notes on the first White House conference on children. *Child Welfare, 49*(7), 365–372.
Trudeau, L., Spoth, R., Mason, W. A., Randall, G. K., Redmond, C., & Schainker, L. (2016). Effects of an adolescent universal substance misuse preventive interventions on young adult depression symptoms: Mediational modeling. *Journal of Abnormal Child Psychology, 44*(2), 257–268.
Turner, K. M. T., Richards, M., & Sanders, M. R. (2007). A randomized clinical trial of a group parent education program for Australian Indigenous families. *Journal of Pediatrics and Child Health, 43,* 243–251.
Walper, S., & Kreyenfeld, M. (2022). The intensification of parenting in Germany: The role of socioeconomic background and family form. *Social Sciences, 11*, 134. https://doi.org/10.3390/socsci11030134

2

WHAT IS SECOND ORDER PARENTING?

Family Development Interventions

First and second order change were terms used by Gregory Bateson (1972), one of the founders of psychotherapy from a systems perspective, to denote the process of change. Each term referred to specific therapy interventions leading to change in the individual or the family system. First and second order change are central concepts that continue in marriage and family therapy models using a systems paradigm. In addition to Bateson's writings, other authors, such as Salvador Minuchin (1974), Jay Haley (Erickson, 1975), and Watzlawick et al. (1979), applied the components of general systems theory and first and second order change to marriage and family therapy.

While both types of change are used by marriage and family therapists, they have a different structure and point to different interventions. First order change comes about because of *direct interventions* that are rational and understood by the participants (Watzlawick et al., 1979). It uses skill-building interventions to improve present functioning and it does not change the overall structure of the problem (Maier, 1986). Consequently, the change is a change within the system and does not alter the system itself. The change typically alters an individual's behavior, but does not impact the overall constitution of the family system. This type of change is referred to as *incremental change* and progresses over time with the goal being to get a different outcome that does not alter the system. As it relates to parenting, first order change would result from new specific skills that are learned to improve parenting effectiveness for a child's misbehavior, but does not change the underlying conception of the meaning of parenting.

Second order change, on the other hand, refers to change that alters the system itself by going beyond individual change (Watzlawick et al., 1979). It is

DOI: 10.4324/9781003381679-3

transformational in nature and may appear irrational and even chaotic. Second order change is change that occurs from indirect, implicit, spontaneous, and even unknowable factors. It is more complex than first order change because it can happen outside of conscious awareness. Second order change is a *qualitative, irreversible change* in which there is a discontinuous process. It goes outside the previous limits and opens new possibilities that were not recognized before. Contrary to first order change, which is referred to as "*change without change*," second order change alters the rules governing the system, creating a fundamental transformation.

Why Transformational Change Is So Difficult

A *system*, such as an individual or family system, is an organized unit which operates to maintain itself through continuation of a functional framework or *schema* (Bartunek & Moch, 1987). Schemas are important to understand because they determine how individuals respond to events associated with change and because they operate outside of consciousness. One's experiences, thoughts, and worldview form a schema by which one understands reality. Thus, a schema is a template or filter that provides a guide for how one views the world. A *parenting schema* is a framework for behaviors toward children, including nurturing and disciplining behavior. A person will develop many schemas that inform decisions and his/her view of reality. In all interactions or conversations with others, each person's schema is activated in this process. Some experiences and cognitive input are emphasized by one's schema, and some input is minimized. Once established, schemas tend to continue and to resist input that would challenge or change the schema's organizing principles. On the other hand, schemas can support and direct change that is consistent with its framework.

In parenting and parent education, first and second order changes are constantly at play. First order change is evident when a skill-building exercise is being practiced, such as improving listening skills. It is considered first order because the value of communication between parent and child is recognized and can be improved, but the overall structure of the relationship remains the same. First order change involves the model and resource materials used by the parent educator to be presented in a stepwise manner so that the parent can quantitatively improve their interactions with their child.

A second order change occurs when a parent changes their attitude from *punitive discipline,* such as corporal punishment, recognizing that it was dysfunctional, in favor of *positive discipline interventions*. In parent education models, most skill-building exercises utilize first order change because the purpose and goal of the interventions are to improve present parenting skills without changing the overall schema. For a new schema to arise, there must be sufficient challenges to the existing schema. The focus in second order parenting is less on *quantitative change* and more on qualitative change where the parent educator is engaged with the participants in searching for unknown answers. Instead of predetermined skills, second order change results from participants learning from observation of the parent educator modeling new input that is experienced as transformational. *Transformational change* requires a change in schema whereby the participants learn from experiencing and through active learning rather than through passive learning. Experiential learning goes beyond doing more or less of some behavior, but encourages the participant to think, process, and value new schema. Second order change is *nonlinear and holistic*, or what Bronfenbrenner (1979) called *ecological learning*, that is, learning takes place within a nested system of influence from the child to the family, to the community, and to the culture.

A second order learning approach necessitates an evaluation process that exceeds merely noting that participants improved. For example, when outcome studies report that parents have more positive feelings toward their child, little can be gleaned from these partial results. What is needed is an evaluation that is based on the participant's ability to perform parenting skills at a higher level in interacting with their child. The question that is always present in reviewing parent education models is whether participants change in linear, incremental ways, or in transformational ways. This question is particularly relevant given that some models utilize *formalized skill-building exercises*, predetermined and packaged modules, that can be done online.

Resistance to Change

While change in mind and behavior is the goal of parent education, change may not be welcomed by all participants. This reaction to the prospect of change was labeled *resistance* by renowned psychotherapist Milton (1975) and his pupil Jay Haley (Erickson, 1975). They viewed second order change as the mechanism to bypass resistance. Unexpected experiences that lead to mental and physical responses tend to trigger a *flight or fight response* (Gordon, 2000). This threat response is stronger in effect and lasts longer than the reward response. The *threat response* occurs because humans desire the status quo and any change to the status quo causes a painful response. Rather than welcoming change, humans seek to maintain a level of *homeostasis*, or equilibrium. This is the way the brain protects a person from experiencing threats.

Recent research sheds some light on what it is so difficult about change (Kaplan et al., 2016). Using an fMRI brain scan procedure, Jonas Kaplan et al. (2016) found that when a person's basic worldview is endangered, the brain functions to protect this self-image. In this way, one's self-image is reinforced by one's worldview and must be maintained. What psychotherapists, such as Milton Ericson (1975), took for resistance can be explained through neuroscience research as the task of the brain to protect the view of the self.

Certain views held by a person that form the meaning of personhood and identity, such as politics and religion, cannot be easily changed. We can assume that along with politics and religion, parenting behavior also fits neatly within the boundary of *self-image* and, therefore, is hard to change. Parent educators must not assume that parents are their allies in changing parenting behaviors by developing new skills. It also means that strategies of interventions need to reflect a diligent understanding of both the child and the parents' beliefs about the self as a prerequisite first step in a training program.

An article on neuroscience and behavior change by Berkman (2018) identifies two processes that occur simultaneously for change to occur—one is *motivation*, referred to as "the will"; the other is *cognition*, or "the way." *Goals* are defined as outcomes that would not have happened unless an intervention occurred. With this definition, goals are viewed as anything we wish to accomplish, but do not have the tools necessary to bring about without help. Berkman combines goal pursuit with the definition of behavior change. To achieve the goal or behavioral change, one must have the means to change and the desire or motivation to change (Berkman & Rock, 2014). When applied to parent education, for parents there must be both the motivation to change and the means for making the change. These two factors Berkman arranged in a four-quadrant design of high skill, low motivation, to low skill, high motivation (see Table 2.1). Regarding specific changes, one must activate the high skill, high motivation quadrant. One of the primary considerations in working with parents is to assess both their skill level and their motivation to change.

There are several factors related to how parents participating in parent education change. The structure of parent education where some parents are under duress to take the course so that they can be reunited with their child suggests that the motivation for change might be low. The motivation would be to get custody of their child rather than to change their behavior. Parents with low motivation for change

TABLE 2.1 Berkman's Four Quadrants of Goals and Behavior Change

Behavior Change Requires Movement along One or Both Axes			
Level of *skill*, *knowledge*, or *ability* required by an action	More	**Complex but Routine Tasks** High skill, low motivation Example: Navigating to a familiar place	**Complex and Novel Tasks** High skill, high motivation Example: Navigating in a new city for the first time
	Less	**Simple and Routine Tasks** Low skill, low motivation Example: Walking to the mailbox	**Simple but Novel Tasks** Low skill, high motivation Example: Changing a diaper for the first time
		Less; feels easy	More; feels hard
		Level of *motivation* required by an action	

Source: Adapted from Berkman, 2018.

Note. The two dimensions (motivational, or the *will*; and cognitive, or the *way*) reflect new Neuroscience studies.

would be going through the motions to achieve a particular outcome. On the other hand, low-skill parents may be too poorly equipped to gain mastery of the skills needed to change.

Initially, it is important for the parent educator to determine if the parent has the skills or motivation needed to bring about behavior change. Also of equal importance is the question of whether the parent is limited by lack of skills or lack of motivation and the capacity to move toward the high skills, high motivation quadrant. What dampens continuation of new behaviors is that there is no reward history related to the new behavior or skill. This means that the *subjective value* of the new behavior must be increased. Determining what limits behavior change will be an individual assessment and will govern the intervention process.

Since behavior change is the foundation of parent education, for without it there is wasted effort, there seems to be little or no development in parent education models of how to motivate behavior change in the parent. The assumption appears to be that when skills are presented, they will be received and put in practice by the parent. According to neuroscience research, there is more to behavior change than meets the eye. Researchers have found that simply weighting firm characteristics of a behavior can amend the worth placed on that behavior (Krajbich et al., 2010). The greater the perceived value of a behavior, the more likely it will continue. For example, a person's motivation to choose a particular behavior will rise as consideration is assigned to it (Krajbich et al., 2010). Based on this information, for first order change it might be necessary to present behavior change skills in small units over a period of time so that the new behavior could be practiced and reinforced. Otherwise, the new behavior lacks the strength to continue. Old behaviors have a history that have been reinforced, continue over time, and may not disappear because new information has been added. As first order change occurs from the introduction of new skills, the new behaviors must be practiced and reinforced in order to continue into the future. Reinforcement is essential to learning new behavior changes in first order change.

Second, the value resulting from self-orienting values identity may claim superior position compared to other values due to the overlay in the brain's neural systems and views of identity and value. Identity and value are attached, leading to the conclusion that the major characteristic of the self is to conceptualize reality by conveying its motivational meaning (Northoff & Hayes, 2011). What this means in simple terms is that for a new behavior to continue, it must be in alignment with the sense of self-identity. For the new behavior to gain traction, it must fit with the core values and the sense of one's identity as a person. For parent education, this means that standardized and preset skills training may not be the most effective way to present new skills to participants for first order change. Rather, what may be more effective is fully understanding what each participant values as their core set of principles and self-image and to devise skills for the new behavior based on that knowledge. A more individualized approach may be needed in contrast to standardized training procedures.

In addition, the value of a skilled behavior can be increased by paying more attention to it, suggesting that value placed on learning a particular skill in parent education may produce greater motivation in participants to change their behavior. According to a research study by Higgins et al. (2003), motivation is increased when there is a fit between the goal type and the process by which the goals are carried out. Applied to parent education, it means that motivation is increased when the skill being taught matches or fits with the process for attaining that skill. For example, learning active listening skills should fit the means of learning that skill, namely, actual experience in attaining listening skill.

Neuroscience Research and the Difficulty of Transformational Change

We can look at other neuroscience research that gives clues as to why transformational change is so difficult. The greatest influence on transformational change is the operational function of the brain (Corr & Perkins, 2006). Neuroscientists have identified three distinct brain functions that are involved in behavior change—the fight or flight system, the *behavior activation system*, and the behavior inhibitory system. The brain's activation system is roughly the reward system of the brain that is stimulated when positive emotions are numerous, and is referred to as the "dopaminergic reward circuits," including the nucleus accumbens, the ventral striatum, and the ventral tegmental area. These brain areas are activated when the brain is engaged in activities such as learning competency skills. The reward system is aroused in areas of the brain where learning and memory formation and storage take place. In fact, researchers have found that the majority of the receptor endorphins can be found in the areas of the brain involved in learning and memory (Biederman & Vessel, 2006). The brain continues to grow through the activation of its reward system.

While the brain has an activation system, it also has an inhibition system that slows things down and even prevents actions from happening (Ippolito, 2020). Brain areas related to this inhibition system include the amygdala, the anterior cingulate cortex, and the septo-hippocampal system. In the activation system, neurons act in a way to transmit information to other neurons, but in the inhibitory system, the tendency to share information across neurons is reduced (Lee et al., 2017). The ideal brain function is for there to be a stable balance between the activation system and the inhibitory system. An imbalance in the activation system and the inhibitory systems is related to several neurological problems, including the development of autism (Pretzsch & Floris, 2020).

The fight or flight brain system is meant to protect us when there is perceived danger. The *limbic system* or emotional system is activated, which floods the neocortex and leads to quick response. In this momentary surge of input into the neocortex, the amygdala overwhelms the neocortex with emotional input resulting in what has been described as the "hijacking of the brain" (LeDoux, 1998). One's action can be either freezing in place or quickly removing oneself from the present context. Along with the emotional reaction, there are internal reactions in higher levels of the stress hormone cortisol, increased blood pressure and heart rate, and suppressed immune reaction (Chancellor-Freeland et al., 2015).

The failure of change to be transformational results from the inhibition to change where the brain is following old patterns that could include a protective function (Bolland, 2021). The adage to practice new behaviors until they become automatic may also not be the route to transformational change. More important than practice of new behaviors is how transformational change takes place. In this case the *how* of behavior change is more important than the *what* of behavior change. While it may be a daunting task to answer the question of how transformational change occurs, the next section of the chapter will attempt to shed more light on this process.

Components of Second Order/Transformational Change

Although neuroscience tends to support incremental change as the dominant form of change, there is also evidence for developing a neuroscience model of transformational change (Reser, 2016). Parent education, like other forms of learning that directly affect self-image and one's behavior, assumes that permanent change is the goal and desired outcome. Determining how transformational change takes place is necessary for educators designing learning experiences for participants. Adequate consideration of this process is needed for parent educators.

Neuroscientist James Zull (2006) believes that transformational change should be the heart of all educational models. How transformational change takes place is more important to Zull than what is being taught. His whole-brained model describes the process by which new experiences become transformational. The first brain area affected by new information or experience is the sensory area; followed by the temporal cortex, which processes critical evaluation; the frontal cortex where dialogue and abstract formalization takes place; and finally, the motor cortex where the new information can be acted upon. While this may seem to be a purely cognitive process, the emotional dimension of learning new behaviors is intertwined.

Emotion and Transformational Second Order Change

According to Immordino-Yang and Damasio (2006) what is generally promoted as cognitive, such as learning, memory, and decision making, are really incorporated under the affective domain of the brain referred to as "emotional thoughts." Immordino-Yang and Damasio stress that for formal learning to be transferred from a classroom setting to practical everyday behavior, the emotional dimension of the brain must be activated. Furthermore, learning and new behavior is typically viewed as a separate disembodied system, when, in reality, there is a cooperative and inclusive connection between the cognitive function of the brain and the emotional and physical functioning. In fact, what appears to be rational or cognitive functions are veiled emotional processes that undergird decision making and learning. What this suggests is that emotional processes are needed for the skills learned to be translatable from the cognitive setting to real-life experiences. Consequently, it also means that role-playing may not adequately allow for a transfer of in-class learned skills to real-life experiences. How emotional processes provide the backdrop for learning has not been adequately developed in the literature, but according to Immordino-Yang and Damasio, emotional processing may act as a kind of rudder that makes possible decision making and ethical behavior.

According to Immordino-Yang and Damasio (2006), while the rational brain can process information for learning, decision making, and memory, it is not useful in the real world of everyday happenings without emotional processing. Emotion acts as a guide for selecting the appropriate reasoning for the situation at hand. Emotional thought is the result of the overlapping of cognition and emotion which can be conscious or unconscious. Emotional thought is the platform where reasoning, emotion, and bodily states come together and where creativity emerges. According to Immordino-Yang and Damasio, educators realize that more is needed than logical or rational thought processes for behaviors to be useful in the real world. When educators disregard or ignore emotions in learning and appeal only to the cognitive, they inhibit the ability to transfer what is learned to real-life situations, thus reducing transformational learning. Lasting transformational change is not possible without emotional grounding.

Other neuroscientists have looked at the role of emotion in learning as well. For example, Zull (2006) found that when engaged in focused cognitive learning, the limbic system, especially activation of negative emotions, are inhibited. When fear or other negative emotions are present in the learning environment, cognitive processes are impeded. The need to reduce fear or anxiety in the learning setting has contributed to educators introducing meditation or mindfulness to help regulate harmful emotions (Quintiliani, 2011).

While negative emotions, such as fear and anxiety, may need to be reduced, other positive emotions, such as attunement in the form of attachment and emotional bonding, should be emphasized. A relationship between the educator and the learner of mutual sharing and empathic understanding can allow for what Immordino-Yang and Damasio called emotional thought, which is necessary for long-term transformational change.

Another critical aspect of transformational change and learning (second order) is a supportive community. Most parent education models are developed with group participation where participants interact in supportive and empathic ways. This structure is very effective because it provides a forum for discussion, sharing, and support. The question could be raised, however, whether the real need to support and strengthen the transformational change happens after the training has ended. In other words, should small group communities be continued after the formal training period has ended? For change to be significant and long-lasting, is there a need for a community that supports that change? The logistics of how such an ongoing small community could continue in the fast-paced and hectic contemporary society may be questionable, but there is no doubt that there would be effective outcomes.

A discussion on second order, or transformational, change would not be complete without including neuroscience research on insight and the *aha experience*. It is common for a person to mull over a decision or have competing ideas about a circumstance and not be able to come to any conclusion. Only after some time has passed where he/she may have not thought of the situation, a person may have a sudden insight and come to a quick decision. In this moment of insight, the solution is crystal clear and effective in determining the course of action. The aha experience moves quickly from lack of insight to amazing new insight on the problem at hand with blinding speed and confidence (Kounios & Jung-Beeman, 2014). Solving a problem is usually accomplished by applying a methodological analysis of the situation and a thorough step-by-step procedure. This process is sidestepped by the aha experience, which can occur without any conscious attempt to solve the problem.

While the aha experience is an unconscious process to provide a sense of insight and confident solution to a problem, it differs from conscious insight derived from reasoning in that the unconscious nature of the Aha experience alters components of the problem which permits the solution to appear (Ohlsson, 2011). Contrary to popular belief, the aha solution does not just appear from nothing. Neuroscience research findings show that the unconscious is busy patching together bits of information gleaned from prior conscious input and puts them together in a unique and creative way that solves the problem at hand (Salvi et al., 2016). Furthermore, the area of the brain most active in an aha experience is the right anterior superior temporal gyrus region of the brain (Sawyer, 2011).

The aha experience is an example of a second order change because the process is unconscious and provides a clear direction for solving the current problem. It is a qualitative change rather than a quantitative change and can be discontinuous from the past. It is not an incremental change, but changes the structure of the problem. It is, therefore, an out-of-the-box solution rather than a first order change that works *within* the box, an older, unhelpful framework. Aha moments occur when the brain has been distracted with other matters with no conscious thoughts about problem resolution (Figure 2.1). Taking breaks during training sessions or giving the brain downtime through meditation or silence are necessary for the aha experience. Researchers have found that the brain produces alpha waves just before the aha experience, which suggests that silence and mediating may help precipitate the aha moment (Raab, 2017). The implication is that deep insight does not occur spontaneously, but results from a particular circumstance in which the unconscious works on the problem outside of an individual's conscious awareness. Furthermore, the implication for parent education is that there should be opportunities

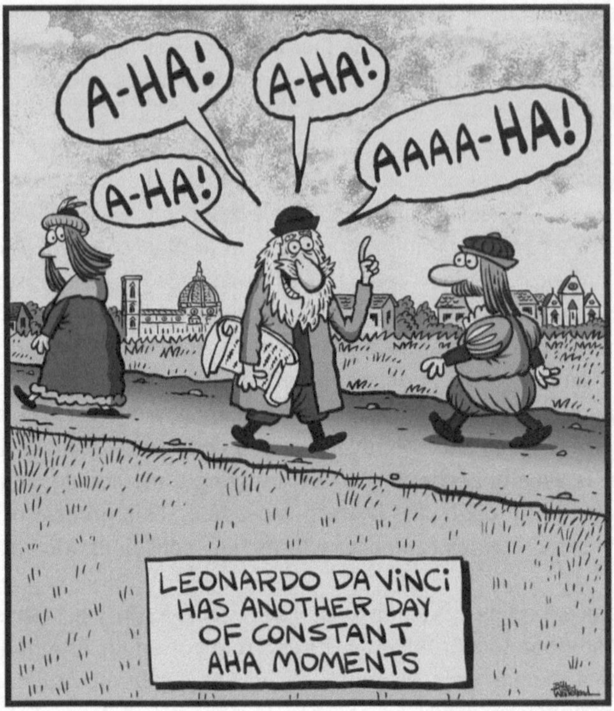

FIGURE 2.1 The unconscious can produce new ideas and resolutions even while being distracted. This is referred to as the "aha moment." (www.CartoonStock.com)

for distraction, silence, or meditation built into the training model to facilitate aha experiences.

How Second Order/Transformational Change Occurs

To this point, we have described how first order and second order changes differ and some of the components of transformational or second order change. Additionally, we have discussed how self-image and schema act to discourage transformational change; learning how to diminish their influence will be necessary for permanent change. This section will discuss in greater depth how second order change occurs. Of particular interest is understanding how change can be long-lasting in a training setting, such as parent education. The question of necessity is: If change is not long-lasting, are we wasting our time with the proliferation of programs? What is clear from research is that permanent change and how to create it are intangible and difficult to operationalize.

Like psychotherapy and other fields of study where serious behavioral change is sought (Kazdin, 2020), parent education models lack a mechanism that explains how change occurs. Even after years of evidence-based research, there does not exist a consensus for how serious change occurs in the field of psychotherapy (Cuijpers et al., 2020) and this seems to also apply to parent education. While the mechanism of long-lasting change has not been studied specifically in parent education, there is enough similarity in attempting to initiate permanent change for applying the findings from psychotherapy to parent education. Like research in psychotherapy (Norcross & Lambert, 2019), parent education researchers have identified contributing factors for change but do not provide a discernible mechanism for how this change occurs. The primary question of concern is assessing how parent education, and for that matter, parenting in general, leads to positive results in developing children.

Factors for Transformational Second Order Change

Factors necessary for effective change in parent education have been proposed. While these factors inform various models of parenting and parent education, they do not explain the mechanism for how change occurs. It seems reasonable that first order and second order change may proceed through different mechanisms because they reflect two different types of change. A closer look at these two types of change may identify the different processes involved. First order change is incremental and over time the problem is expected to decline during training or long-term reinforcement. On the other hand, second order change occurs at the point of training and results in transformation change in which the problem has disappeared.

Instead of changing old memory systems, first order change simply creates a separate memory alongside the old memory without changing the original memory. This mechanism can produce change, but the change tends to be partial and incomplete. Some partial changes might be long lasting, however, depending on the type of skill and the experience in using the skill. Conscious practice is required for first order change to be long lasting.

On the other hand, second order transformational change alters the memory system of parenting schema entirely and replaces it with a new memory. Rather than competing with an old implicit memory, second order change is transformational. The new skill will not need practice to be effective. It is effective because it replaces the old memory on which the ineffective behavior relied. While there are many memory systems, the one that concerns parenting and parent education are semantic and related to schema formation and self-image. Transformational change is contrasted with partial or incomplete change and is the underlying standard to measure effective change.

As stated earlier, two components of the brain's implicit memory system that are prominent in parenting behavior are self-mage and schema. Both of these processes are actively involved in maintaining the status quo and, therefore, are resistant to new input. Prior to 2000, neuroscientists believed that implicit memory could not be intentionally changed (Ecker & Bridges, 2020). So, this leads to the major question of how to change these implicit schemas that are the basis for dysfunctional parenting behavior and will allow for new skills be to accepted leading to permanent change.

Changing Implicit Schemas

Since 2000, neuroscientists have discovered more regarding how implicit memory can be changed through different processes, such as *memory reconsolidation*, the process of replacing old memory that affects current functioning (Ecker & Bridges, 2020). While memory reconsolidation is only one of a number of mechanisms by which memory can be removed and new memories created to replace them, it is a decent starting point for understanding how transformational second order change can occur.

Prior to understanding how memory reconsolidation is possible, the general procedure for changing implicit memories was to have new experiences, causing the old implicit memories to fade or be less bothersome. In order to make the new experiences significant, there was a need to practice the new behaviors until they became automatic (Papastamatis & Panitsides, 2014). While this was the goal, it seldom worked well and failed to produce long-term change. The idea that memory could effectively be erased was not known and it took numerous research studies and brain imaging experiments to discover it.

But, why should we be concerned about erasing memories in a discussion about parenting and parent education training? This question and its answer are especially pertinent for any endeavor meant to produce permanent change in belief systems and behaviors. As noted in an earlier part of the chapter, parenting behaviors emerge from the implicit memory system that was developed without conscious awareness. There exists a schema about values and beliefs about how to parent that emerge without conscious effort or thinking. Therefore, to create long-term second order change, the schema for parenting behavior hiding out in the implicit memory system must be changed. This might seem like a daunting task for parent educators and beyond their scope of work, but if second order change is necessary for more than partial effective outcomes, it is suggested that a new mechanism for producing change be instituted.

Memory Reconsolidation

Neuroscience research over the past two decades has opened a new approach to transformational learning through the process of memory reconsolidation (Mezirow et al., 1990). The belief that memory was malleable was a new concept. When memories are recalled with their original emotion, they are present in consciousness and amenable to change. This recalling of the memory and the emotion is then contradicted or disconfirmed, which challenges the legitimacy of the original memory. This new information changes the original schema and is consolidated into the memory system, resulting in new behaviors.

While this process of memory reconsolidation was mainly a conscious cognitive process, identifying the emotional content in the original memory was necessary to change or erase the memory when disconfirmed (Ecker & Bridges, 2020). The disconfirming is necessary to be able to implant a new memory. The process of memory reconsolidation is appropriate not only for erasing traumatic memories but also for changing worldviews that are no longer helpful.

Carruthers (2017) used the term "*predictive mind*" to refer to the automatic function of the mind. The predictive mind theory embraces the idea that the major brain orientation is about future social and personal outcomes, which occurs automatically, and consciousness is only activated when predication fails. Implicit processes guide and direct all thoughts, beliefs, and perceptions. Research by Nicolas Schuck et al. (2015) found that the frontal lobe is activated before a decision is made, implying that the unconscious processes had made the decision before the conscious decision was made.

Recently, the process of memory reconsolidation as a central component in transformational learning has been challenged based on more recent neuroscience research findings of the relationship of emotions and implicit processes and rationality. For example, Solms and Friston (2018) found that the brain acts to restrict consciousness, which appears as conscious awareness only when there is a predictive failure. What this means is that consciousness has less involvement in thinking, setting goals, and creating belief systems than unconsciousness.

One area of research that sheds light on the relationship of the conscious and unconscious conundrum is in the area of "goal pursuit," and being able to determine a future outcome. The belief previously was that goal pursuit was only possible in consciousness and, therefore, was not possible in the unconscious. According to Bargh and Marsella (2008), it is an undisputed fact that goal pursuits originate in the unconscious and are taken over by the conscious as if it originated in consciousness. This means what is thought to be cognitive mental processes occur first in the unconscious but the conscious mind obscures awareness of this, which results in the feeling a person is always consciously aware of decisions.

The view that the brain functions automatically with consciousness accounting for only a small part of brain functioning turns much behavioral science theory on its head. It means that far too much consideration has been given to rationality and the neocortex and far too little emphasis has been put on implicit and unconscious processes.

Other researchers such as Daniel Kahneman (2011) have emphasized that consciousness and unconsciousness work together and are not separate entities, but that the unconscious is the driving force behind what was thought of in the past as being the function of consciousness and the neocortex. The implication of this research is that all cognitive functions that were once believed to be the product of the conscious brain are instead processes of the automatic unconscious system.

In sum, the above discussion stresses the importance of implicit learning that is outside of cognitive awareness. Cognitive and rational approaches to transformational change have been overemphasized in the literature and implicit processes have been underemphasized. While the central role of unconscious and implicit processes is evident, learning new skills related to transformational change can occur on both conscious and unconscious levels (Taylor, 2001). Neuroscience research has demonstrated that transformational change can occur without conscious reflection. When skills are taught, such as in parent education, it is not necessary to reflect on them to ensure transformational change occurs. In fact, it is well-noted that persons cannot explain skills involved in learning explicitly and critical reflection of them may be frustrating and unproductive (Wilson & Schooler, 1991). While it may seem counterintuitive to place less emphasis on conscious rational reflection, the implication for parent education is that more attention should be given to how implicit learning takes place, as well as how emotional content is the foundation for transformational change.

Applying Secord Order/Transformational Change to Parenting and Parent Education

Parent education models have evolved over the years and continue to do so, but major findings in neuroscience research have made little headway into the conceptualizing or practice of parent education. Books on parenting primarily written for parents, teachers, and clinicians have made inroads into applying neuroscience to parenting, but questionably may not have addressed the underlying structure of how neuroscience transforms the parenting process. This topic will be addressed more thoroughly later on.

Issues related to parent education structure reveal a decidedly cognitive process. It reflects a learning model that focuses on gaining new skills and insights that can be consciously practiced and that change ingrained and automatic parenting behaviors. However, outcomes of parent education training typically are small and partial, and long-term effects are questionable at best. The obvious question is: Why are the outcomes of parent education not more robust? (See Table 2.2.)

The answer to this question may primarily lie in what is known about neuroscience research on transformational change. So far, the phrases "transformational change" and "second order change" have been used interchangeably. Both refer to qualitative change that radically impacts the structure of the situation and creates a new pathway for a worldview or filter to process thoughts and behaviors. Second order change begins with an understanding that parenting behaviors are the outward expression of one's unconscious automatic and implicit brain functions and, therefore, are not the primary focus of change.

TABLE 2.2 Enhancing Transformational Change

Second Order/Transformational Parenting
Utilizes interventions that are creative, intuitive, and implicit
Begins training with didactic material and follows with experiential implicit interventions
Allows confusion to happen, but provides a path of clear understanding
Facilitates recall of memories associated with parenting schemas and reflects on new information
Infuses training with emotional content
Develops follow-up supportive communities for parent education participants
Allows for distractions to facilitate aha learning
Increases complexity

If the primary focus of change is transforming unconscious processes, the question arises: How are unconscious processes changed? In answering this question, the tendency is to brush it off by exclaiming that a person must become consciously aware of the hidden unconscious beliefs that affect their behavior and then be open to new skills that will take the place of the old dysfunctional ones. The assumption is that the trainee is open to change—that is, motivated to change, and has the cognitive capacity to change. Motivation to change and the capacity to change generally are not assessed in models of parent education. Neuroscience has determined that the self-image and the value placed on it are resistive to change. This means that the trainer must address that each trainee has a self-image that is not threatened by new skills and beliefs and is typically addressed through goal setting. Conscious goal setting coupled with a positive self-image can unconsciously change or alter old and dysfunctional schemas, and this is seen in many parent education models.

How the unconscious can be a greater focus in parent education models could greatly impact the long-term positive effects of parent training. One innovation that has not been incorporated into parent education models is implicit interventions that may allow for change in unconscious processes. Much has been noted about the overreliance of cognitive content, the lack of emotional content, and little or no implicit interventions in the field of transformational learning (Taylor, 2001). The infusion of implicit processes into parent education training could be brought about by several effects. First, increase emotional content. As stated earlier, cognitive learning does not occur without emotions. Emphasizing how one feels as they are engaged in remembering old parenting behaviors and how they feel in learning a new skill may provide an avenue for how the unconscious comes into play.

It could well be the case that what we consider conscious insight is informed by the unconscious and in becoming conscious has fooled the trainee into believing that the insight is the product of the conscious mind. Because the conscious and unconscious work together rather than act as two separate and independent systems, it changes the way transformational change takes place. For example, the aha experience is a good metaphor for how transformational second order change occurs. The aha experience results from confusion, dilemmas, or information overload leaving a person unable to consciously move toward a resolution. After a period of distraction or engrossing oneself in other, unrelated thoughts or activities, the solution seems to suddenly come without further reflection. What is known is that, while the conscious mind is preoccupied with other thoughts or activities, the unconscious mind keeps working on the problem and when a resolution happens, the solution bursts forth into consciousness. For parent education training models, this fact suggests that dilemmas, confusion, or information overloading may be an effective way to facilitate transformational change.

Although it is well documented that learning can take place outside of conscious awareness, utilizing implicit techniques in educational training is undeveloped in the literature. Apart from *priming*, the presentation of information that is not consciously perceived by the subject, there exist both a dearth of research and the use of implicit techniques. The preponderance of neuroscience research on explicit and implicit memory is that they collaborate. Implicitly learned information can become explicit through intuitions that can guide thoughts and behaviors, and explicitly learning information can become implicit and acquire an automatic response (Epstein, 2010). Researchers have noted that in training educational settings, such as parent education, explicit learning takes place early in the process, while implicit learning is more present later in the process as one has increased proficiency in the learning exercise (Posner & Rothbart, 2014). It is the implicit shift in the learning setting that provides for transformational change in thoughts and behaviors. This shift from the explicit to the implicit is not consciously recognized and is mistakenly ascribed to the explicit system. When parent educators shift from didactic presentation to role-play or reflective responses, the shift from explicit to implicit learning takes place. The implication for parent education is that there should be ample attention on how to enhance implicit learning by incorporating activities that make implicit learning possible.

One final consideration in applying transformational second order change to parent education training is utilizing interventions that are creative, intuitive, and implicit. Parent educators have not developed interventions that focus on implicit, creative, or intuitive ways of knowing despite numerous research studies that support them. For example, research in creativity shows that divergent thinking can enhance learning experiences because it allows for competing ideas and novel solutions (Brenner, 2018). Creativity results from spontaneous, out-of-the-box thinking and not from attempting to be spontaneous (Runco, 2015).

Implicit and intuitive interventions could further enhance learning and contribute to second order transformational change. Future chapters will explore in depth how intuitive and implicit interventions can be used to broaden the mechanism for creating second order change.

References

Bargh, J. A., & Marsella, E. (2008). The unconscious mind. *Perspectives on Psychological Science, 3*(1), 73–79.

Bartunek, J. M., & Moch, M. K. (1987). First-order, second-order, and third-order change and organization development inventions: A cognitive approach. *The Journal of Applied Behavioral Science, 23*(4), 483–500.

Bateson, G. (1972). *Steps to an ecology of mind*. Chandler.

Berkman, E. T. (2018). The neuroscience of goals and behavior change. *Consulting Psychology Journal, 70*(1), 28–44. https://doi.org/10.1037/cpb0000094

Berkman, E. T., & Rock, D. (2014). AIM: An integrative model of goal pursuit. *Neuro Leadership Journal, 5,* 1–11.

Biederman, I., & Vessel, E. A. (2006). Perceptual pleasure and the brain: A novel theory explains why the brain craves information and seeks it through the senses. *American Scientist, 94*(3), 247–253.

Bolland, S. (2021). *The science of transformational change*. https://www.linkedin.com/pulse/neuroscience-transformational-change-learning-soar-dr-scott-bolland/

Brenner, G. H. (2018). *Inhibition: The counterintuitive key to creativity: Research on intelligence and creativity inspires release of divergent thinking*. Retrieved May 12, 2021, from https://granthbrennermd.medium.com/grant-h-brenner-185fdf1cfeb9

Bronfenbrenner, U. (1979). *The ecology of human development*. Harvard University Press.

Carruthers, P. (2017). The illusion of conscious thought. *Journal of Consciousness Studies, 24*(910), 228–252.

Chancellor-Freeland, C., Chang, A., & Szabo, Y. Z. (2015). Locus of control predicts cortisol reactivity and speech performance in response to acute stress in undergraduate students. *College Student Journal, 49*(2), 225–236.

Corr, P., & Perkins, A. M. (2006). The role of theory in the psychophysiology of personality: From Ivan Pavlov to Jeffrey Gray. *International Journal of Psychophysiology, 62,* 367–376.

Cuijpers, P., Reijnders, M., & Huibers, M. J. (2020). The role of common factors in psychotherapy outcomes. *Annual Review of Clinical Psychotherapy, 15,* 207–231. https://pubmed.ncbi.nlm.nih.gov/305507

Ecker, B., & Bridges, S. K. (2020). How the science of memory reconsolidation advances the effectiveness and unification of psychotherapy. *Clinical Social Work Journal, 48,* 287–300. https://doi.org/10.1007/s10615-02-00754-z

Epstein, S. (2010). Demystifying intuition: What it is, what it does, and how it does it. *Psychological Inquiry, 21*(4), 295–312. https://doi.org/10.1080/1047840X.2010.523875

Erickson, M. H. (1975). The varieties of double bind. American Clinical Journal of Hypnosis, 8, 57–65.

Gordon, E. (2000). *Integrative neuroscience: Bringing together biological, psychological, and clinical models of the human brain*. Harwood.

Haley, J., & Hoffman, L. (1973). *Techniques of family therapy*. Basic Books.

Higgins, E. T., Idson, L., Freitas, A. L., Spiegel, S., & Molden, D. C. (2003). Transfer of value from fit. *Journal of Personality and Social Psychology, 84*(6), 1140–1153.

Immordino-Yang, M. E., & Damasio, A. (2006). We feel, therefore we learn: The relevance of affective and social neuroscience to education. *Mind and Education, 1*(1), 3–10. https://doi.org/10.1111/j.1751-228X.2007.00004.x

Ippolito, K. (2020). Balancing act in the brain: Excitatory and inhibitory activity. *Max Blanck Institute for Neuroscience*. https://mpfi.org/balancing-act-in-the-brain-excitatory-and-inhibitory-activity/

Kahneman, D. (2011). *Thinking, fast and slow*. Farrar, Straus, and Giroux.

Kaplan, J. L., Gimbel, S. I., & Harris, S. (2016). Neural correlates for maintaining one's political views in the face of counterevidence. *Scientific Reports, 6,* 39589. https://www.ncbi.nlm.nih.gov/pmc/articles/PMC5854216/figure/F1/

Kazdin, A. E. (2020). *Single-case research design* (3rd Ed.) Oxford, UK: Oxford University Press.

Kounios, J., & Jung-Beeman, M. (2014). The cognitive neuroscience of insight. *Annual Review of Psychology, 65*, 71–93. https://doi.org/10.1146/annurev-psych-010213-115154
Krajbich, I., Armel, C., & Rangel, A. (2010). Visual fixations and the computation and comparison of value in simple choice. *Nature Neuroscience, 13*(10), 1292–1298.
LeDoux, J. (1998). *The emotional brain: The mysterious underpinnings of emotional life*. Simon & Schuster.
Lee, H. J., Lin, F. H., & Kuo, W. J. (2017). The neural mechanism underpinning balance calibration between action inhibition and activation initiated by reward motivation. *Scientific Reports, 7*, 9722. https://doi.org/10.1038/s41598-017-10539-z
Maier, H. (1986). First and second order change: Powerful concepts for preparing childcare practitioners. In K. Vander Ven & E. Tillnich (Eds.), *Competent caregivers—competent children: Training and education for childcare practice* (pp. 36–45). Haworth.
Mezirow, J. (Ed.). (1990). *Fostering critical reflection in adulthood*. Jossey-Bass.
Minuchin, S. (1974). *Families and family therapy*. Harvard University Press.
Norcross, J. C., & Lambert, M. J. (Eds.). (2019). *Psychotherapy relationships that work: Vol. 1. Evidence-based therapist contributions*. Oxford University Press.
Northoff, G., & Hayes, D. J. (2011). Is our self nothing but reward? *Biological Psychiatry, 69*(11), 1019–1025.
Ohlsson, S. (2011). *Deep learning: How the mind overrides experience*. Cambridge University Press. https://doi.org/10.1017/CBO9780511780295
Papastamatis, A., & Panitsides, E. A. (2014). Transformational learning: Advocating for a holistic view. *Review of European Studies, 6*(4), 74–81. https://doi.org/10.5539/res.v6n4p74
Posner, M. I., & Rothbart, M. K. (2014). Attention to learning of school subjects. *Trends in Neuroscience and Education, 3*(1), 14–17. https://doi.org/10.1016/j.tine.2014.02.003
Pretzsch, C. M., & Floris, D. L. (2020). Autism: Balancing excitation and inhibition in autism. *eLife*. https://doi.org/10.7554/eLife.60584
Quintiliani, A. R. (2011). Developing mindfulness and emotional self-regulation. In A. N. Johnson & M. W. Neagley (Eds.), *Educating from the heart: Theoretical and practical approaches to transforming education* (pp. 25–36). R&L Education.
Raab, D. (2017). *Writing for bliss*. Loving Healing Press.
Reser, J. E. (2016). Incremental change in the set of coactive cortical assemblies enables mental continuity. *Physiology and Behavior, 167*(1), 222–237.
Runco, M. A. (2015). The standard definition of creativity. *Creativity Research Journal, 24*(1), 92–96.
Salvi, C., Bricolo, E., Kounios, J., Bowden, E., & Beeman, M. (2016). Insight solutions are correct more often than analytic solutions. *Thinking and Reasoning, 22*(4), 443–460. https://doi.org/10.1080/13546783.2016.1141798
Sawyer, K. (2011). The cognitive neuroscience of creativity: A critical review. *Creativity Research Journal, 23*(2), 137–154. https://doi.org/10.1080/10400419.2011.571191
Schuck, N. W., Gaschler, R., Winke, D., Heinzle, J., Frensch, P. A., Haynes, J.-D., & Reverberti, C. (2015). Medial prefrontal cortex predicts internally driven strategic shifts. *Neuron, 86*(1), 331–340. https://doi.org/10.1016/j.neuron.2015.03.015
Solms, M., & Friston, K. (2018). How and why consciousness arises: Some considerations from physics and physiology. *Journal of Consciousness Studies, 25*(5–6), 202–230.
Taylor, E. W. (2001). Transformational learning theory: A neurological perspective of the role of emotions and unconscious ways of knowing. *International Journal of Lifelong Education, 20*(3), 218–238.
Watzlawick, P., Weakland, J., & Fisch, R. (1979). *Change: Principles of problem formation, and problem resolution*. Norton.
Wilson, T. D., & Schooler, J. W. (1991). Thinking too much: Introspection can reduce the quality of preferences and decisions. *Journal of Personality and Social Psychology, 60*(2), 181–192. https://doi.org/10.1037/0022-3514.60.2.181
Zull, J. (2006). *The art of changing the brain: Enriching the practice of teaching by exploring the biology of learning*. Stylus.

3

SYSTEMS/DIALECTICAL THEORY

Theoretical Foundation of Second Order Parenting

To better analyze and dissect the nuances of neuroscience research focusing on implicit, intuitive, and creative components of second order parenting, a theoretical foundation is needed. The challenge is to apply a theoretical model that describes the parenting process and considers stability and change over time. The systems/dialectical model will be used as the theoretical framework for understanding this process because it can explain both how persons interact within a family system and how persons and systems change over time. The author has applied the systems dialectical framework to parenting (Roberts, 1994), marriage, and family therapy training (Roberts et al., 1999), and to social policy for child and family development (Roberts, 2019). A systems/dialectical perspective addresses both ontology, or content, and epistemology, that is, by what means the content is expressed. The purpose of this chapter is to illustrate that, in terms of systems, a family system, including parenting behaviors, is an interacting whole that changes through a dialectical process of contradictions. A corollary purpose is to demonstrate how the systems/dialectical framework might establish a defensible model of parent education.

Ludwig von Bertalanffy (1972), a biologist by training, founded general systems theory to explain how living organisms interact. He attempted to develop principles of common characteristics of all living organisms in both plant life and animal life. While this description emphasized how organisms are interconnected and illustrate wholeness, it did not necessarily show *how* interacting parts of a system change. *Dialectical thinking* shares the concept of wholeness with systems theory and describes a process for change through contradiction, conflict, and oppositions (Basseches, 1984). This chapter will review the main trends of systems theory and

DOI: 10.4324/9781003381679-4

dialectical theory, and how combining them can provide a framework for understanding the nuances of parenting and parent education. Systems theory is a general theory that could be thought of as an umbrella theory that lacks specifics and concrete behavior (Turner & Baker, 2019). Its strengths outweigh this weakness, however, because it provides a way to decipher and understand complex interactions. The components and general method of analyzing interactions will be discussed later.

Systems Theory

Wholeness

As mentioned earlier, one of the major characteristics of systems theory is **wholeness** (von Bertalanffy, 1972). Interactions and behaviors within the family are interrelated, rather than isolated, and represent a bidirectional link. The concept of wholeness depicts the family as a unit of interactional parts that mutually affect each other. Any behavior within a family, including parenting, must be viewed from the perspective of shared causality. Parenting is a behavior based on history and the ongoing interactional dynamic of parent and child. Both child and parent contribute to the outcome of interaction between them and any change in either will result in a response in the other. The parent–child interaction cannot be understood from the standpoint of only one member of the dyad. While one parent may be in a close relationship with the child, the partner or other persons involved in parenting exert significant influence on parenting that cannot be ignored.

Boundaries

Boundaries define barriers between individual parts of a system that determine its function and composition (Goldenberg & Goldenberg, 2008). In families, boundaries are set by communication patterns which are described as open, closed, or diffuse. Open boundaries allow for free exchange of information across various parts of the system. Closed boundaries allow for little information to be shared between parts of the system, and diffuse boundaries are difficult to identify. For example, a family with a closed boundary would restrict certain people or experiences from entering the family system, and a family with a diffuse boundary would allow anything in. *Subsystems* are created in the family to regulate emotional closeness and distance, which include the spousal subsystem, the sibling subsystem, and the parent–child subsystem. Each subsystem has different functions within the family unit and contributes to the overall quality of family relationships.

Closeness and distance among family members are ongoing concerns because too much or too little closeness can result in dysfunctional relationships (Bowen, 1978). Families with too much closeness are described as *emotionally fused* where members do not develop functional self-awareness. Families with too little closeness are described as *disengaged*, which is characterized by lack of intimacy and emotional support. The balance between fusion and disengagement is labeled *differentiation*, the ability to emotionally separate while maintaining closeness.

The term "boundary," used to describe various aspects of family relationships, has been challenged by several writers (Baptist & Hamon, 2022). Montgomery and Fewer (1988) preferred the phrase "*relative openness*" to "boundary" because "boundary" carries many different meanings in the literature and "relative openness" refers to a more precise meaning. Fused and enmeshed boundaries have been criticized for not being cross-culturally relevant (Goldenberg & Goldenberg, 2008). However, a recent cross-cultural study found Bowen's concept of differentiation to be validated and cross-culturally relevant (Lampis et al., 2019).

In terms of parenting, appropriate boundaries are necessary to ensure that assigned roles and behaviors are conducted as needed and that a clear boundary exists between parent and child. The relationship can also be assessed for enmeshment, which is implicated in parental overreaction to strivings for normal independence exerted by the child.

Rules

Rules refer to repeatable patterns of interaction that occur without conscious awareness, referred to as the *redundancy principle* (Day, 2009). Rules govern how humans interact in reciprocal ongoing relationships that occur and cannot be viewed as happening accidently (Shannon et al., 2019). Family rules delineate expected behaviors of family members and can be passed down through generations and encapsulated in cultural norms. Rules are considered normative because they regulate expectations on such matters as division of labor, patterns of closeness and distance, and the allocation of resources.

Rigid family rules correspond to complementary *roles* that are acted out between partners. These are complementary in that the partners do not perform the same role. While this may create a distinct division of labor and on the surface appear to be working, over time it can lead to over-functioning of one partner and under-functioning of the other partner (Dallos & Draper, 2010). In parenting, roles can be explicit or implicit, the same or complementary. Unacknowledged rules set the tone for roles, such as nurturing and disciplining behaviors, which tend to be complementary.

In parenting, rigid complementary roles lead to one parent being overinvolved in a particular role and the other parent being overinvolved in a different role and the outcome is one of dissatisfaction with each other. An escalation of anger and dissatisfaction arises because the solution tends to be "doing more of the same," or trying to solve the problem by doing the same behavior repeatedly with the same poor results. Consequently, doing more of the same can lead to complete rejection of the partner's role.

Hierarchy

Hierarchy is a principle of systems theory that demonstrates the organizational structure of a system, that is, a system is organized from the least to the most complex (Goldenberg & Goldenberg, 2008). In families, this refers to an organization beginning with a simple unit consisting of limited complexity, then to a subsystem consisting of two or more units, next to a larger family system, followed in complexity to the community, the state, the nation, and the world.

Within the family hierarchy, a generational hierarchy exists whereby parents have more authority and power to make family decisions and set rules or guidelines for behavior (Thornton, 2017). While parents may not have equal power in parenting, a shared sense of power between parents maintains a hierarchical position over children. The hierarchy between parent and child demands that parents are in a hierarchical level of complexity over the child, which does not necessarily mean that the children have no input or voice in the decision making process. It refers to taking responsibility and not abnegating their role of leadership to the child or the children. In the three styles of parenting, *authoritarian*, *authoritative*, and *diffuse*, the most functional family is the authoritative style and the least functional is when the hierarchy is undermined, meaning when a child or children are at the head of the hierarchy. When the child becomes the head of the hierarchy and parents assume a child position in the family, dysfunction in the family will occur.

Homeostasis

Homeostasis, or equilibrium, defines the desire and attempt on the part of a system to maintain a steady state (Figure 3.1) (Hammond, 2010). When stress enters the family system, the system responds in ways to return it to the prestress level. The analogy for understanding the homeostatic function of the family is a thermostat regulating the airflow in a house. For example, when the air becomes too hot, cool air begins to circulate to return the air temperature to the desired temperature. Thus, the dialectic involved with homeostasis and *morphogenesis*, or change, is a constant and ongoing process that explains much of the behaviors within the family. The force to change and the opposing force to maintain the status quo is the dialectic that is played out in different contexts within and outside the family.

In parenting, a source of stress is when a child is misbehaving and the parent feels irritated at not being able to get compliance from the child. The parent responds automatically to regain control, which can result in a visceral action that reduces the misbehavior but sets in motion actions that create negative interactional patterns. In addition, the misbehaving of the child can return the family to stability (Haley & Hoffman, 1973). For example, the parents argue in a manner that is chaotic and potentially violent, which is followed by the child acting out and demanding attention. The parents are diverted from their destructive argument and instead focus on controlling the child's misbehavior.

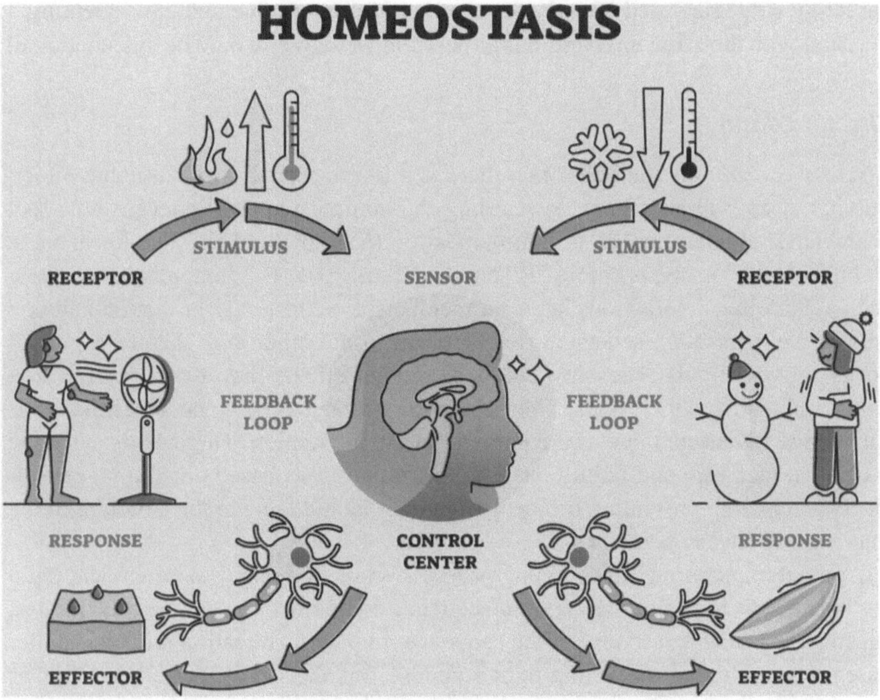

FIGURE 3.1 Homeostasis maintains the status quo via feedback loops, though change can be necessary.

Feedback Loops

Feedback loops between the system and the environment provide both new input from the environment and the system's response to the new input (Zelenska, 2019). Feedback from and to the environment and within the family is an ongoing process that is both explicit and implicit. Feedback can be either positive, change is occurring, or negative, change is not occurring. The dual response of maintaining homeostasis and allowing for change acts as a self-correcting mechanism that ensures that the system will function adequately. Therefore, the main function of feedback loops is self-correcting to maintain the system. Feedback loops represent an ongoing evaluation of the system's ability to function in times of challenges and stress.

Applied to parenting and parent education, feedback loops account for how new input in the form of the child's behavior is responded to by the parent. Sometimes the same behavior in the child can produce new responses from the parent and other times new input from the child can precipitate new behavior in the parent. As the child ages and goes through various developmental stages, new responses are needed by the parent. A major consequence of parenting is continuing the same parenting strategies used in early development for later development. Parenting a teenager with the same interventions as parenting a toddler would be dysfunctional.

Circular Causality

Circular causality is the belief that there is a linear progress of cause and effect; this is not appropriate for understanding the complex interactional patterns that characterize human nonlinear communication (Mantova, 2022). The linear view claims that "A" happens before "B" and is the cause of "B." In nonlinear systems, such as families, interactions between members are constantly in motion and one part of the interaction sequence is antecedent to the other and, therefore, cannot be its cause. Circular causality points to mutual effects that a person exerts on another person and vice versa. The interaction between the two becomes the focus for change rather than one of the partners in the interaction. Therapeutic systemic models in marriage and family therapy utilize questions based on circular causality to reframe the presenting problem from individual blame to the structure of the interaction between persons.

Applied to parenting, the ongoing progression of exchanges of parent and child are antecedent to each other, and no sequence of interactions can be identified as causing a particular response in the sequence. In parent education models, neither parent nor child can claim that their response was caused by the other. Circular causality is very helpful in parent education models because parents participate in training for one of two reasons: (1) They believe that their child has a conduct disorder (the child is the problem). (2) They have abused their child and must attend parent education to be reunited (they are the problem). Circular causality allows intervention in the parent–child problem situation without blaming the individual (parent or child), but instead focuses on the maladaptive interrelationship.

Morphogenesis

Morphogenesis depicts change within the system and is the opposite of homeostasis (Zastrow & Krist-Ashman, 2010). These two forces, morphogenesis and homeostasis, activate each other to keep the system stable. For example, when too much change enters the system, the homeostatic function kicks in to return it to balance or equilibrium. This dynamic of change versus homeostatic function in the family is useful to family therapists. Family systems therapists not only embrace change but believe that the systems must be shaken up to acquire a higher level of functioning. Increasing the tension in the family by introducing unexpected change provides an opportunity to reorganize the system and increase its functionality (Minuchin, 1998). On the other hand, too little change results from doing more of the same, which leads to stagnation and lack of growth.

In parenting, too much change in the child's behavior can destabilize the balance in the relationship with the parent, which results in inactivating homeostatic efforts to reduce the effects of the change. The purpose of parent education is to facilitate change in the parent–child relationship by changing the underlying system that supports it. This change in the system is referred to as second order change.

Equifinality

Equifinality is a principle of systems theory based on the knowledge that a particular starting point can produce many outcomes or vice versa, that many starting points can produce a single outcome (Goldenberg & Goldenberg, 2008). Applied to families, equifinality means that in open systems there are more than one functional path. Behavior within the family cannot be reduced to a simple formula but represents complexity (Dauchot, 2018). The tendency to eliminate options in decision making to find the right option may reduce rather than enhance decision making. Equifinality supports a dialectical view because more than one solution is viable.

Applied to parenting, equifinality implies that a single parenting behavior can lead to many outcomes, some of which may not be desired. On the other hand, it reflects that there are numerous parenting behaviors that could have positive outcomes. Applied to parent education, equifinality suggests that the tendency to predetermine specific training modules may artificially limit the effectiveness of the program by not allowing spontaneity and flexibility.

Systems theory has a long history of being applied to family dynamics (see Table 3.1). It is the most used theory for understanding communication patterns, roles, rules, and dysfunction in family relationships. A cardinal belief in family systems theory is that families "cannot communicate" and that family members are constantly attempting to explain the composition of their relationship (Johnson & Ray, 2016).

The shortcomings of systems theory include being too general and lacking specific interventions (Murphy & Callaghan, 1988). While systems theory emphasizes change, it does not describe the process whereby change happens. It also has been criticized by some scholars for the nebulous description of domestic violence (Yllo, 1993). These shortcomings are offset by combining systems theory with dialectical theory, which will be discussed later in this chapter.

Dialectical Theory

Dialectical theory is based on how change takes place and represents a number of applications. This book focuses on dialectics as developed by Georg Hegel (1830/1991), Klaus Riegel (1976, 1979), and the writings of Baxter and Montgomery (1998). Georg Hegel believed that the process of competing phenomena, a *thesis*, and its *antithesis* or opposite, leading to a *synthesis* described how change in humans and society took place. This process repeats with the synthesis becoming the new thesis pitted against its antithesis, followed by the synthesis.

TABLE 3.1 Components of Systems Theory

Systems Theory	
Wholeness	The concept of wholeness depicts the family as a unit of interactional parts that mutually affect each other. Interactions and behaviors within the family are interrelated, rather than isolated, and represent a bidirectional link
Boundaries	Boundaries define barriers between individual parts of a system that determine its function and composition. In families, boundaries are set by communication patterns which are described as open, closed, or diffuse. Open boundaries allow for free exchange of information across various parts of the system. Closed boundaries allow for little information to be shared between parts of the system, and diffuse boundaries are difficult to identify
Rules	Rules refer to repeatable patterns of interaction that occur without conscious awareness, referred to as the redundancy principle. Rules govern how humans interact in reciprocal ongoing relationships that occur and cannot be viewed as happening accidently. Family rules delineate expected behaviors of family members and can be passed down through generations and encapsulated in cultural norms
Hierarchy	Hierarchy is a principle of systems theory that demonstrates the organizational structure of a system, that is, a system is organized from the least to the most complex. In families, this refers to an organization beginning with a simple unit consisting of limited complexity, then to a subsystem consisting of two or more units, next to a larger family system, followed in complexity to the community, the state, the nation, and the world
Homeostasis	Homeostasis, or equilibrium, defines the desire and attempt on the part of a system to maintain a steady state
Feedback loops	Feedback loops between the system and the environment provide both new input from the environment and the system's response to the new input
Circular causality	Circular causality is the belief that there is linear progress of cause and effect; this is not appropriate for understanding the complex interactional patterns that characterize human nonlinear communication
Morphogenesis	Morphogenesis depicts change within the system and is the opposite of homeostasis
Equifinality	Equifinality is a principle of systems theory based on the knowledge that a particular starting point can produce many outcomes or vice versa, that many starting points can produce a single outcome. Applied to families, equifinality means that in open systems there are more than one functional path

Klaus Riegel

Klaus Riegel (1976, 1979) developed the dialectical theory of child development based on Hegel's dialectical process. He believed that development lacked predictable stages but reflected an interplay of internal and external occurrences. For Riegel, as it was for Hegel, change is the product of a synthesis formed from opposite positions. Riegel revised the stage theory of child development by replacing it with the view that development occurred by the interface of four dimensions—the inner/biological, the individual/psychological, the outer/physical, and the social/cultural (see Table 3.2). The inner/biological dimension explains biological and physical maturity, which does not occur at the same time in everyone. The outer/physical refers to the world outside of the individual that interacts and creates a dialogue. The individual/psychological dimension refers to emotional and mental maturity. The social/cultural aspect refers to the social environment the child is born into. *Contradictions* within a dimension or between dimensions lead to developmental change. Breaking with Piaget (1926), Riegel did not believe in an equilibrium period in which change is dormant, but instead postulated that development was always in flux because of contradictions. Furthermore, the dialectic for Riegel, contradictions between one or more of the four dimensions of development, differed from Piaget who believed that the dialectic was between the individual and the environment.

Baxter and Montgomery

The relational dialectical view of Baxter and Montgomery (1998) also influenced the development of systems/dialectical theory presented in this book. *Relational dialectics* refers to how contradictions and conflicts are structurally engrained in interpersonal interactions, especially in romantic and marital relationships. Baxter and Montgomery discuss four concepts that describe dialectics in intimate relationships—totality, change, contradiction, and praxis— that must be viewed as a whole. One-sided or partial views of an interaction between individuals within a family are prone to be misunderstood and provide misinformation. The parent and child relationship cannot be understood from the standpoint of either the parent or the child.

TABLE 3.2 Klaus Riegel (1976, 1979) Developed the Dialectical Theory of Child Development

Inner/Biological	Individual/Psychological
Biological and physical maturity	Emotional and mental maturity
Outer/Physical	Social/Cultural
The world outside of the individual	Social environment the child is born into

When Baxter and Montgomery (1998) use the word *change*, they mean that things are always in flux. This tendency for relationships to always be in flux requires much flexibility and the ability of systems and subsystems to adjust and move forward. One of the ongoing issues in parenting is that children change frequently due to ongoing psychological, emotional, and physical development, which alters and redefines the relationship with the parent who might also be changing. Change is not a value term and can be positive or negative depending on the circumstances.

Contradiction refers to the acknowledgment that any given point of view, belief, perspective, assumption, and the like have opposing positions that are equally valid (Baxter, 2004). For parenting, it means that there are many parenting behaviors that are equally adequate and appropriate. It also suggests that the parent and the child may have opposing assumptions, beliefs, and behaviors that are valid. Power assertions by either the parent or the child leads to reduced intimacy and a strained relationship.

Praxis states that human relationships are composed of actions and reactions which tend to be understood as circular causality. Human relationships are nonlinear and nonrecursive, which explains how escalation of conflict occurs. In terms of parenting, there can be no action that does not produce a reaction.

Combining systems theory and dialectical theory provides for a unique theory that can be applied to many human entities, including parenting and parent education. How systems/dialectical theory can be applied to parenting and parent education models will be discussed later.

The Systems/Dialectical Model

One of the hallmarks of combining systems theory and dialectical theory is the dynamic view of human relationships. Change is the cornerstone on which relationships are built. Michael Basseches (1984) believed that dialectical thinking was to adult's development what Piaget's (1926) *formal operations stage* was to a child's development. In other words, dialectical thinking is more complex and takes off where the formal operations stage stopped. For Basseches, development occurred from changes that were transformational since the change process is ongoing through integration and change. Developmental change is transformational in that there is both recognizing similarities among elements and concurrently recognizing differences. Basseches labeled transformational change as *constitutive change* because it was a fundamental change in the composition of a person in contrast to being only an *add-on change* which does not become the nature of the person. For parenting, changes that do not change the underlying structure of the parent–child relationship are considered first order changes, or what Basseches called add-ons. On the other hand, changes that are constitutive are transformational and second order because they change the very nature of the relationship.

Thinking from a Systems/Dialectical Perspective

Critical thinking is the ability to think rationally by weighting alternative positions and ideas and determining the most appropriate and useful position. Critical thinking requires an unbiased mind that is open to all possibilities (Horvath & Forte, 2011). It involves more than accumulating facts and involves evaluating alternative solutions and choosing the best option (Reynolds, 2011). This means that other options are discarded in favor of the best option. While critical thinking is a fundamental component of education and teaching, according to Basseches (1984), it does not go far enough. Dialectical thinking is needed to complement critical thinking because it assumes that many viable options exist and that the best option may not continue in perpetuity. As time passes and new input is introduced, new options will appear that will challenge the old position and a new best option will emerge. Because dialectical thinkers assume everything is in flux, no decision is final.

The position that new input that better addresses the original problems will replace the old solutions is similar to the writings of Thomas Kuhn (1962). Kuhn's theory of scientific revolution is based on the view that a paradigm, or structured belief system, does not change by linear accumulation of facts. For Kuhn, scientific knowledge changes because an accepted paradigm is challenged by new ideas that give better answers than the old paradigm. The paradigm shift may alter the old paradigm or completely replace it, depending on its ability to address all the issues involved. Thus, *paradigm shifts* explain how transformational scientific theories emerge.

Systems/dialectical thinking is grounded in Kuhnian logic. For example, systems/dialectical thinking values critical thinking and is aware that the nature of change occurs via competing information and contradictions that give rise to an ongoing process. Contradictions and debate are not oppositional; rather, they are complementary, and the change process is characterized as a debate in which different views can be synthesized into a new position that is uniquely different from the opposing views. Therefore, a new option is created by the synthesis of the opposing views that may be different or can have features of both views (Roberts, 2019).

A systems/dialectical approach postulates that opposites are bound together, much in the fashion of the yin/yang (Roberts, 2019). The phrase "*unity of entities*" describes how things are bound together and cannot be separated into individual parts. This means that there is fluidity in the change process in which movement occurs back and forth between positions. A position and its opposite are different sides of the same coin and are inclusive, not mutually exclusive. Attempting to eliminate the opposite alternative will ensure that at some point in the future, it will emerge (Roberts, 2019). A basic difference between critical thinking and systems/dialectical thinking is that critical thinking attempts to find the right position, while systems/dialectical thinking acknowledges that change is inevitable,

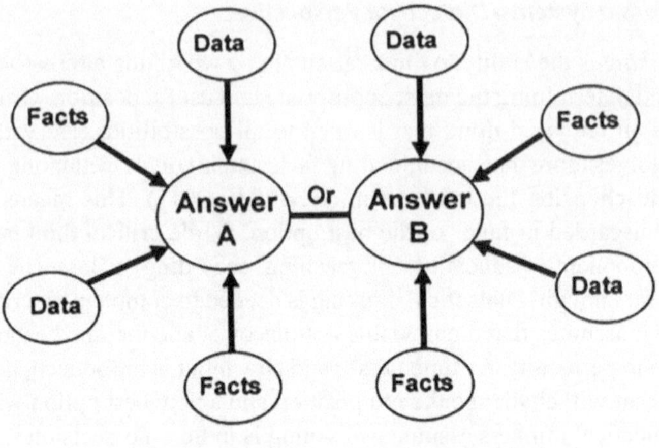

FIGURE 3.2 Convergent thinking differs from divergent thinking because, in divergent thinking, many solutions are possible. (CC BY-SA 3.0)

and no position is final. Systems/dialectical thinkers view the present and the future concurrently.

The procedure for finding a position in critical thinking is *convergent thinking*, or the endeavor to logically determine a path to the best position by eliminating alternative positions and converging on the best choice (Figure 3.2). Once a best choice is made, other options are no longer considered valuable. The decision process for the best choice is linear and leaves no room for ambiguity. *Divergent thinking* takes a 90-degree turn from convergent thinking. While both convergent and divergent thinking have the common goal of finding the most appropriate option, divergent thinking uses a process that is more creative than logical. Divergent thinking entails an open mindset and a recognition that the starting point can be seen from multiple points of view similar to generating multiple options.

Convergent and divergent thinking have not been applied to parenting or parent education models and doing so makes assumptions that would need verification (Figure 3.3). It seems reasonable, however, to note that there are many parenting behaviors that are appropriate and helpful in raising successful children. The danger in prescribing particular parenting behaviors and not prescribing others is to limit and perhaps reduce the effectiveness of interventions. This type of self-imposed limitation on teaching parenting behaviors lacks creativity and spontaneity to address unexpected child behaviors.

A Systems/Dialectical Perspective of Parenting and Parent Education

A systems/dialectical perspective of parenting attempts to understand group behavior within the family. The child's behavior cannot be understood apart from the

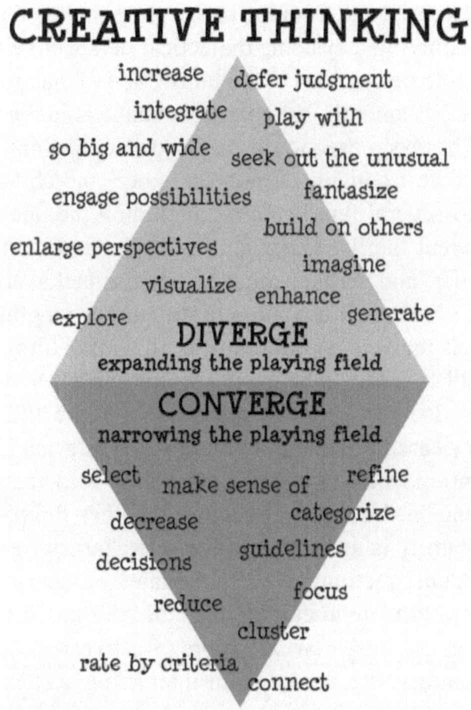

FIGURE 3.3 Convergent and divergent thinking are nearly opposite approaches to decision making.

reciprocal and nonrecursive interaction patterns among family members. In fact, the misbehaving of the child should not be the focus of parent education interventions, but rather be viewed as a symptom of the organizational structure of the family system. The goal of parenting and parent education from a systems perspective is, as in most parent education models, to develop functional families, not to merely help parents get control of acting-out or noncompliant children. The systems/dialectical principle of circular causality debunks the belief in cause and effect thinking and instead emphasizes the complexity of family relationships. The interaction in the family is more than a collection of dyadic relationships. It is a total ecosystem that must be addressed to affect long-lasting change. A single interaction may result in a multitude of responses leading to multiple outcomes. The systems/dialectical perspective does not focus on blaming any member of the family for problems within the family, but recognizes a shared responsibility. The interactional patterns within the family are bidirectional, which means that the parents affect the child, and the child affects the parents. The focus is on how shared responsibility results from the family's organization.

A systems/dialectical perspective would teach parents about family dynamics and an understanding of their own contribution to that dynamic, which would facilitate a transfer of knowledge from the parent training to their everyday interactions. The results of applying a systems/dialectical perspective would be to better understand what needs to be changed in the family and to make second order transformational change. Consequently, the locus of change is in the family.

The term "family" has been used to this point to refer to a unit of related persons with the assumption that it contains a mother, father, and children. However, the family today refers to several family forms, including the nuclear family, remarried family, single-parent family, foster families, homeless families, gay, lesbian, and transsexual families, and perhaps other family forms that are yet to be named. Different family forms have their own unique structure, strengths, weaknesses, and challenges. Given that there is a proliferation of family forms in contemporary society, the family will continue to be the basic unit of child and personal development. While this book does not delineate the nuances of the different family forms, it will make note of research pertaining to them when relevant.

The focus of parenting from a systems perspective is to enact transformational second order parenting in the family structure. Neither the parent nor the child is the problem. The family is an interacting whole characterized by bidirectional interaction patterns. A unidirectional view of the family assumes that the parent has acted either too early or too late in guiding the child through developmental stages and then needs help in learning new and more effective ways of interacting with their child. To the contrary, the family is an interacting system that goes beyond its boundaries to interact with other systems such as the school and governmental agencies. A systems/dialectical perspective would consider the influence of these interacting hierarchy roles that affect family interactions.

The parent education program intrudes into the family system having the same interactional effect on the family as any external system. The question is: Does the parent education program establish a unidirectional or a bidirectional relationship with the family? The answer is that most parent education programs do not consider this question. Typically, the parenting program is developed with this consideration: The program is based on the latest research in identifying characteristics of healthy families and skills that are needed to achieve a healthy family. The program leaves little room for spontaneity and flexibility in educational content. A systems/dialectical parent education program based on neuroscience research on learning, on the other hand, would look significantly different. For example, learning should not be merely thought of as requiring conscious cognitive awareness that is rational and logical. Learning also occurs from unconscious processing and from contradictions and illogical input.

Although change is inevitable within families, too much change in an individual can destabilize the family because of the reciprocal nature of interaction. A healthy family is one that can adapt to both *normative change*, expected developmental change, or *nonnormative change*, unexpected change, such as caused by accidents, illness, or economic status changes. The family unit consists of two interwoven developmental processes related to change within the family—the development of the child, and the development of the family beginning with the onset of the relationship.

Parenting is a stage in normative family development that can be very stressful for some parents, which can lead to a disruption in the partners' relationship. Each parent has an unconscious schema of what parenting entails that could conflict with the other's, resulting in a strained relationship. The parenting role is affected by the relationship factor with their partner, coupled with extrafamilial factors, such as social standing, community, poverty, quality of education, and violence (Kerig, 2019). More will be stated about the extrafamilial factors in other chapters.

Components of a Systems/Dialectical Parent Education Model

The benefits of applying a systems perspective to parenting was first suggested by Getz and Gunn (1988). Unfortunately, their work was not expanded, and little development has occurred since. A more developed model proposed by this author was not empirically tested (Roberts, 1994). It is hoped that with the grounding in neuroscience, a more comprehensive and useful model will arise. The rationale and structure of that model is presented later. The content and interventions will be presented in Part II of this book.

Basic Prerequisites

To change the family in the most effective way, adult participants should include anyone who is involved in parenting. In some families this may include grandparents, in others it may include a parent's live-in boyfriend or girlfriend. There is some evidence that not including participation by all adults in the family who have a parenting role can be detrimental to family relationships (Getz & Gunn, 1988). It is also important to include in parent education to assess asymptomatic children in the family. Systems theory assumes that all members of the family are affected by problems in any part of the system.

Assess the Family Dynamics

To accomplish the goal of changing the family structure, a thorough evaluation of the interactional patterns, hierarchy, rules, feedback loops, and the like must be done individually with each family. Only this type of individual assessment can reasonably be assumed to determine the types of interventions that are needed. Families are already equipped with some skills that they do not need help with. Thus, predetermined generic interventions are hit or miss and may not be the interventions needed. *We cannot assume that there is an undisputed healthy model of family relationships that can be applied to all families.*

Assessing the family dynamics is not unique to a system/dialectical perspective since most current models initially assess family strengths. The difference is after assessing the family dynamics, most models would find specific interventions to address problem areas taken from their repertoire of interventions. In contrast, a systems/dialectical perspective maintains the bidirectional nature of the system, which now includes the parent educator. Parents and educators could brainstorm options in a dialectical manner to generate options for changing behaviors.

Involving parents in a brainstorming exercise is a unique way of enhancing the strengths of parents. Creating options is generally the prerogative of the parent educator who presents to parents a best option to address their concerns. When parents are invited to participate in this process, their strengths are put into action, and they are less resistant to transformational change. Recent research supports the view that learning takes place via taking action rather than via abstract thinking (Paul, 2014). Parents' involvement in the process of creating options enhances their learning and reduces their resistance to change.

Involving parents in creating options for new interventions will affect both the motivation to change and the cognitive ability to change (Berkman, 2018). In terms of Berkman's model, parents that participate in identifying how they need to change and brainstorm with the educator how to change will move toward Berkman's quadrant of high motivation and high knowledge (see Table 2.1). Change is enhanced because participants have increased the subjective value of the learning experience by being participants rather than being only observers. As one places higher value on the behavior, they have higher motivation to perform it (Krajbich et al., 2010). Neuroscience has demonstrated that plasticity of the brain is increased by action. Neurons form new connections from doing an activity that are not evident when there is passive involvement.

In assessing the family dynamics, parents become aware of their behaviors and interventions that do not work, which can present some uneasy responses. They recognize that other interventions are needed to change the parent–child dynamic, including a change in their frame of reference (Sawatsky et al., 2018). Implicit self-assessment at this point could stimulate negative emotions such as anger and guilt.

The family assessment phase includes scrutiny of the function and role of subsystems (see Table 3.3) (Mandak et al., 2017). Questions arise as follows: Is there a strong functional parental subsystem? Are there marital problems that affect parenting? Are there clear boundaries between parents and children? Does triangulation occur that might be transferred into the training experience (Fosco & Bray, 2016)? The answers to these questions and others help to determine the whole family system, which is the goal of systems/dialectical parenting.

Emotions

As has been previously noted, emotions are necessary for transformational change, and parent educators would be good to acknowledge emotions. In typical learning

TABLE 3.3 Contributions of a Systems/Dialectical Parenting Approach

Based on neuroscience findings of implicit learning
Includes parents in determining training needs
Focuses on family transformational/second order change
Does not prescribe predetermined skill-building modules
Uses contradiction and novelty to increase dialectical and divergent thinking
Recognizes the role of implicit schemas in parenting
Includes structured downtime in training sessions
Empowers parents to be their own change agents
Trainer uses spontaneous, creative, and implicit interventions
Trainer forms a bond with trainees
Trainer incorporates emotions to enhance learning

environments, emotional responses are expected to be minimized because they are perceived to be a distraction. Training models emphasize rational content, and the display of emotions is viewed as interfering with the acquisition of knowledge. According to neuroscientist James Zull (2006), learning is both a cognitive and an emotional experience. In fact, learning cannot happen without the emotional areas of the brain being involved. Contrary to popular belief, when one attempts to problem-solve by using logical arguments, the area of the brain that is active is the emotional or limbic system and not the neocortex (Immordina-Yang & Damacio, 2006). Learning, memory formation and recall, and making decisions fall under the rubric of what Immordino-Yang and Damasio called emotional thoughts. What has been perceived to be the domain of the logical thinking brain is now viewed as the domain of the emotional processes of the brain. This conclusion does not mean that the emotional brain replaces or is dominant over the neocortex but points to the intricate collaboration of the emotional and the rational brain functions that in the past were separated to the degree that the emotional brain was subordinate to the rational brain.

There should be ample connection between what one is learning cognitively and what one is feeling in parent education training if the training is to be effective. If the emotional brain is activated in the learning experience and not the neocortex, it would be helpful for the educator to inquire of the trainees what they are feeling. Making this connection between the cognitive input and the emotional processes taking place would provide a needed bridge between the explicit and implicit mental processes. The knowledge that the emotional brain is activated in learning and decision making could be incorporated into the training model periodically. For example, after teaching a basic communication skill, such as listening, the educator could ask trainees what they are feeling. Some introduction to emotions should be a prerequisite before the training begins.

Emotional responses can be positive or negative, depending on the individual response to the training. Negative emotions can hamper learning, while positive emotions can enhance learning (Zull, 2006). While parent education is distinct from therapy, some overlap exists because of the importance of processing cognitive and emotional input that is meant to produce transformational change. To deal with the possible negative fallout, the educator should be familiar with interventions aimed at increasing positive emotions.

It should also be noted that, paradoxically, negative emotions can lead dialectically to resolutions that could not be attained otherwise. In the sense of creating wholeness, it is important not to hide or minimize negative emotions. A systems/dialectical perspective posits that negative and positive emotions are intertwined like the yin and yang symbol. Acknowledging the presence of negative emotions with a degree of acceptance leads to greater unity and wholeness.

Antithesis

The learning environment typically uses a critical thinking process for presenting information that is logical, conscious, and explicit. The goal is to eliminate ambiguity and unclear thinking. The last thing educators want to do is to confuse trainees or present information that has multiple meanings. Recent neuroscience research demonstrates that the very opposite may be true, namely, for deep learning to take place, multiple points of view increase learning (Kovač et al., 2023). Learning does not have to be conscious, logical, or explicit. Consequently, the learning process should expose the trainee to both thesis and antithesis. Contradictions can improve deep learning and lead to spontaneous insight for trainees, such as the aha experience.

Downtime

Planned downtime for strategic purposes is not a typical aspect of training programs and learning environments, perhaps partly because of the emphasis on conscious cognitive learning. Recent neuroscience studies contradict this popular belief and foster an environment that recognizes that learning can be both conscious and unconscious (Fukuta & Yamashita, 2021). In fact, studies show that learning is heightened by periods of distraction in a learning environment. The research on the aha experience illustrates how downtime following an ambiguous cognitive input can facilitate a spontaneous and sudden understanding that could not be reached before. Strategically placed downtime within a parent education model in the form of a distraction may facilitate deep learning. A distraction, such as playing an unrelated game, gives the unconscious an opportunity to continue working on the issue at hand to find a solution.

Creativity and Novelty

Research studies in several disciplines confirm the overall benefits of active learning (Begus & Bonawitz, 2020). Active learning promotes creativity and novelty and increases self-efficacy (Sawyer, 2017). The ability to learn stretches over the entire lifespan and reflects both maturational processes and experiences. While learning is generally thought of as related to the brain's reward system and increase in dopamine (Dayan & Daw, 2008), recent research found that novelty of the learning experience increased the motivation to learn. According to Dyan and Daw, novelty increased dopamine levels that activated the hippocampal network, which acted to increase motivation for novelty-seeking experiences. From this perspective, models of learning that continue to treat a dualism of rational and emotional brain processes and limit emotional expression will be less effective. To stimulate novelty, educators should provide opportunities for trainees to offer suggestions and engage in the divergent process of skill development.

Joining

One of the most celebrated beliefs of systems family therapy is that the therapist cannot change the family from outside the family but must join with the family as an insider (Minuchin, 1998). *Joining* the family system means that the therapist must adopt their language and style and be able to play a role in the family. The concept of joining may be difficult to operationalize in parent education training, but the trainer–trainee relationship is unique and requires forming a bond. Research has demonstrated that patients value their therapy experience based on how they feel about the therapist and not the actual, specific interventions (Norcross & Lambert, 2018). In other words, the personal attachment and attunement with the therapist provides the healing that takes place rather than any explicit behavior models or interventions employed by the therapist (Stern, 1998). The process of therapeutic change involving implicit knowledge has relevance for parent training in a number of ways.

Applying this to parent education, it means that in behavior change, especially as it leads to second order change, the relationships between the trainer and the trainee trump using the cognitive content. Attunement with the family is not something that the educator can script beforehand. It must occur spontaneously in the interchange between the educator and members of the family and must reflect genuine concern by responding to verbal or nonverbal information and gut feelings. It can be assumed that lecturing and presenting didactic material without joining the family and attuning to their concerns would not be very successful in producing behavioral change. It can also be assumed that online parent education may be less effective because there is no relationship with the trainer.

In sum, a systems/dialectical model of parenting based on second order change emphasizes the interaction and communication patterns within the family. The child's misbehavior is viewed in the context of family, which is a rule-governed system. Any change in one part of the system sends waves throughout the system. The focus is not for parents to learn skills to control or change the child's behavior, but to form a deeper and more meaningful relationship. The systems/dialectical parent educator attempts to empower the family to be its own change agent. Trainees would be encouraged to bring their own personal meanings into the training situation and in doing so would be their own change agents. Emotional content would be emphasized. Recognizing that one's personal schema may require altering to make changes in the family system would influence how the educator addresses the problem behavior.

References

Baptist, J., & Hamon, R. R. (2022). Family systems theory. In K. Adamsons, A. L. Few-Demo, C. M. Proulx, & K. Roy (Eds.), *Sourcebook of family theories and methodologies* (pp. 209–223). Springer.

Basseches, M. (1984). *Dialectical thinking and adult development*. Ablex.

Baxter, L. A. (2004). Relationships as dialogues. *Personal Relationships, 11,* 1–22.

Baxter, L. A., & Montgomery, B. M. (1998). *Dialectical approaches to studying personal relationships*. Erlbaum.

Begus, K., & Bonawitz, E. (2020). The rhythm of learning: Theta oscillations as an index of active learning in infancy. *Developmental Cognitive Neuroscience, 45,* 1–10. https://doi.org/10.1016/j.den.2020.100810

Berkman, E. T. (2018). The neuroscience of goals and behavior change. *Consulting Psychology Journal, 70*(1), 28–44. https://doi.org/10.1037/cpb0000094

Bowen, M. (1978). *Family therapy in clinical practice*. Jason Aronson.

Dallos, R., & Draper, R. (2010). *Introduction to family therapy: Systemic theory and practice*. Open University Press/McGraw Hill.

Dauchot, N. (2018). Systems theory for designers: Equifinality, multifinality, unifinality, and counterfinality. *Medium*. https://medium.com/@nickuxd/finality-constructs-in-design-systems-466ae4c2c06c

Day, R. D. (2009). *Introduction to family processes*. Routledge.

Dayan, P., & Daw, N. B. (2008). Decision theory, reinforcement learning, and the brain. *Cognitive, Affective, and Behavioral Neuroscience, 8,* 429–453.

Fosco, G. M., & Bray, B. (2016). Profiles of adolescents' triangulation and appraisals of interparental conflict: Implications for adjustment. *Journal of Family Psychology, 30,* 524–537.

Fukuta, J., & Yamashita, J. (2021). The complex relationship between conscious/unconscious learning and conscious/unconscious knowledge: The mediating effects of salience in forming meaning connections. *Second Language Research*. https://doi.org/10.1177/02676583211044950

Getz, H., & Gunn, W. B. (1988). Parent education from a family-systems perspective. *The School Counselor, 35,* 331–336.

Goldenberg, H., & Goldenberg, I. (2008). *Family therapy: An overview* (7th ed.). Thomson.

Haley, J., & Hoffman, L. (1973). *Techniques of family therapy*. Basic Books.

Hammond, D. (2010). *The science of synthesis: Exploring the social implications of general systems theory*. The University Press of Colorado.

Hegel, G. W. F. (1991). *The encyclopedia logic* (T. F. Geraets, Trans.). Hackett. (Original work published 1830)

Horvath, C. P., & Forte, J. M. (Eds.). (2011). *Critical thinking*. Nova. https://doi.org/10.38146/bsz.spec.2022.2.6

Immordina-Yang, M. E., & Damacio, A. (2006). We feel, therefore we learn: The relevance of affective and social neuroscience to education. *Mind and Education, 1*(1), 3–10. https://doi.org/10.1111/j.1751-228X.2007.00004.x

Johnson, B. E., & Ray, W. A. (2016). Family systems theory. In *Encyclopedia of family studies*. https://doi.org/10.1002/9781119085621.wbefs130

Kerig, P. K. (2019). Parenting and family systems. In M. H. Bornstein (Ed.), *Handbook of parenting: Being and becoming a parent* (pp. 3–35). Routledge/Taylor and Francis Group. https://doi.org/10.4324/9780429433214-1

Kovač, V. B., Nome, D. Ø., Jensen, A. R., & Skreland, L. L. (2023). The why, what, and how of deep learning: Critical analysis and additional concerns. *Education Inquiry*. https://doi.org/10.1080/20004508.2023.2194502

Krajbich, I., Armel, C., & Rangel, A. (2010). Visual fixations and the computation and comparison of value in simple choice. *Nature Neuroscience, 13*(10), 1292–1298.

Kuhn, T. (1962). *The structure of scientific revolutions*. University of Chicago Press.

Lampis, J., Rodríguez-González, M., Cataudella, S., Relvas, A. P., Neophytou, K., & Agus, M. (2019). Cross-cultural validity of Bowen theory in southern European countries. *Australian and New Zealand Journal of Family Therapy*, *40*(4), 457–482. https://doi.org/10.1002/anzf.1394

Mandak, K., O'Neill, T., Light, J., & Fosco, G. M. (2017). Bridging the gap from values to actions: A family systems framework for family-centered AAC services. *Augmentative and Alternative Communication, 33,* 32–41.

Mantova, K. S. (2022). Theoretical overview of circular questions in family and systemic therapy. *Knowledge: International Journal, 54*(1), 187–191.

Minuchin, S. (1998). *Family healing: Strategies for hope and understanding*. Free Press.

Montgomery, J., & Fewer, W. (1988). *Family systems and beyond*. Family Science Press.

Murphy, J., & Callaghan, K. A. (1988). Systems theory and the family: A critique. *Early Child Development and Care, 39*(1), 163–176. https://doi.org/10.1080/0300443880390113

Norcross, J. C., & Lambert, M. J. (2018). Psychotherapy relationships that work 111. *Psychotherapy*, *55*(4), 303–315. https://doi.org/10.1037/pst0000193

Paul, L. A. (2014). *Transformational experience*. Oxford University Press.

Piaget, J. (1926). *The language and thought of the child*. Harcourt Brace.

Reynolds, M. (2011). Critical thinking and systems thinking: Toward a critical literacy of systems thinking in practice. In C. P. Horvath & J. M. Forte (Eds.), *Critical thinking* (pp. 37–68). Nova.

Riegel, K. F. (1976). The dialectics of human development. *American Psychologist, 31,* 689–700.

Riegel, K. F. (1979). *Foundations of developmental psychology*. Academic Press.

Roberts, T. W. (1994). *A systems perspective of parenting: The individual, the family, and the social network*. Brooks/Cole.

Roberts, T. W. (2019). *Social policy for child and family development: A systems/dialectical perspectives*. San Diego, CA: Cognella.

Roberts, T. W., Winek, J., & Mulgrew, J. (1999). A systems/dialectical model of supervision: A symbolic process. *Contemporary Family Therapy, 21,* 291–302.

Sawatsky, A. P., Nordhues, H. C., Merry, S. P., Bashir, M. U., & Hafferty, F. E. (2018). Transformational learning and professional identity formation during international health electives: A qualitative study using grounded theory. *Academic Medicine, 93,* 1380–1391. https://doi.org/10.1097/ACM0000000000002230

Sawyer, K. (2017). The development of creativity. *Imperial Studies of the Arts*, *38*(1), https://doi.org/10.11770276237419868958

Shannon, S., Sutton, J., Simmons, B., & Holowacz, E. (2019). Family rules. In J. Lebow, A. Chambers, & D. Breunlin (Eds.), *Encyclopedia of couple and family therapy*. Springer. https://doi.org/10.1007/978-3-319-15877-8_268-1

Stern, D. (1998). The process of therapeutic change involving implicit knowledge: Some implications of developmental observations for adult psychotherapy. *Infant Mental Health Journal, 19*(3), 300–308.

Thornton, J. (2017). *Family structure*. Foundations Family Counseling. https://www.foundationsfamily.com/post/family-structure

Turner, J. R., & Baker, R. M. (2019). Complexity theory: An overview with implications for the social sciences. *Systems, 7*(1), 4. https://doi.org/10.3390/systems7010004

von Bertalanffy, L. (1972). The history and status of general system theory. In G. Klir (Ed.), *Trends in general systems theory* (pp. 21–41). Wiley.

Yllo, K. (1993). Through a feminist lens: Gender, power, and violence. In R. Gelles & D. Loseke (Eds.), *Controversies on family violence* (pp. 19–34). SAGE.

Zastrow, C., & Krist-Ashman, K. K. (2010). *Understanding human behavior and the social environment*. Brooks/Cole.

Zelenska, M. (2019). Feedback loops in systems. *Medium*. https://medium.com/@myroslavazel/feedback-loops-in-system-thinking-7ef06e2ff310

Zull, J. (2006). *The art of changing the brain: Enriching the practice of teaching by exploring the biology of learning*. Stylus.

4

FACTORS THAT IMPACT PARENTING

Attachment

Attachment theory describes both the relationship of parent and child in the child's early years and development of relationships over the life course (Bowlby, 1988). Attachment is a bond between child and caregiver, usually the mother, which results from the quality of the caregiving. Attachment in infants is evident by their proximity to the caregiver, displaying distress when separated, and is stress-free when the caregiver is nearby (Ainsworth, 1973). During the first year of life, attachment develops through a series of states. Initially, the infant is equipped from birth to have a proclivity for generalized excitement that is manifested in positive and negative features. For example, smiling signifies a wish for communication and reflects one of three circumstances—an internal state, an external stimulus, or engaging a familiar person. Anxiety, distress, or fear can be present during the first year of life from separation from the mother, introduction of a stranger, or unfamiliar circumstances (Jones & Raag, 1989).

The initial testing of Bowlby's attachment theory was done by Ainsworth et al. (1978) through the *stranger situation paradigm* with infants 12–18 months old. Several scenes occur where the mother is present with the infant and is replaced by a stranger and then returned to the room. Of prime concern in this stranger situation test was how the infant reacted when separated from and reunited with her. They described three scenarios—*secure infants* who are in proximity with their mothers for a secure base and are quickly comforted on her return; *avoidant infants* who are not in proximity with their mothers and are not comforted on her return; *resistant infants* who fail to search their environment and react with ambivalence on the mother's return.

DOI: 10.4324/9781003381679-5

Attachment theory has been applied to human relationships across the lifespan, most notably in romantic and intimate pair bonding (Shaver et al., 2000). Early attachment, which develops implicitly before the rational center of the brain develops, becomes an unconscious internal working model for relationships across the lifespan. A plethora of research findings support the relation between attachment and relationship outcomes. For example, insecurely attachment children develop secondary attachment tactics because closeness with the caregiver is futile (Mikulincer et al., 2003). Anxiously attached children develop strategies to repetitively screen their environment for threats and overreact to minor risks to their sense of security. This hyperactive scrutiny of their environment for threats resulted from parenting that was intrusive and prevented the child from learning self-monitoring skills.

Securely attached children have mothers who emphasize emotional awareness and accurately respond with emotional support to their children's verbal interactions, which leads to *emotional self-regulation*, the ability to control emotional arousal so that a subdued response can be made in the child (Figure 4.1) (Chen et al., 2012). Researchers have found that securely attached young children express less negative emotion (Smith et al., 2006), and securely attached adolescents show higher levels of empathy (Murphy et al., 2015). These findings suggest that emotional regulation is a primary characteristic of securely attached and insecurely attached children; for insecurely attached children, poor emotional regulation is related to the development of psychological problems. For example, Brenning and Braet (2013) found that lack of self-regulation is related to adolescent aggression.

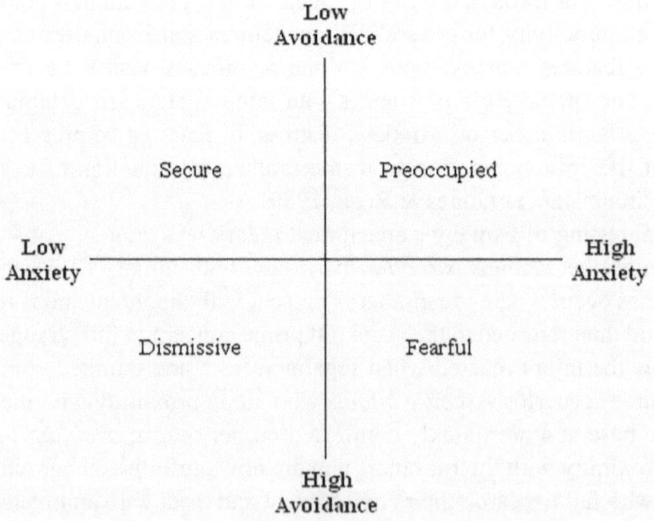

FIGURE 4.1 Securely attached children display low anxiety and low avoidance, while insecurely attached children display high anxiety and high avoidance.

Furthermore, research has found differences in avoidantly attached and anxiously attached individuals. Avoidantly attached individuals suppress emotional response, while anxiously attached individuals have problems with regulating their emotional responses (Sutton, 2019).

Neuroscience research has demonstrated that *dysregulation of emotional development* occurs because of attachment disorder (Schore, 2010). The evidence for dysregulation is based on the knowledge that experiences are related to brain development (Hart, 2008). According to Schore (2011), the mother acts as the executive control for the infant brain and is the neurobiological base for the interaction with the external world. Secure attachment with the mother is prerequisite for normal brain development and will determine how the brain will deal with trauma and stress as the child ages. This suggests that attachment is the foundation for the development of the right brain which is associated with implicit and unconscious processes that are operative throughout the lifespan.

Beginning in childhood and continuing throughout the lifespan, the *right lateralized brain* components are integral in unconscious affective processes. Research using Functional Magnetic Resonance (fMRI) found that anatomical changes in the brains of persons diagnosed with *borderline personality disorder* are related to attachment issues (Bernheim et al., 2022). This research demonstrates the brain activation associated with loneliness and abandonment that is associated with borderline personality disorder is labeled disorganized attachment.

Studies show that childhood maltreatment and trauma are associated with the degree of activity in the amygdala. For example, anxiety in children is related to an increase in amygdala responses, whereas depressed children have a decrease in the amygdala response (Thomas et al., 2001).

While research has demonstrated the relation of attachment and emotional dysregulation, some research has demonstrated that attachment reparative interactions can alter emotional dysfunctions resulting from attachment disorder (Tronick, 2007). Psychotherapy grounded in nonverbal and implicit methods demonstrate that some level of *brain plasticity* continues throughout life and can amend earlier neural connections (Hart, 2008). The therapeutic process in which change occurs in the attachment disorder is a nonverbal re-attuning that replaces the early mother–child dynamic (Siegel, 2010). Misaligned attachment lends itself to being altered by the same means by which it was formed, namely, by implicit and unconscious means instead of verbal and explicit means. The process of change occurs in the here and now through implicit nonverbal communication. The here and now is referred to as *felt moments*, where the goal of the intervention is to move the patient from this dyadic relationship with the therapist to a state of self-regulation (Figure 4.2).

On the surface, attachment theory is relatively unassuming and easy to grasp. It paints a picture of the enormous influence of the early relationship of the mother (or the primary caregiver to the infant) and child and how the quality of this relationship endures through implicit and unconscious processes throughout the

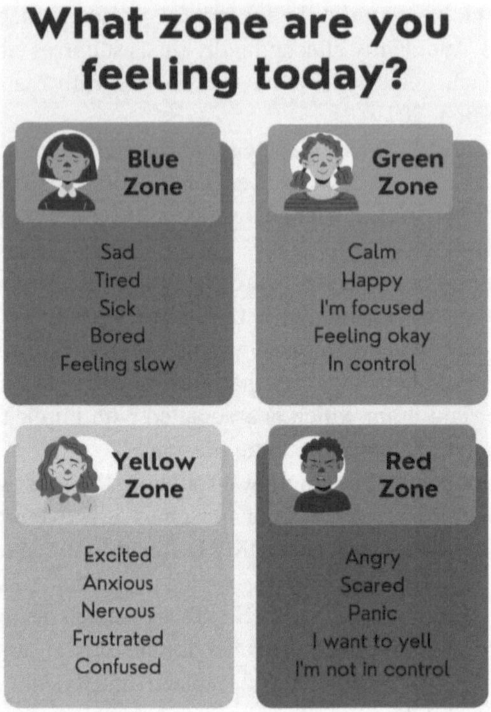

FIGURE 4.2 Attachment styles and temperament impact a child's ability to emotionally self-regulate.

lifespan. Ongoing research over past decades has confirmed the basic premise of attachment theory and demonstrated how psychobiological processes determine affective responses and early brain development (Schore & Schore, 2008). With the psychobiological underpinnings and neuroscience findings of early brain development, attachment theory can be described as a regulation theory.

Research on the attachment relationship has, for the most part, focused on the mother–child relationship. While it is acknowledged that fathers have a role in attachment, there is a paucity of research on father–child attachment (Jones et al., 2015). While it has been noted for some time that fathers can be as nurturing as mothers and a capable attachment figure for a child (Lamb, 1977), societal constraints and employment outside the home hampered a more focused observation of the father's role in attachment.

In studying parent–child attachment of both mothers and fathers, researchers found that each parent has an independently structured attachment with the child which is supported by different interactional patterns (Grossmann & Grossmann, 2019). Thus, it seems plausible to assume that different styles of relating to the infant may influence different spheres of development. Generally, mother–child

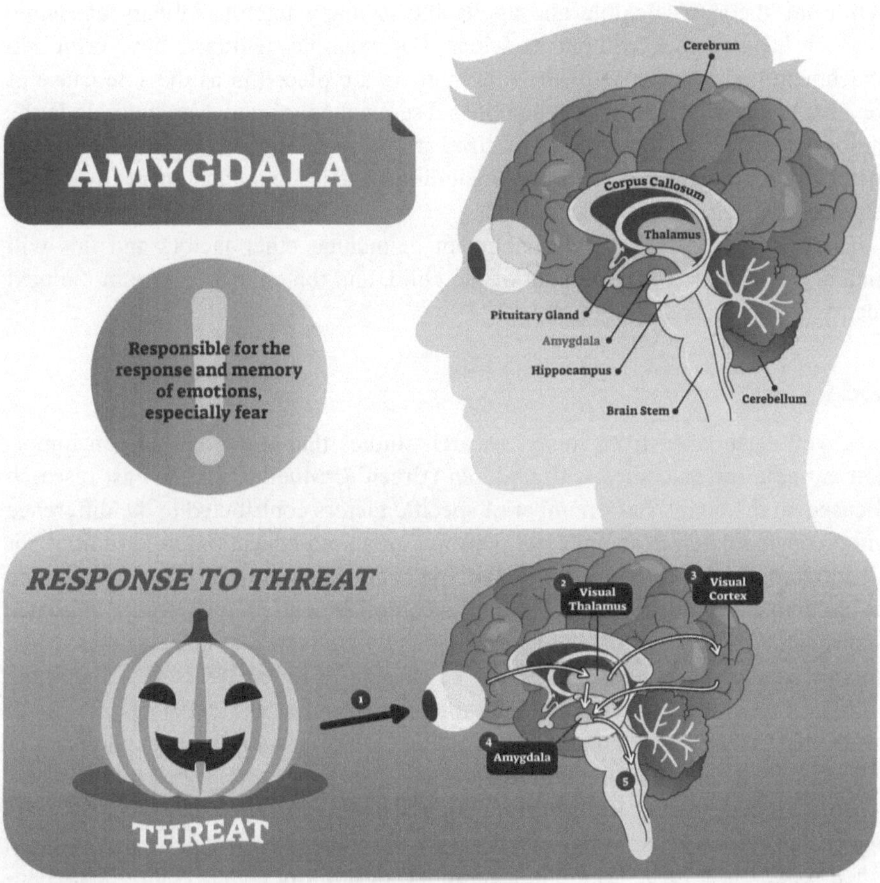

FIGURE 4.3 As the brain center for learning and decision making, the amygdala is also highly involved in emotional processing.

attachment consists of warmth, calm, and reassuring exchanges, while father–child interactions are characterized by more excitable exchanges. Some recent studies have looked at the joint effect of both the mother and the father on the attachment outcome of the infant (Cowan & Cowan, 2019). A recent study found that emotional regulation in preschool children was predicted by the father–child attachment but not the mother–child attachment (Fernandes et al., 2021). Furthermore, the researchers found the combined mother–father attachment provides a higher prediction of emotional regulation than either one alone (Figure 4.3).

In addition to attachment theory's application to parent–child relationships, attachment theory is also applicable to the study of sociology, social work, biology, anthropology, and pediatric sciences. Sroufe et al. (2005) described it as the most important developmental construct for determining child self-regulation outcomes.

While the theory is flexible and applicable to many interdisciplinary academic fields, it has not gone without its critics. For example, feminists have criticized attachment theory because of the role mothers are placed in as the sole cause of the misalignment of attachment and the subsequent emotional dysregulation in the child (Allen, 2020). Others have criticized attachment theory on the basis that other factors affect outcomes in children, including genetics and attachment to siblings and peers (Harris, 1998).

There is a need to expand attachment to include other factors and this will include social class, temperament of the child, and the child's culture in the next section of the chapter.

Social Class

It is well established from many research studies that social class is an important variable for outcomes with children (Breen & Mueller, 2020). Past research focused on the belief that a number of specific factors contributed to the difference in outcomes related to social class. Despite increased education opportunities for all children, the family's economic standing continues to be of primary importance in children's overall development and accomplishments. How parents influence their children's success has not been completely addressed in these studies. Most notably, studies have concentrated on the amount of time parents spend with the child and their support for the child's interests (Cano et al., 2019). Based on the research on social class and children's outcomes, higher status affluent parents provide more resources for their children.

Both mothers and fathers spend more time with their children today than 50 years ago (Ishizuka, 2019). Nevertheless, there are differences in the outcome of children when social class variables are looked at. According to Lareau (2000), discrepancies in outcome are not so much due to working-class and middle-class parents' lack of interest in helping or providing resources to their children. Rather, Lareau states that the culprit is in the type and breadth of resources and the type of interactions that they engage in. Upper-class parents have more professional careers and use this status to provide their children with greater advantages. Furthermore, higher status parents allow more self-direction and flexibility in making choices than lower status parents (Kohn, 2006).

The involvement of parents to hold the outcomes of their children in high regard is referred to as *parental values* (Baker & Barg, 2019). According to Kohn (2006), the higher the social class status of the parents, the more likely they are to allow for self-direction on the part of their children. While the specific parental behaviors toward their children may vary in different cultures, the premise remains that higher status parents allow more self-direction, and lower class parents expect greater conformity to their views across different cultures. This means that higher status parents allow their children more freedom to think for themselves.

In recent years, several circumstances have altered the traditional views of social class difference on outcomes with children. A major factor is that families have changed over the past few decades. The erosion of the nuclear family and the high number of single-parent families change the dynamic within the family, such as time spent with the children. Other changes include the fading of distinct social class stratification due to changes in the economics of the family (Gallie et al., 2018). In addition, increased immigration has produced a more diverse population in many Western countries around the globe. Diversity in the population reduces the social/cultural values and religious practices within the society and creates a smorgasbord of values (Bruce, 2016). The recent loosening of legal marriage laws where gay marriage is openly accepted and transgender persons are finding support and encouragement may further impact the development and outcome of children.

In investigating contemporary social class variables as they relate to outcomes in children in the United Kingdom, Baker and Barg (2019) found support that values continue to be important. Further, they found that, in the United Kingdom, parental values are affected by educational level, racial and cultural heritage, and religion. In addition, Baker and Barg found support for older research that higher status parents encourage their children to be self-reliant, while lower status parents wish their children to be compliant to their authority. A surprising finding was that the parents' educational level was a stronger predictor of parenting values than was social class.

Additionally, Baker and Barg (2019) found that religion for church attenders plays an important role in the parent's values and how those values are transferred to their children. Religious experience varied, especially for a person with an immigrant status, and so did the values emphasized by parents. An inference is that religious parents influence their children and their socialization can easily be made, but the values religious parents hold vary according to their particular religious beliefs. In the United States, a study by Alwin (1986) on the influence of religion on parental values found that religious practices, such as regular church attendance, was a more significant factor affecting parental values than was denominational differences.

Good parenting is related to positive outcomes in children which prepares them to function effectively within their sphere of influence of family and friends (Darling & Steinberg, 1993). The exact definition of *good parenting* is nebulous, but some characteristics of the meaning of good parenting can be identified. It seems rather clear that the foremost cause of child problems which are readily identified in adolescence at the leaving-home stage are due in part by the parents' style of parenting (Haley, 1997).

Parenting styles and their effects on children's behavior have been well researched and documented by Baumrind (1991). According to Baumrind, there are four distinct styles of parenting—*authoritative, authoritarian, permissive*, and *uninvolved* (see Table 4.1). These four styles are associated with particular parenting strategies

TABLE 4.1 Baumrind's Four Parenting Styles

Authoritarian	*Authoritative*
One-way mode of communication Parent establishes strict rules No room for negotiations or errors Mistakes lead to punishments Parents are less nurturing, have high expectations, and low flexibility	Close, nurturing relationship with children Clear guidelines Reasons are explained Disciplinary methods are a way of support Children have input into goals and expectations Appropriate levels of communication
Permissive	*Uninvolved*
Parents are warm, nurturing Minimal to no expectations Limited rules on children Rare use of discipline Parents act like friends	Children have a lot of freedom Parents fulfill children's basic needs Parents are detached from child's life No particular discipline style Limited communication Low nurturing Few or no expectations

Source: Adapted from Sanvictores & Mendez, 2022.

which produce distinct behaviors in children. Authoritative parenting is the most effective because it fosters trust, bidirectional open communication patterns, and emotional attunement. Parents respond to the child's misbehavior in a firm but warm manner. Authoritarian parenting, on the other hand, seeks to maintain control by closed and rigid communication patterns. In permissive parenting style, parents allow for open communication but do not exert control over the child's behavior. In uninvolved parenting, children tend to be on their own because their parents offer no guidance. These parenting styles are associated with different outcomes in children. For example, children raised by authoritative parenting tend to have fewer behavior problems and be more socially competent and more successful in school. Authoritarian parenting leads to children who lack initiative and have more problems at home and in a school setting. Permissive parenting allows children to make decisions for themselves and can have positive effects in that they develop confidence in their abilities. The downside, however, is they have issues with authority figures and may refuse to take responsibility for their actions. Children of uninvolved parents lack self-control and have more behavior problems than children raised by parenting using the other three styles.

These parenting styles appear to be related to the social class of parents. For example, the higher the social status of the parents, the more likely they will use authoritative or permissive styles of parenting and children are more likely to have children who are successful and have fewer behavioral problems. Working-class parents use either more control methods of authoritarian style or are uninvolved in discipline and are less emotionally attuned with their children and their children have poorer outcomes (Bradley & Corwyn, 2002).

Other research on parenting style and social class have found interesting findings. For example, in a study conducted in the United Kingdom, Chan and Koo (2011) concluded that authoritative style was used more by two-parent families than single-parent families or step-families. Furthermore, the highest social classes used authoritative parenting style significantly more than others and the use decreased significantly when compared to lower class. Permissive parenting style tended to be in vogue when going down the social status ladder, but the relation between social class and parenting became less distinct at the lower class level. Chan and Koo also found that social class had no association with a child's sense of well-being, while parenting style does have a significant relation.

In a recent study, Elena van Stee (2022) found that social class differences continue into adulthood, noting that most studies on social class and advantages for children focus on children to adolescence, but not into adulthood. This past research emphasizes economic differences but not other aspects of social class, such as leaving home, finding a career, getting married, and establishing a family. The finding concluded that understanding the transition into adulthood requires knowledge of the relationship and status of parents.

The global pandemic from late 2019 to 2022 provided another setting for research on social class and educational attainment of children. A recent study by Sanrey et al. (2021) on the effects of social class on homeschooling during the COVID-19 pandemic revealed interesting findings. Since parents had to increase their involvement in their child's education during the pandemic, it provided a perfect lab for analyzing how social class affected the parents' involvement with their children. Subjects consisted of 360 parents who answered a questionnaire on their involvement and the technical support at their disposal to do homeschooling. Findings indicated that all parents, regardless of social class, were involved in homeschooling but some differences were found. For example, the lower the social class, the more the time spent with their children. Although lower status parents spent more time with their children, they had less technical equipment and were less confident in their ability to provide quality educational support. On the other hand, higher social class parents had more technical equipment and felt more confident in their role of *self-schooling*, and their children were engaged in more activities that were conducive to learning. The researchers concluded that social class differences during the COVID-19 would result in long-term educational accomplishments. Other studies have also concluded that the pandemic exacerbated the educational differences resulting from social class (Goudeau et al., 2021).

Temperament

Temperament is the contribution that children make to the interactions they have with parents resulting in their own developmental trajectories (see Table 4.2) (Rothbart & Bates, 1998). In the study of infants, temperament is considered biological

TABLE 4.2 Nine Temperament Traits of Children

Temperament Traits of Children	
Active	Level of motor activity
Regularity	Pattern of sleep waking and sleep cycle, eating eliminating
Initial reaction	Response to new people and things
Adaptability	Adjusting to changes
Sensitivity	Reaction to stimuli
Intensity	Strength of reaction
Mood	Cheerful or cranky
Distractibility	Ability to stay focused
Attention span	Level of attention and persistence in an activity

Source: Adapted from Thomas et al., 1963.

in nature and emanating from the infant's moods and activities. For example, *infant sociability* refers to the degree to which infants respond to their parent. In addition, another characteristic of temperament is positive and negative emotionality. *Positive emotionality* refers to the infant's ability to interact with the parent and the environment free of apprehension and fear, while *negative emotionality* refers to the infant having predominantly fear, anger, and distrust in the relationship with the parent. Finally, temperament refers to how the infant responds to new situations as either positive or negative reactivity.

Generally, research on temperament in children has coalesced around fears, inhibitions, anger, and irritability. The concept of temperament as an important component for understanding child development was slow to develop because the focus was mostly on the parents' contribution to child development. One of the first researchers to identify how children contributed to their own development was the research team of Chess et al. (1963). Following this seminal work, there was a quick acknowledgment that children are not passive observers in their development, but active participants from the beginning of life who can wield influence on how parents respond to them (Rothbart, 1989).

The longitudinal study of Chess et al. (1963) was the first in-depth analysis regarding the child's own contribution to their development, which described two categories of temperament—difficult and easy. *Difficult temperament* was defined as the child having poor adaptability, a negative mood pattern, being withdrawn, and slowness in being calmed. On the other hand, the *easy temperament* was characterized as being adaptable, having a positive mood pattern, and easily soothed. These initial studies found that temperament, parental behavior, and culture combined to determine problem behaviors in children. Subsequent research on temperament found the terms *difficult temperament* and *easy temperament* were problematic to operationalize (Bates, 1989) and lacking in consistency across time (Rothbart & Bates, 1998).

Temperament of the child is influenced by the parent's behavior, and vice versa. It does not represent nature versus nurture, but a combination in which nature and nurture interact to produce the outcomes. This *bidirectional relationship* with the parent is complex and means that some behaviors of the parent can result in better or worse outcomes for the child depending on temperament, and some characteristics of the child's temperament can result in healthier or poorer development depending on the quality of parenting (Rothbard, 2007). The kind of reciprocity with the parent will continue to affect development at all periods. While this much is known, research on child temperament and developmental trajectories is fraught with difficulties.

One of the main concerns with research on child temperament is *continuity over time*. Because temperament has a genetic component, it is reasonable to assume that research conducted in one time frame would apply to later research, but this assumption is somewhat nebulous. This is mainly true because the child's interaction with parents, who also have a specific temperament that may be different from the child, may change over time (Feldman, 2015).

An association between parenting, child temperament, and developmental outcomes is well represented in the extant literature (Sacchi et al., 2018). Researchers have found that negative emotions in children are associated with authoritarian, controlling parenting (Laukkanen et al., 2015). Anxiety problems in children have been associated with overprotective parenting behaviors. On the other hand, some research shows that parents of children with difficult temperaments exhibit more positive behaviors toward their children perhaps in a way to reduce the child's negativity (Sanson & Rothbart, 1995).

Goodness of Fit

In their seminal study, Chess et al. (1963) defined the mother–child interaction pattern, which leads to stability, as *goodness of fit*. This concept suggests that the fit of the child with its environment, particularly the relationship with the caregiver, should allow for expected growth and development. Attachment of mother–infant is based on analyzing the patterned interactions between them as either being in or out of sync. Goodness of fit shows congruity with the environment, while poorness of fit would constitute lack of congruity. The fitness with the environment can be affected by other factors as well, including culture and economic status. If the parent is responsive to the child's temperament, later development is assumed to be adequate and adaptive.

While goodness of fit is an important concept in understanding the child's genetic disposition for responding to its total environment, including the relationship with parents, operationalizing it for research purposes has presented challenges. While the methodology of Lerner and Lerner (1987) focusing on the child's temperamental features as evident in actual behavior and how well it corresponded to parents' expectations generated much research, it failed to provide an unambiguous data base. Typically, research models on goodness of fit have not identified specific traits of children but rather have used desirable genetic traits. Consequently, researchers have not identified the specific pattern of child interaction related to goodness of fit with its environment (Dong et al., 2022).

Researchers have typically used one of two models for testing goodness of fit. One method that has been used by several researchers including Chess et al. (1963) is labeled person-centered, identifying the elements of the child's temperament, and matching or not matching with parental practices. The other method, *variable-centered method*, has two derivatives—*expectation-behavior* and behaviors matching approach. For the expectation-behavior approach, the differences were found between the expected points and the actual points and considered the goodness of fit categories which predict outcomes in children (Windle & Lerner, 1986). In the behaviors matching method, the prediction of outcomes in children is made from the exchanges of factors measuring the level of socialization and the children's temperament characteristics (Suor et al., 2019).

In the parent–child relationship, goodness of fit refers to how well the child's temperament fits with the temperament of the parent. Goodness of fit comes into play in several disparate situations in the family. For example, when one child believes that they are not the favorite child of the parent and acts out negatively as a result, or when a child feels more comfortable with one parent compared to the other parent, this is considered "poorness of fit." Poorness of fit between the parent and the child is associated with problems at some point in the relationship.

Goodness of fit applies beyond the parent–child relationship and encompasses how the child interacts with the larger social network of extended family and school. Similar responses of the child to the parent may be acted out in other settings, such as with teachers. In later development, this early temperament morphs into "personality." *Personality* is the term that is most often used for temperament as the child matures, and refers to the internal characteristics of a person including his/her psychological makeup, moods, and disposition. The development of personality over time is a complex process that remains relatively stable throughout the lifespan.

Temperament-Based Parent Education Training

The Preventative Ounce Temperament Program was developed at the University of Wisconsin for providing an individualized educational program based on improving goodness of fit between parent and child (Ostergren, n.d.). This program is a skills-based program that evaluates both the parents' temperament and the child's temperament. Participating parents complete questionnaires to determine their own temperament and receive a report on their child's temperament. The strength of this program is the individualized aspect, making it applicable to the unique issues of a family. The program can have a profound impact on improving the interactions between parent and child and can lead to less tension and anger.

A systems/dialectical approach to temperament suggests that the parent–child relationship is fueled by each one's temperament and is primarily an unconscious process. Children are not consciously aware of their temperament and its effect on others. Additionally, the parent generally would lack conscious awareness of their own temperament, which in the literature is usually referred to as "personality." Parents and researchers generally mislabel parental temperament as personality because their behaviors are more complex and harder to define. The question that follows is one that this book has raised before: How do you change an unconscious process?

We are aware that the conscious, over-analyzing brain distrusts the unconscious, although the unconscious, in recent research, has been found to be the driving force in consciousness (Barge, 2014). The unconscious is the organizing, problem-solving component of the brain that works on unsolved issues while we sleep, or in the background while we attend to other conscious tasks. Because the unconscious is better at assessing vast amounts of information (Payne et al., 2008), goodness of fit might be well served by implicit interventions rather than conscious, direct ones. Taking the perspective of the other in an interaction allows a person full reign to respond from the wellspring of its unconscious mind. The goodness of fit between parent and child need not be a complex analytical process. By restricting the conscious, analytical mind, one can give the mind permission for the unconscious to emerge. Not unlike a therapist, the parent needs to be present, accepting, and empathetic to the child's point of view.

Culture

Children grow and develop in a particular culture that is shared by their parents and community. They learn expectations and rules from parents and authority figures. Ultimately, the child will become socialized, and their adult behavior will reflect the culture in which they were raised. Consequently, the culture will be preserved and passed on to the next generation (Kuczynski & Knafo, 2014). This process of *socialization* is fluid and continually changing and adapts over the lifespan.

Parents in different cultures tend to relate in different ways with their children (Novianti & Nur Islami, 2023). For example, Chinese parents use methods that foster more compliance from children and more submission to authority. Children raised in a culture that demands obedience are less likely to resist authority even when they oppose the authority. In contrast, Euro-American children resist authority and are more independent in thinking and have parents that support self-direction than children raised in authoritarian cultures.

The parents' role in socializing their child has been central to understanding the child's responses to individual and familial changes. Until recently, the role of the parent in socialization of the child has been prominent and created a unidirectional posture for analyzing developmental outcomes in children. In giving parents the major responsibility for socialization, other important facets of the child's environment have been ignored (McHale & Cowan, 1996).

In the first few years of life, parents play a major role in their children's development and many of their interactions with their child are predicated on who they are, their sense of self-identity, and their values and goals, much of which is not in their conscious awareness. Children raised in different cultures will be exposed to different values, beliefs, and customs that influence how they think and make decisions. In fact, children raised in the same country but to parents of different cultural backgrounds will differ on many cognitive and behavioral indices. Different cultures are set apart by different languages, customs, food, and rituals. All these carry meanings for the child that make them unique and different from each other (McHale & Cowan, 1996).

Language is one of the greatest demarcations of culture because language provides for the sharing of symbols and meanings that have special significance for those within the culture. One of the major characteristics of language is how it is used in interpersonal communication. From the beginning of life, parents use language to communicate with children. Research indicates that parents from different cultures talk differently to their infants, which is instrumental to their development of self-identity. Generally, in Western societies that emphasize greater individual freedom, language includes more open-ended interactions, while in collective cultures mothers encourage child to think more in terms of their social obligations. Over time, these differences affect how children will interact with others, plan, and engage in intimate relationships.

The use of language by children of different cultures is reflected in memorization of stories and their recall. For example, Han et al. (1998) conducted a memory recall of a narrated story with 58 4- to-–6-year-old Korean, Chinese, and American children and found differences related to culture. The first day of the study, the researchers presented a narrative story and the next day the children were interviewed about the contents of the story. The researchers found that Asians, when compared to Americans, were less descriptive in their recall of the story, used less evaluative terms, made less reference to past happenings, and used less personal references. A sex difference was found in American children, while an age difference was found with Asian children.

Another study by Fivush and Wang (2005) found interesting differences in how Asian and Euro-American mothers interact with their 3-year-old toddlers. In describing a positive and a negative experience, researchers found that in both cultures, mothers used less positive and more negative words and descriptions. Chinese mothers used more negative total words than Euro-American mothers, who verbalized more negotiated interactions. Overall, gender showed no differences.

Measuring early memory recall in European, Canadian, and Chinese children, 8-, 11-, and 14-year-olds, was conducted by Peterson et al. (2009). Older children had less recall of earlier memories than younger children, and Canadian children were more likely to recall memories and earliest memories than Chinese children. By age 14, Chinese children have much less recall of childhood memories than European and Canadian children.

An interesting endeavor to determine how cultural differences affect child development has been investigating developmental milestones and culture (Kelly et al., 2006). Studying developmental milestones and culture is important because it could answer some questions about child development that linger. Kelly et al. reviewed studies that have found differences in the physical development of children due to cultural practices and more. Furthermore, they cite studies that show different explanations for the difference in physical development ranging from genetics to cultural considerations. The research by Kelly et al. attempts to fill the gap in the literature regarding the effects of race and ethnicity, and specific socialization within cultures on developmental delays. Kelly et al. (2006) found that Black Caribbean, Black African, and Indian were not as likely to have gross motor delays, while White infants showed more delay. This difference could not be explained by their methodology. Socioeconomic factors explained the finding that Pakistani and Bangladeshi infants were delayed in fine motor and communication milestones which raises some concerns for behavioral and cognitive delays. While this research did not answer all the questions about ethnic and racial cultures and developmental milestones, it did place a spotlight on a neglected area of research and reiterate the need to take cultural considerations and child outcomes seriously.

It should be noted from the outset that socialization is not unidirectional, from the parent to the child. A systems/dialectical approach to culture emphasizes that the change process is not continuity so much as it is contradictions. Changes in the environment lead to changes in the child, and vice versa. The parent–child relationship takes place within a cultural background where parents and children are viewed as coequal in interactions, but with unequal power, in the interactional dynamics, which may reflect different perspectives. Inevitable contradictions and conflicts arise which create the opportunity for further developmental change.

References

Ainsworth, M. D. (1973). Patterns of infant-mother attachment. In B. M. Caldwell & H. N. Ricciuti (Eds.), *Review of child development research* (Vol. 3). University of Chicago Press.

Ainsworth, M. D. S., Blehar, M., Waters, E., & Wall, S. (1978). *Patterns of attachment: A psychological study of the strange situation*. Erlbaum.

Allen, D. M. (2020). Attachment theory and feminist politics. *Psychology Today*. https://www.psychologytoday.com/us/blog/matter-personality/202012/attachment-theory-and-feminist-politics

Alwin, D. F. (1986). Religion and parental child-rearing orientations: Evidence of a catholic-protestant convergence. *American Journal of Sociology, 92*(2), 412–440. https://doi.org/10.1086/228506

Baker, W., & Barg, K. (2019). Parental values in the U.K. *British Journal of Sociology*. https://ore.exeter.ac.uk/repository/bitstream/handle/10871/36449/Accepted%20manuscript%20Baker%20Barg%202019%20BJOS.pdf?sequence=1; https://doi.org/10.1111/1468-4446.12658

Barge, J. A. (2014). Our unconscious mind. *Scientific American, 310*(1), 30–37. https://doi.org/10.1038/scientificamerican0114-30

Bates, J. E. (1989). Applications of temperament concepts. In G. A. Kohnstamm, J. E. Bates, & M. K. Rothbart (Eds.), *Temperament in childhood* (pp. 321–355). Wiley.

Baumrind, D. (1991). Parenting styles and adolescent development. In J. Brooks-Gunn, R. M. Lerner, & A. C. Petersen (Eds.), *The encyclopedia on adolescence* (pp. 746–758). Garland Publishing.

Bernheim, D., Buchheim, A., Domin, M., Mentel, R., & Lotze, M. (2022). Neural correlates of attachment representation in patients with borderline personality disorder using a personalized functional magnet resonance imaging task. *Frontiers in Human Neuroscience, 16*, 810417. https://doi.org/10.3389/fnhum.2022.810417

Bowlby, J. (1988). *A secure base: Clinical applications of attachment theory*. Routledge.

Bradley, H. R., & Corwyn, F. R. (2002). Socioeconomic status and child development. *Annual Review of Psychology, 53,* 371–399.

Breen, R., & Mueller, W. (Eds.). (2020). *Education and intergenerational social mobility in Europe and United States*. Stanford University Press.

Brenning, K. M., & Braet, C. (2013). The emotion regulation model of attachment: An emotion-specific approach. *Personal Relationships, 20,* 107–123. https://doi.org/10.1111/j.1475-6811.2012.01399.x

Bruce, S. (2016). The sociology of late secularization: Social divisions and religiosity. *British Journal of Sociology, 67*(4), 613–631.

Cano, T., Perales, F., & Baxter, J. (2019). A matter of time: Father involvement and child cognitive outcomes. *Journal of Marriage and Family, 81*(1), 164–184.

Chan, T. W., & Koo, A. (2011). Parenting styles and youth outcomes in the UK. *European Sociological Journal, 27*(3), 385–399.

Chen, F. M., Lin, H. S., & Li, C. H. (2012). The role of emotion in parent-child relationships: Children's emotionality, maternal meta-emotion, and children's attachment security. *Journal of Child & Family Studies, 21,* 403–410. https://doi.org/10.1007/s10826-011-9491-y

Chess, S., Thomas, A., Rutter, M., & Birch, H. G. (1963). Interaction of temperament and environment in the production of behavioral disturbances in children. *American Journal of Psychiatry, 120,* 142–148.

Cowan, P., & Cowan, C. (2019). The role of parental relationships in children's well-being: A modest set of proposals for improving the lives of children. *Human Development, 62,* 171–174. https://doi.org/10.1159/000500173

Darling, N., & Steinberg, L. (1993). Parenting style as context: An integrative model. *Psychological Bulletin, 113,* 487–496.

Dong, S., Dubas, J. S., & Dekovic, M. (2022). Revisiting goodness of fit in the cultural context: Moving forward from post hoc explanations. *Child Development Perspective, 16*(2), 82–89. https://doi.org/10.1111/cdep.12446

Feldman, R. (2015). Mutual influences between child emotion regulation and parent–child reciprocity support development across the first 10 years of life: Implications for developmental psychopathology. *Development and Psychopathology, 27,* 1007–1023.

Fernandes, C., Fernandes, M., Santos, A. J., Antunes, M., Monteiro, L., Vaughn, B. E., & Verissimo, M. (2021). Early attachment to mothers and fathers: Contributions to preschoolers' emotional regulation. *Frontiers in Psychology, 12*, 660866. https://doi.org/10.3389/fpsyg.2021.660866

Fivush, R., & Wang, Q. (2005). Emotion talks in mother-child conversations of the shared past: The effects of culture, gender, and event valence. *Journal of Cognition and Development, 6,* 489–506. https://api.semanticscholar.org/CorpusID:35298275

Gallie, D., Felstead, A., Green, F., & Henseke, G. (2018). *Participation at work in Britain. First findings from the skills and employment survey 2017.* Centre for Learning and Life Chances in Knowledge Economies and Societies, UCL Institute of Education.

Goudeau, S., Sanrey, C., Stanczak, A., Manstead, A., & Darnon, C. (2021). Why lockdown and distance learning during the COVID-19 pandemic are likely to increase the social class achievement gap. *Nature Human Behavior, 5,* 1273–1281. https://doi.org/10.1038/s41562-021-01212-7

Grossmann, K., & Grossmann, K. E. (2019). Essentials when studying child-father attachment: A fundamental view on safe secure base phenomena. *Attachment in Human Development, 22,* 9–14. https://doi.org/10.1080/14616734.2019

Haley, J. (1997). *Leaving home: The therapy of disturbed young people* (2nd ed.). Brunner-Mazel.

Han, J. J., Leichtman, M. D., & Wang, Q. (1998). Autobiographical memory in Korean, Chinese, and American children. *Developmental Psychology, 34*(4), 701–713. https://doi.org/10.1037/0012-1649.34.4.701

Harris, J. R. (1998). *The nurture assumption: Why children turn out the way they do.* Simon & Schuster.

Hart, S. (2008). *Brain, attachment, personality: An introduction to neuroaffective development.* Karnac.

Ishizuka, P. (2019). Social class, gender, and contemporary parenting standards in the United States: Evidence from a national survey experiment. *Social Forces, 98*(1), 31–58. https://doi.org/10.1093/sf/soy107

Jones, J. D., Cassidy, J., & Shaver, P. R. (2015). Parents' self-reported attachment styles: A review of links with parenting behaviors, emotions, and cognitions. *Personality and Social Psychology Review, 19*(1), 44–76.

Jones, S. S., & Raag, T. (1989). Smile production in infants: The importance of social recipient for the facial signal. *Child Development, 60,* 811–818.

Kelly, Y., Sacker, A., Schoon, I., & Nazroo, J. (2006). Ethnic differences in achievement of developmental milestones by 9 months of age: The millennium cohort study. *Developmental Medicine and Child Neurology, 48,* 825–830.

Kohn, M. L. (2006). *Change and stability: A cross-national analysis of social structure and personality.* Paradigm.

Kuczynski, L., & Knafo, A. (2014). Innovation and continuity in socialization, internalization, and acculturation. In M. Killen & J. G. Smetana (Eds.), *Handbook of moral development* (2nd ed., pp. 93–112). Taylor & Francis.

Lamb, M. E. (1977). The development of mother-infant and father-infant attachments in the second year of life. *Developmental Psychology, 13*(6), 637–648.
https://doi.org/10.1037/0012-1649.13.6.637

Lareau, A. (2000). *Home advantage: Social class and parental intervention in elementary education.* Rowman and Littlefield.

Laukkanen, J., Ojansuu, U., Tolvanen, A., Alatupa, S., & Aunola, K. (2015). Child's difficult temperament and mother's parenting styles. *Journal of Child and Family Studies, 23,* 312–323.

Lerner, R. M., & Lerner, J. V. (1987). Children in their contexts: A goodness-of-fit model. In J. B. Lancaster, J. Altmann, A. S. Rossi, & L. R. Sherrod (Eds.), *Parenting across the lifespan: Biosocial dimensions.* Aldine de Gruyter.

McHale, J. P., & Cowan, P. A. (Eds.). (1996). *Understanding how family-level dynamics affect children's development: Studies of two-parent families.* Jossey-Bass.

Mikulincer, M. P., Shaver, P. R., & Pereg, D. (2003). Attachment theory and affect regulation: The dynamics, development, and cognitive consequences of attachment-related strategies. *Motivation & Emotion, 27*(2), 77–102.

Murphy, T. P., Laible, D. J., Augustine, M., & Robeson, L. (2015). Attachment's links with adolescents' social emotions: The roles of negative emotionality and emotion regulation. *The Journal of Genetic Psychology, 176*(5), 315–329. https://doi.org/10.1080/00221325.2015.1072082

Novianti, R., & Nur Islami, S. (2023). Parenting in cultural perspective: A systematic review of parental roles across cultures. *Journal of Ethics and Cultural Studies, 10*(1), 22–44. https://doi.org/10.29333/ejecs/1287

Ostergren, C. (n.d.). *A family perspective on a temperament based parenting program*. Department of Human Development & Family Studies, University of Wisconsin. https://www.purdue.edu/hhs/hdfs/fii/wp-content/uploads/2015/06/fia_analyses_fptbpp.pdf

Payne, J. W., Samper, A., Bettman, J. R., & Luce, M. F. (2008). Boundary conditions on unconscious thought in complex decision making. *Psychological Science, 19,* 1118–1123.

Peterson, C., Wang, Q., & Hou, Y. (2009). "When I was little": Childhood recollections in Chinese and European Canadian grade school children. *Child Development, 80*(2), 506–518. https://doi.org/10.1111/j.1467-8624.2009.01275.x

Rothbard, M. K. (2007). Temperament, development, and personality. *Current Directions in PsychologicalScience,16*(4),207–212.https://doi.org/10.1111/j.1467-8721.2007.00505.x

Rothbart, M. K. (1989). Temperament and development. In G. A. Kohnstamm, J. E. Bates, & M. K. Rothbart (Eds.), *Temperament in childhood* (pp. 187–247). Wiley.

Rothbart, M. K., & Bates, J. E. (1998). Temperament. In W. Damon (Series Ed.) and N. Eisenberg (Vol. Ed.), *Handbook of child psychology: Vol. 3. Social, emotional and personality development* (5th ed., pp. 105–176). Wiley.

Sacchi, C., De Carli, P., Vieno, A., Piallini, G., Zoia, S., & Simonelli, A. (2018). Does infant negative emotionality moderate the effect of maternal depression on motor development? *Early Human Development, 119,* 56–61.

Sanrey, C., Goudeau, S., Stanczak, A., & Darnon, C. (2021). A two-sided lockdown? Social class variations in the implementation of homeschooling during the COVID-19 lockdown. *Frontiers in Psychology, 12,* 670722. https://doi.org/10.3389/fpsyg.2021.670722

Sanson, A., & Rothbart, M. K. (1995). Child temperament and parenting. *Handbook of Parenting, 4,* 299–321.

Sanvictores, T., & Mendez, M. D. (2022). *Types of parenting styles and effects on children*. Retrieved April 4, 2024, from https://www.ncbi.nlm.nih.gov/books/NBK568743/

Schore, A. N. (2010). Relational trauma and the developing right brain: The neurobiology of broken attachment bonds. In T. Baradon (Ed.), *Relational trauma in infancy*. Routledge.

Schore, A. N. (2011). The right brain implicit self lies at the core of psychoanalysis. *Psychoanalytic Dialogues, 21,* 75–100. https://doi.org/10.1080/10481885.2011.545329

Schore, J. R., & Schore, A. N. (2008). Modern attachment theory: The central role of affect regulation in development and treatment. *Clinical Social Work Journal, 36*(1), 9–20. https://doi.org/10.1007/s10615-007-0111-7

Shaver, P. R., Belsky, J., & Brennan, K. A. (2000). The adult attachment interview and self-reports of romantic attachment: Associations across domains and methods. *Personal Relationships, 7,* 25–43. https://doi.org/10.1111/j.1475-6811.2000.tb00002.x

Siegel, D. J. (2010). *Mindsight: The new science of personal transformation*. Norton.

Smith, C. L., Calkins, S. D., & Keane, S. P. (2006). The relation of maternal behavior and attachment security to toddlers' emotions and emotion regulation. *Research in Human Development, 3*(1), 21–31. https://doi.org/10.1207/s15427617rhd0301_3

Sroufe, A., Egeland, B., Carlson, E., & Collins, A. (2005). Placing early experiences in developmental context. In K. Grossman, K. Grossman, & E. Waters (Eds.), *Attachment from infancy to adulthood* (pp. 48–77). Guilford.

Suor, J. H., Sturge-Apple, M. L., Davies, P. T., & Jones-Gordils, H. R. (2019). The interplay between parenting and temperament in associations with children's executive function. *Journal of Family Psychology, 33*(7), 841–850. https://doi.org/10.1037/fam0000558

Sutton, T. E. (2019). Review of attachment theory: Familial predictors, continuity and change, and intrapersonal and relational outcomes. *Marriage & Family Review, 55*(1), 1–22. https://doi.org/10.1080/01494929.2018.1458001

Thomas, A., Chess, S., Birch, H. G., Hertzig, M. E., & Korn, S. (1963). *Behavioral individuality in early childhood*. New York University Press.

Thomas, K. M., Drevets, W. C., Dahl, R. E., Ryan, N. D., Birmaher, B., Eccard, C. H., Axelson, D., Whalen, P. J., & Curry, B. J. (2001). Amygdala response to fearful faces in anxious and depressed children. *Archives of General Psychiatry*, 5810571063.

Tronick, E. (2007). *The neurobehavioral and social-emotional development of infants and children*. Norton.

van Stee, E. G. (2022). Parenting young adults across social class: A review and synthesis. *Sociology Compass*. Published online August, 11 2022. https://doi.org/10.1111/soc4.13021

Windle, M., & Lerner, R. M. (1986). The 'goodness of fit' model of temperament-context relations: Interaction or correlation? In J. V. Lerner & R. M. Lerner (Eds.), *New directions for child development: No. 31. Temperament and social interaction in infants and children* (pp. 109–119). Jossey-Bass. https://doi.org/10.1002/cd.23219863108

5

PARENTING AND NEUROSCIENCE

Approaches to Parenting

Parenting has clearly evolved over the years and with that process, changes have occurred in what constitutes adequate parenting. In the 1950s, parenting was influenced by schools of psychotherapy that were applied to the parent–child relationship. For example, the person-centered approach of Carl Rogers (1961) was applied to parenting where active communication and empathy were the cornerstones of purposeful parenting. This emphasis is strongly represented in the writings of Thomas Gordon (1975) and the parenting model of Parent Effectiveness Training (PET).

Other models began to proliferate, such as Dreikurs' (1979) parenting model based on Adlerian therapy. Behavior modification developed from behavioral psychotherapy and was explained by social learning theorists, such as Gerald Patterson (1971). As research began to accumulate on the development of the brain in the 1900s, a major shift occurred toward research in biology and sociology and away from psychotherapy models. In place of the psychological components of the parent–child relationship, parenting professionals were influenced by an array of social, economic, and environmental issues and the effects of these issues on the child's developing brain (Macvarish et al., 2014).

Neuroscience Findings

Attachment

One of the earliest to apply brain research to parenting was Daniel Siegel (2010), a psychiatrist by training. He focused on bringing more clarity to the early attachment

DOI: 10.4324/9781003381679-6

period and the developing brain. Siegel discovered that the most important factor in why parents behave in certain ways with their children is due to how they make sense of their experiences. *Secure attachment* in one's children, as it turns out, is highly correlated with how the parents positively dealt with and processed their upbringing. On the other hand, children with *insecure attachment* have parents who have not dealt with their upbringings and tend to make the same mistakes that their parents made with them. The key to making sense of one's past is described through the process of telling one's past life story, referred to as *life narrative*. If a person can tell their life story, showing both positive and negative events and connecting them to their later development, they tend to develop a secure attachment style.

Mindfulness

Siegel (2010) espouses the concept of *mindfulness*, the art of being present in the moment. Research has generally supported the benefits of focusing on present thoughts, feelings, and perceptions (Siegel, 2007). The neural benefit of mindfulness is shown in the redundant patterns of synaptic activation that occur with these states and lead to long-term reinforcement of certain synaptic patterns. Siegel believes that mindfulness techniques provide an avenue for certain neural pathways that focus on present moments, which changes the flow in the brain and ultimately transforms the mind. Thus, the intentional attention of the mind on itself can alter some neural pathways and strengthen others.

Siegel (2010) believes that through mindfulness practice, the brain can form new pathways that will disrupt and eliminate old and dysfunctional pathways. The brain regions affected by mindfulness include the middle prefrontal area which includes the medial and anterior cingulate. Studies have found that these areas of the brain are thicker in persons with long histories of mindfulness practice (Cahn & Polich, 2006). The effects on the brain from the practice of mindfulness are deeper and more involved than merely a present mental focus and include thickening of brain areas related to executive and cognitive functions of the prefrontal cortex. Furthermore, the practice of mindfulness allows for integration of differentiated components, which may be the key to well-being (Siegel, 2010). Mindfulness practice alters the way we view our own mind and opens new possibilities for different behavior.

Siegel (2010) applies mindfulness to children in how parents respond to them. Creating a "*yes*" *environment* opens their brain to receiving new experiences, while saying "no" inhibits their brain. Using a "yes" response to a child goes beyond the word and carries the connotation of a whole atmosphere of emotional support. The way parents interact with the child can open them up to new experiences rather than close them down. According to Siegel, the parents' major role is to create the yes response to life in their children. The children with parents who encourage a yes environment are creative and take initiative in new situations.

A strength of Siegel's (2007) approach is the interdisciplinary focus. The integration of biology, anthropology, sociology, behavioral genetics, developmental psychology, and cognitive neuroscience converges to provide an expanded understanding of how human development takes place. According to Siegel, taken separately, none of these disciplines can provide a coherent answer to the question of how the mind develops in a social context.

What is clear from an interdisciplinary approach is that the mind develops within a specific social context of other interacting persons and according to the timing of neural pathways laid down in the early brain (Siegel, 2010). What is generally thought of as the mind, including memory, cognition, emotion, and the like, cannot be studied as concrete entities, but their activity can be noted through the study of the brain. According to Siegel, it is now apparent from the integration of various disciplines studying the brain that early brain activity within a social context is directly related to the development of the mind.

The brain contains billions of neurons that form connections with each other through synapses where a neurotransmitter allows or denies the connection across neurons (Siegel, 2010). Thus, the nature of this connection will determine the mind process that follows. The connection that occurs, coupled with the location within the brain, will determine the specific nature of the process that follows. For example, if the connection takes place in the sensory region of the brain, the specific nature of the connection will produce an activity that could be visual, auditory, and the like. These connections are experience-dependent in that the connections rely on repeated experience to continue over time. Since these initial connections occur early in life, early experiences are crucial to the formation, maintenance, and later development of neural connections. Experiences accomplish the creation of new neural connections and their maintenance through the activation of *genes* and the proteins that they release across synapses. Consequently, the early experiences with the major caregiver, generally the mother, will have exponential influence on the developing brain and mind of the infant.

From the earliest moments in the infant's life, there is a dance with the caregiver of sending and receiving messages. The flow of information back and forth between the infant and the caregiver is not perfectly congruent, but a secure attachment can occur when the parent responds to the infant's signals with like-kind gestures. The idea behind attachment theory is that the communication of verbal and nonverbal signals between caregiver and infant will have some long-term effects on the infant's development.

Attunement

Allan Schore (2000) has written and researched exclusively on attachment and the formation of the unconscious that takes place primarily in the *right hemisphere.* The right hemisphere has long been associated with the formation and memory development of implicit and nonconscious processes. It is also well-known that the right hemisphere of the brain develops first and is associated with the development of attachment between infant and caregiver. The quality of the parent–infant relationship provides a good understanding for how the right brain develops and affects the person's relationship development throughout their lifecycle. Central to this early relationship with the mother is the concept of self-regulation.

According to Schore (2000), the primary caregiver must be competent to understand the nuances of the infant's gestures. The caregiver facilitates emotional regulation for the infant by responding with emotional attunement through gaze, facial expression, body posture, and tone of voice. If the caregiver can stay attuned to the infant in periods when the infant is disengaged, reengagement will be quicker and less disruptive to their relationship. In this sequence of mis-attunement to re-attunement, the caregiver provides for the regulation of emotion. This process has been referred to in the literature as "good enough" parenting, which is considered to be the bare minimum effort needed for the child to develop. This process where the caregiver regulates the infant's emotional responses will pave the way for the developing child to self-regulate.

This view of attunement, which is so necessary in the infant–caregiver relationship, becomes a prototype for other relationships as the infant advances through the life cycle. Adult relationships reflect this unconscious and implicit dynamic established prior to the development of the left brain and rational thought. The implicit processes in the formation of the right brain are centrally the most important aspect of the development of a self. The implicit processing in the right hemisphere is present in decision making and mainly operates outside of conscious attention. Recent neuroscience research reveals that all decision making is an emotional response and not a rational response. Although it is a common understanding that selection of one decision over another is a rational process, the part of the brain that is activated in decision making is the emotional center. One makes a decision on the basis of how something feels emotionally, not on the basis of purely rational thought, even when individuals utilize more rational techniques, such as pro and con lists, the establishment and organization of 'pro' and 'con' features occurs via an unconscious, emotional process. What this means is that consciousness takes a back seat to unconscious and implicit processes that were laid down in the brain's pathways through the activation of the right hemisphere.

Allan Schore (2000) has investigated attachment theory from the perspective of the developing child's ability for emotional regulation. The major accomplishment for the infant in the first year of life is the regulation of the affective domain that occurs within the relationship between the infant and the caregiver. Consequently, emotional development is related to this early period which then has consequences for the rest of the life cycle.

Schore's (2000) work describes both secure and insecure attachment and the outcomes of both styles. While much work has been done on secure attachment, it is the insecure attachment style and the poor outcome for children that Schore addresses in detail. Two factors, *child neglect* and *abuse*, exist prominently in most mental disorders, including depression, suicide, personality disorders, and borderline personality. According to Schore, neglect of an infant is a particular problem because the neural wirings that promote emotional regulation do not develop, or develop atypically. What results from this complete mis-attuning is described by Schore as emotional trauma or *attachment trauma.*

Attachment trauma results from the caregiver not creating an optimum environment for attunement and persists because the caregiver does not repair the mis-attunement. According to Schore (2000), severe psychopathologies develop from this failure of the caregiver to repair negative affect. Since the left brain is not developed during the first year of life, all the stored experiences and the dysregulation experienced during the first year is stored in the right brain. As a result, implicit memory stored in the right brain becomes the focal point for psychopathology. The right brain has greater connections to the *hypothalamic pituitary axis*, which regulates stress in the body.

Nondeclarative Memory Network

The brain is composed of two memory systems—*declarative* and *nondeclarative memory* (Camina & Guell, 2017). Declarative memory is conscious memory of past events and can be recalled from conscious awareness. This type of memory is not present during the first years of life when the infant is forming attachment relationships. Nondeclarative memory is present from birth and is characterized as learning that takes place outside of conscious awareness.

The infant brain is particularly tuned in to receiving language sounds (Kuhl, 2004). This sensitivity to language development aids in native language acquisition. In the first year of life, the infant begins to distinguish between certain sounds of the native language while decreasing its ability to distinguish sounds of non-native language during the second half of the first year. At the same time, facial processing by the infant can determine two different faces by six months of life and is tuned in to observing them.

The Bucharest Early Intervention Project (BEIP) demonstrated that experiences affect the development of the brain (Zeanah et al., 2003). This study was a landmark study that began in 2001. After communism was defeated in Romania, many children were abandoned by their parents and were placed in orphanages. The sheer number of children compared to available childcare providers contributed to wide-scale neglect. No foster home system was in place at this time until researchers at the University of North Carolina conducted a research project that created a network of adequate foster home placements. Some of the children were removed from the orphanage and placed in these high-quality foster homes. The BEIP study demonstrated that children who were institutionalized as infants experienced deprivation, which had long-term negative effects. Both physical and cognitive delays were noted in the group of children who were institutionalized when compared to children who were not, but when these children were placed in foster homes at 2 years of age, subsequent findings yielded little difference with children not institutionalized (Sheridan et al., 2022). However, the longer the children were institutionalized past 2 years of age, the greater the degree of deprivation, which included both cognitive and language development.

Brain Plasticity

Brain plasticity has been a popular topic in studying the brains of children. Brain plasticity typically refers to the ability of the neural pathway connections in the brain, particularly those related to emotion and thought, to be altered by interactions with the environment or through implicit psychobiological processes. A new study, focused primarily on when plasticity decreases as the child ages (Sydnor et al., 2023), built on prior research that associated brain plasticity with exclusive patterns of intrinsic brain activity and the neural activity when the brain is at rest. Neurons in this part of the brain tend to be more connected and synchronized. When there is less activity in a brain region, the brain is more plastic and is more malleable from stimuli. Plotting these regions of the brain, researchers were able to locate areas that are more likely to be plastic. Using MRI scans, researchers were able to determine that brain plasticity was decreased in the sensory–motor regions in early childhood, but not in adolescence. The areas of the brain in early childhood related to these brain regions associated with plasticity are associated with cognitive development, social relationships, and emotional health.

Certain brain regions remain plastic longer—from early childhood to adolescence—and are more susceptible to environmental influences (Sydnor et al., 2023). The implication from this research is that plasticity continues at least into the adolescent period of development, which supports the view that interventions addressing deficiencies in children's development through adolescence are beneficial.

Parental Behavior

Another recent study shows that communication with parents during the adolescent years is a protective factor against overeating and alcohol or drug consumption (Holmes et al., 2018). This longitudinal study was conducted on rural Black children beginning at age 11 and concluding at 25. The implications of this research reinforce the critical role of parents in the development of their children. The study concluded that the interactional frequency and pattern between parent and child can affect neural wiring in the brains of children. At age 25, a subsample of the participants were studied using functional magnetic resonance imaging (fMRI). The researchers were especially interested in a specific brain network called the anterior salience network (ASN). Results demonstrated that there was increased connectivity in the ASN of participants whose parents provide high-quality communication patterns. Furthermore, decreased alcohol use and overeating occurred in participants with increased connectivity in the ASN.

Other recent research suggests that some common social and cultural norms used by parents may, in fact, negatively affect the child's development. These widely accepted practices include feeding infants formula, leaving children alone and isolated for periods of time, and letting infants cry it out at night instead of comforting them. According to Narvaez (2017), research demonstrates that responding to infant crying and physical touch with infants is positively associated with several good outcomes, including development of empathy and higher IQ. Narvaez believes that current parenting practices do not emphasize these healthy patterns of parental behavior, which is leading to increased psychosocial problems in children. Lack of contact with extended families is another problem according to Narvaez that reduces the feeling of connectedness, resulting in isolation and loneliness. The end result are children who are more aggressive and who lack empathy and compassion.

A recent study by Suffren et al. (2021) sheds more light on the detrimental effects of harsh parental discipline techniques. *Harsh parental behavior*, such as hitting, yelling, and constant anger at a child, result in smaller brains in adolescence and derailed social and emotional development. According to Suffren et al. (2021), these parental practices are widely accepted by most parents. The conclusion of this research is noteworthy because the parenting techniques isolated for this study and used often by most parents result in the same damage to the prefrontal cortex and the amygdala as more severe forms of child abuse and neglect.

This research by Suffren et al. (2021) for the first time demonstrates that even accepted social practices of harsh parenting not characterized as abuse can lead to reducing the size of the prefrontal cortex and the amygdala affecting the very structure of the brain. Children in this study were 2–9 years of age and anatomical MRIs were conducted when the same children were 12–16 years of age.

Parental use of corporal punishment has come under new scrutiny from a recent study. Burani et al. (2022) highlighted how corporal punishment affects neural pathways in children's brains. The use of physical punishment on a child sets in motion a myriad of emotions that can have detrimental effects on children. Participants in the study included 149 males and females of 11–14 years of age who underwent electroencephalography (EEG) while completing a reward-based video game. In this study, the EEG measured brain waves that were instrumental in obtaining data associated with rewards in completing a task and errors in completing a task. The longitudinal study followed up two years later with questionnaires to determine the presence of depression and anxiety and parents' methods of discipline. The findings indicate that a decrease neural response to reward and an increase in neural response to error means that corporal punishment leads to poor behavior and altered brain chemistry (Burani et al., 2022). The long-established belief that corporal punishment has detrimental effects on neural development and behavior is proven by this study. The implication of this study is that the increase in neural responsiveness to error and a decrease in responsiveness to reward may create a pattern of undue focus on errors, leading to depression throughout the lifespan.

What has been learned from neuroscience research is that the brain develops from lower to higher processes (Ayre & Krishnamoorthy, 2020). Sensory and perceptual development is the foundation for language acquisition. This internal predisposition for language and recognition for faces is met with input from the environment, consisting of interactions between the infant and others, which determine the specific outcome. Early interactional experiences either build on these predispositions or, if the environment is deprived, fail to continue developing. Based on neuroscience research, recommendations for optimum infant brain development suggest that both genetic predispositions and the quality of the interactional environment of the child should be taken into consideration.

Animal studies show that maternal contact with their pups influenced gene activity affecting brain cells, learning, and memory (Hackman et al., 2010). Research using rats shows that the mother's licking of pups during early development affects gene activity that then influences brain development. According to Hackman and colleagues, these studies conclusively demonstrate how parental behavior affects brain development, learning, and memory formation in children.

Childhood and Infant Depression

While research has long established the anatomical connection between depression and the adult brain, only recently has research established the same connection in infants (Morgan et al., 2021). The specific area of the brain associated with depression in adults is the ventral striatum (VS), which is allied with pleasure, and goal-direction activities. Adolescent depression has been related to reduced activity in the ventral striatum. The study by Morgan and associates demonstrate that brain effects of depression originated in childhood. The research consisted of 49 children 6–8 years of age who had no known mental concerns. Mothers of half of the participant children had a history of depression. Functional magnetic resonance imaging (fMRI) was conducted on the children as they were engaged in a video game. Mothers of the children completed questionnaires regarding vignettes of emotional outbursts in children and their reaction was analyzed. Results showed that children of mothers who were not depressed had expected levels of reward-related brain stimulation in the VS, while children of depressed mothers had reduced brain activity in the VS if the mother responded with less excitement to the child's positive emotional response. This study is noteworthy because it demonstrates that the reduced VS activity is related to the mother's show of support and not merely the mother's history of depression.

Lack of Sleep

Lack of sleep has been studied for some time particularly in relation to sleeping patterns of children (Figure 5.1) (Kurth et al., 2016). Lack of sleep in the adult brain leads to a brain response for more deep sleep, which can be measured by an electroencephalography (EEG). The *prefrontal cortex* known for cognitive functions is

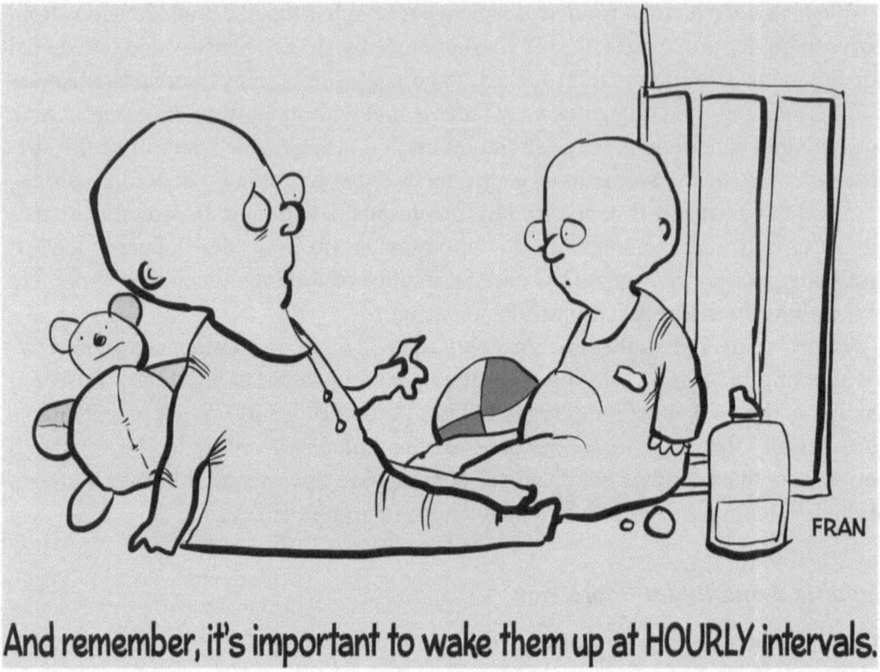

FIGURE 5.1 Lack of sleep for all family members is common with infants. While not intentional, an infant's inability to sleep through the night can have detrimental effects for parents and the developing child. (www.CartoonStock.com)

the most affected brain region from sleep loss. In children, brain regions affected by sleep differ from adults in that the affected brain regions are the parietal and occipital lobes in the back of the brain. In addition, Kurth et al. (2016) found that in children the increased need for deep sleep because of loss of sleep is related to myelin content in brain areas associated with the visual system. Measuring the myelin content provides a boilerplate for brain maturity that surges during childhood into adolescence. Moreover, this new research reveals that the more the myelin content in children's brains, the closer their deep sleep pattern to adults.

The procedure in this study was to allow the children participants to sleep their regular amount of sleep using EEG measurements and fMRI to determine the myelin content (Kurth et al., 2016). This was repeated for the second night when the children were awakened halfway into their sleep. The study showed that the deep sleep effect is related to a myelin content in a specific part of the brain. The study concluded that the amount and quality of sleep are necessary for the child's brain to develop normally. The recommended amount of sleep for the developing child was 9–11 hours of sleep per night.

Stress

Studies focused on how stress affects children's brain development have found similar findings to past research on animal brains. The prefrontal cortex appears vulnerable to stress during the developing period, particularly in the spatial working memory (Hanson et al., 2012). The stress level was determined by interviews with children 9–14 years of age and their parents. The researchers aimed to get a broad spectrum of the stress experienced by the children instead of a narrow focus on particular stressors. MRI scans revealed that the area of the brain involved in spatial working memory is smaller in children exposed to long-term and severe stressful situations, which results in spatial memory deficits. What is not known from this research is whether the deficits continue or are reversible at a later point in development. Hansen and colleagues speculated that it is very likely that, over time, these brains will develop fully, but more research is needed to make that conclusion. Puberty, as would be expected, revealed the most stress, but there was no difference in younger and older children regarding accumulated stress.

One interesting finding was a reduction in both gray matter and *white matter* from stress experiences (Hanson et al., 2012). This finding is important because white matter is necessary for forming connections across the brain, and gray matter is important for processing the information from the connections in the brain. Gray matter seems especially important early in development. The researchers emphasized a need to develop interventions that could address ways to manage stress to reduce and repair the effects.

Poverty

Poverty has been linked to many concerns for the developing child's brain (Gur et al., 2019). Children raised in poverty are typically exposed to more trauma than other children. The combination of poverty and the experience of trauma are highly associated with abnormal brain development; mental health issues, such as depression and psychosis; and early puberty. Gur and associates used data from the Philadelphia Neurodevelopmental Cohort consisting of a large pool of participants 8–21 years of age. Researchers found that, compared to subjects who did not experience poverty or a traumatic experience, subjects who did had greater psychiatric problems and poorer cognitive performance. Gender was a factor in that females were more affected by poverty and traumatic experience than males.

Another study on the effects of poverty was conducted by Boyce et al. (2012), which investigated the effects of hierarchy in a kindergarten setting. The findings concluded that children lower in a classroom hierarchy had more depression, fewer friends, and reduced academic success. In fact, the researchers concluded that the lower the socioeconomic status of the children, the more likely they were to have the aforementioned deficits. The study also found that teachers who used child-centered methods played a pivotal role in reducing the severity of the deficits.

Researchers at the Canadian Institute for Advanced Research (CIFAR), a global research organization, released a report on the evolving science of developmental studies and childhood harsh conditions. The findings in the report have important implications for childhood learning, interventions for behavioral problems, and governmental policymaking. The research emphasizes the essential periods of development that are necessary for optimum development throughout the lifespan. The research is interdisciplinary, bringing together biology, neuroscience, genetics, and behavioral sciences in an effort to create a broad template for understanding and addressing development concerns that have enormous influence on the life course.

Neuroparenting

As noted earlier, Daniel Siegel (2007), Alan Schore (2023), and Schore and Schore (2007) were at the forefront of a movement that soon developed intending to apply neuroscience to parenting, which created a new focus labeled *neuroparenting* (Hughes & Baylin, 2012). While Siegel and Schore were most concerned about emotion regulation and the implicit brain processes that support it throughout the lifespan, neuroparenting—which is based in part on research cited earlier —is more narrowly focused on teaching parents how to use neuroscience to enhance their children's development and attachment style in the present. The endeavor to apply neuroscience to parenting has resulted in many books aimed at helping parents use insights from neuroscience to parent their children; this is labeled *brain-based parenting* (Snoek & Horstkötter, 2021).

Neuroparenting is defined as child-rearing practices that are based on neuroscience research (Macvarish, 2016). A similar term for applying neuroscience to parenting is brain-based parenting. It assumes that applying neuroscience research to specific parenting behaviors will result in better outcomes for children. Neuroscience research has helped parents learn more about their child's development than was thought possible just a few decades ago. Two of the earliest developmental milestones for infants are forming a secure attachment with the caregiver and the self-regulation of emotion.

While in the past, research on parenting as it affected the developing child was mainly conducted on at-risk, abusive, or neglectful parents, the current trend in applying neuroscience research investigates parenting for both clinical and nonclinical parents (Belsky & de Haan, 2011). The rationale for broad application of neuroscience to parenting interventions is that all parents can improve their parenting by applying scientific insights and better tailor their parenting behavior to their child's age and developmental stage. Private child welfare agencies, government agencies, clinicians, authors of parenting books, and online bloggers offer counsel on how to be a better parent using neuroscience research.

The neural network for the infant's attachment to the caregiver has received much focus in recent years (Hughes & Baylin, 2012). The application of interventions based on neuroparenting can be summarized in a few descriptive statements: Parents should (1) be sensitive to their child's emotions; (2) consistently comfort their child when they are stressed; (3) be a good model for developing cooperative endeavors; (4) know how and when to let children struggle so that they can learn self-reliance; and (5) be the regulator of emotions and gradually allow this to shift to the child. Hughes and Baylin detail skills that parents need to provide for optimum development of their child. Of primary importance is the functioning of the parent's brain, which is the essential element for good parenting. According to Hughes and Baylin (2012), parents must learn to regulate their own dysregulation before they can be effective at regulating the child. Hughes and Baylin (2012) developed a method for ameliorating the blocks for good parenting called PACE, an acronym for playfulness, acceptance, curiosity, and empathy (PACE, A brain-based parenting program, n.d.) (see Table 5.1).

In addition to PACE, Hughes and Baylin (2012) identified five domains of parenting that are necessary for good parenting. The first parental system is the *approach system*. The brain secretes bonding hormones, such as oxytocin, that make it rewarding for parents to provide caregiving behaviors to their young child. The parents' approach/avoidance brain systems are involved based in part on their own upbringing and experiences. Parents need to be evaluated to determine which system dominates to enhance attachment.

The *parental reward system* is activated by the release of oxytocin which stimulates the production of dopamine and the orbitofrontal cortex and the nucleus accumbens (Hughes & Baylin, 2012). Because the reward system can be activated by a wide and diverse range of experiences, parents need to be aware of the activities they engage in that are rewarding, some of which may be detrimental and block rewarding experiences with their child. When the parent does not project a positive expectation on an interaction with their child, the defensive reaction of avoidance emerges, and negativity follows.

The third domain to good parenting is the *parental reading system*, or how adequately the parent can understand verbal and nonverbal communication

TABLE 5.1 Hughes and Baylin (2012) Developed a Method for Ameliorating the Blocks for Good Parenting Called PACE

	PACE
Playful	Parents are taught to be playful rather than punishing when interacting or disciplining
Acceptance	The parent teaches unconditional acceptance so that the child will learn to fully trust in the parent
Curiosity	In place of being stressed by the child's behavior, the parent learns to encourage a wider range of behaviors
Empathy	An important parenting behavior that takes patience is developing excellent communication skills

(Hughes & Baylin, 2012). The temporal lobe is activated in processing verbal and nonverbal cues and, in turn, activates the limbic system. What follows is the activation of either the reward center of the brain or the avoidance center, which determines how the parent will respond to the child.

The *parental meaning-making domain* is the fourth system discussed by Hughes and Baylin (2012). Parents need to have a good sense of themselves and be comfortable with who they are. According to Hughes and Baylin, if parents lack maturity and self-awareness, they will inevitably negatively affect their children. For example, a parent who cannot control their temper models poor behavior that the child copies. Finally, the *parental executive system* is based on the belief that parents can make conscious efforts to control negative and emotional responses. Parents use explicit first order change to change specific child behaviors. For example, a parent decides to ground their children breaking curfew.

Applying Neuroscience to Parenting: A Critical Analysis

In summary, neuroparenting or brain-based parenting relies on research that openly associates parenting behaviors with various negative outcomes in children, such as mental and emotional illness, behavioral, and cognitive deficits. The belief is that parents can be taught the best way to parent, which will lead to children with more competence and positive behavioral outcomes. Consequently, good parenting in the early years will reduce the occurrence of lifelong personal and social problems.

For the most part, brain-based parenting rejects the well-known phrase of Winnicott (1960) that "good enough" parenting will lead to good enough outcomes in children. Snoek and Horstkötter (2021) point out that child abuse and neglect that is perpetrated by mothers is an affront to attachment and the well-being of children. They argue that if the concept of "good enough" mothers was valid, there would be much less abuse and neglect by mothers. Conversely, mothers should be targeted to learn skills made possible by neuroscience research. Further, Snoek and Horstkötter argue that parenting would be broadened by neuroscience applications because of the interdisciplinary nature of the research, which combines genetics, behavioral sciences, past parenting, and environmental circumstances into the interventions.

While Snoek and Horstkötter (2021) favor parents using insight on child development, especially brain development gleaned from neuroscience, they do acknowledge that a few drawbacks in applying neuroscience findings to parenting behavior exist. For example, claims of the benefits of neuroscience on child development can be exaggerated and based on no direct evidence of the benefits. Snoek and Horstkötter cite an illustration of the misuse of neuroscience when the governor of the state of Georgia encouraged parents to buy CDs of Mozart music for their infants. Only one study existed suggesting a link between Mozart and brain development at the time and none on improving infants' cognitive development. Likewise, Disney's campaign to promote "baby Einstein" animated DVDs meant to increase language and cognitive ability was not supported by subsequent research, which forced Disney to recount those claims and reimburse parents for the cost of the CDs.

Neuroscience research is generally conducted within a specific domain but can be applied to other domains that cannot be verified. Application of neuroscience findings varies according to the beliefs and orientation of the applicator. Neuroscience can also be used to justify and support existing theories or interventions with children that have not been specifically studied. For example, the PACE parenting program of Hughes and Baylin (2012) is based in communication theory and is not unique to neuroscience findings. Neuroscience is an evolving science and new discoveries tend to overturn or alter previous conclusions. Consequently, the time is not right to draw conclusive precepts from this developing field of study, unless the research and its application are specific and limited.

The above sentiment is reflected in an analysis of the application of neuroscience to parenting by van de Werff (2017), who points out that applying neuroscience to parenting is guided by values and, therefore, is not an objective endeavor. A close observation of the application of neuroscience to parenting reflects popular established views of what constitutes good parenting. The question at hand is: Does neuroscience provide evidence across the board for all families that enhances developmental outcomes, or do they point to what is already accepted as good parenting? If these ideas of what constitute good parenting implicitly represent accepted views of the normative family, does it equally apply to all families of various racial, ethnic, and economic statuses? For example, the concept of bonding is central to applying neuroscience to parenting, but in terms of culture and diverse types of family units, bonding may not involve a mother and child, and may instead take different familial forms.

Perhaps the most grievous pitfall in neuroparenting is the overemphasis on mothers, which neglects fathers and even the use of the term "parents." Even when the word "caregiver" is used, it is assumed to refer to the mother. Macvarish (2016) refers to the focus on the mother in neuroparenting as "neuromothering" because it ignores the parenting unit of two individuals. This overfocus on the mother does not reflect the history of parenting or current parenting practices where fathers are more involved and the couple's relationship is viewed as egalitarian. In times past, fathers had a greater role in the economic standing of the family and in household management. Even in Western societies, as late as the early modern period, fathers oversaw the child's socialization and education (Furedi, 2001).

Another concern in the literature of neuroparenting is the term itself (Snoek & Horstkötter, 2021). For example, what does "neuro" mean? If it means any intervention that is believed to influence cognitive and behavioral development in children, that paints a broad spectrum of observation, which may not be supported by specific research. On the other hand, if it refers to specific research using the latest technology, such as brain imaging procedures, it is a much smaller pool of research with specific application. Common parenting practices that are believed to enhance infant cognitive learning need to be validated by current research procedures to be considered neuroparenting. According to the critics, the consequences of labeling parenting practices that lack research validity as neuroparenting is not only confusing but undermines the very meaning of neuroparenting.

Snoek and Horstkötter (2021) review various studies on neuroparenting that highlight concerns affecting applicability to parenting practices. For example, Wall (as cited in Snoek & Horstkötter, 2021) concluded in a study on parenting that neuroscience made parents more vigilant in parenting, increasing their stress level, but used insights gained from neuroscience research in a flexible way rather than in an inflexible or dogmatic manner. Chen (as cited in Snoek & Horstkötter, 2021) found that parents using *Herbaika cards,* created to increase cognitive development, used the cards to play with their children, not to increase cognitive development. As a result, parents exposed to neuroscience research on parenting interventions pick and choose the information based on their own needs in parenting (Broer et al. as cited in Snoek & Horstkötter, 2021).

Some parenting suggestions based on neuroscience may be summarily rejected by parents based on not being applicable to their situation. What this means is that parents are cautious to use neuroscience techniques touted by experts that do not apply to them, or that seem ideal or unrealistic. Taken collectively, parents seem uninterested in neuroscience finding on parenting. If parents tend to tailor neuroscience findings to their own needs, it suggests that parenting training models based on neuroscience should cautiously advise parents and provide flexible applications.

Macvarish (2016) has written extensively about the dangers of how neuroparenting has been used by governments and policymakers in the United Kingdom. Government programs and social policy on child welfare, according to Macvarish and Lee (2019), go far beyond their ability to help parents, creating a kind of magic bullet mentality that promises to solve child development problems, particularly regarding cognitive development. Furthermore, Macvarish (2016) believes the "*zero to three*" *movement* in both the United States and the United Kingdom reiterate common beliefs about the long-term effects of early experiences and reify them with isolated research findings. They further argue that while it may be true that severe emotional damage can be inflicted on children during the first three years, which have long-term effects, to believe this is true for all children, or needs to be prevented, pathologizes normal child-rearing practices.

Macvarish (2016) believes that the zero to three movement is a global focus on perceived parental failure that is promoted by international agencies and governmental programs. The programs put parents in the central role of responsibility for outcomes with their children, while at the same time requiring parents to follow rigid parenting practices to demonstrate their competence as parents. Consequently, the source of child problems and later adult problems is the quality of the parenting, which can be referred to as *parental determinism*. The quality of the parent–child relationship depends on the mother's mental and emotional states pre- and post-delivery. From this perspective, attachment is compromised when the quality of parenting is poor. While programs for zero to three heavily focus on the mother, little is directed at the father except for interventions to help fathers be more present or involved with their children and their potential to act out in violence due to prolonged stress. What is missing in these parenting programs is any biological or genetic connection to the father (see Table 5.2).

Macvarish (2016) noted that although there is considerable criticism of the zero to three literature and parental determinism, there has been little overall slowing of this parenting movement. Macvarish et al. (2014) raised the question: How can parents who are viewed as the problem also be viewed as the solution? A similar question is how can the child be expected to have different outcomes if their brain is determined along a certain pathway so early in life? The answers to these questions lack specificity and range from reducing stress to remediating attachment. From this perspective, a therapist is needed to intercede to become the advocate both for the child and for parents becoming better parents. In placing the therapist in the role of being the means for positive change, parents become less influential in the sphere of influence.

According to Macvarish and Lee (2019), the zero to three movement has pathologized parents and politicized the early years of parenting. It has fomented an intrusion of the state into family life but has not answered the question of how the state can blame parents for the child's problems, on the one hand, and expect parents to be purveyors of competent parenting, on the other hand. The upshot of this kind of public policy according to Macvarish and Lee (2019) is to reduce natural, spontaneous parenting to a technical and mechanistic endeavor.

The focus on neuroparenting may, in fact, be paradoxical in that parents attempting to be better parents by learning how to be more loving may produce the opposite effect brought about by increased parenting stress and feeling incompetent in that role (Macvarish, 2016). Government programs aimed at improving all parenting creates a reinterpreted family where one size fits all lacking flexibility by rejecting the long-held notion that there is more than one way to raise a competent child into adulthood. The constant vigilance on parenting in the right way changes the phrase of "good enough" parenting to "not good enough, period." Parents who lack confidence in their parenting skills are not motivated for change. According to Macvarish and Lee (2019), the spontaneous and unrehearsed happenings within

TABLE 5.2 Criticism of Parental Determinism

Focuses on neuromothering, which minimizes father involvement
Zero to three movement has pathologized parenting
Fosters an intrusion of the government into family life
Reduces natural spontaneous parenting
Creates a reinterpreted family where one size fits all
Lacks flexibility
Cultures differ on what is effective parenting
Only a small number of parents need help

the family give way to mechanized procedures of how to enhance the brain of the child.

According to Faircloth (2017), these mechanized behaviors prescribed by experts for parenting today have not always been touted by experts and parents functioned just as well in their everyday routines in spontaneously showing love and nurturance to their children. Further, societies differ on expected parental behavior, which results in no significant increase in negative outcomes in the child's development.

In short, the critics of neuroparenting are cautious of government intrusion into family life through various parenting advice and reject parental determinism in child development. They believe that the overemphasis on attachment theory paradoxically undermines the spontaneous display for parental nurturance. Much can be said for the caution these critics pose for mandating early childhood parenting practices for all parents, when only a small percentage of parents need help. The critics themselves, however, can be critiqued on several fronts. For example, their arguments are based on observation and not founded in rigorous research evidence. What is the evidence that early trauma does not have long-term effects across the lifespan? Are parents genuinely paranoid about neuroparenting or do they accept parenting advice because of a desire to be the best parents they can be?

While the debate over the effects of neuroparenting on the parent–child relationship continues, a systems/dialectical position would welcome the various arguments in the belief that debate allows for divergent thinking, which is most important for finding solutions. Part II of the book will describe in greater detail how second order parenting from a systems/dialectical approach can shed light on neuroscience research on neuroparenting.

References

Ayre, K., & Krishnamoorthy, G. (2020). *Trauma informed behaviour support: A practical guide to developing resilient learners*. University of Southern Queensland. https://usq.pressbooks.pub/traumainformedpractice/

Belsky, J., & de Haan, M. (2011). Annual research review: Parenting and children's brain development: The end of the beginning. *Journal of Child Psychology and Psychiatry, 52*, 409–428. https://doi.org/10.1111/j1467-8721.2007.00525.x

Boyce, W. T., Obradović, J., Bush, N. R., & Adler, N. (2012). Social stratification, classroom climate, and the behavioral adaptation of kindergarten children. *Proceedings of the National Academy of Sciences (PNAS), 109*(2), 17168–17173. https://doi.org/10.1073/pnas.1201730109

Burani, K., Brush, C. J., Spahr, C., Slavich, G. M., Meyer, A., & Hajcak, G. (2022). Corporal punishment is uniquely associated with a greater neural response to errors and blunted neural response to rewards in adolescence. *Biological Psychiatry: Cognitive Neuroscience and Neuroimaging*. https://doi.org/10.1016/j.bpsc.2022.09.004

Cahn, B. R., & Polich, J. (2006). Meditation states and traits: EEG, ERP, and neuroimaging studies. *Psychological Bulletin, 132*(2), 180–211. https://doi.org/10.1037/0033-2909.132.2.180

Camina, E., & Guell, F. (2017). The neuroanatomical, neurophysiological, and psychological basis of memory: Current models and their origins. *Frontiers in Pharmacology, 8*. https://www.frontiersin.org/articles/10.3389/fphar.2017.00438/full; https://doi.org/10.3389/fphar.2017.0043

Dreikurs, R. (1979). *The challenge of parenthood*. Dutton.
Faircloth, C. (2017). 'Natural' breastfeeding in comparative perspective: Feminism, morality, and adaptive accountability. *Ethnos*, *82*(1), 19–43. https://doi.org/10.1080/00141844.2015.1028562
Furedi, F. (2001). *Paranoid parenting: Why ignoring the experts may be the best for your child*. Chicago Review Press.
Gordon, T. (1975). *P.E.T. parenting renting effectiveness training*. Plume.
Gur, R. E., Moore, T. M., Rosen, A. F. G., Barzilay, R., Roalf, D. R., Calkins, M. E., Ruparel, K., Scott, J. C., Amasy, L., Satterthwaite, T. D., Shinohara, R. T., & Gur, R. C. (2019). Burden of environmental adversity associated with psychopathology, maturation, and brain behavior parameters in youths. *JAMA Psychiatry*. https://doi.org/10.1001/jamapsychiatry.2019.0943
Hackman, D. A., Farah, M. J., & Meaney, M. J. (2010). Socioeconomic status and the brain: Mechanistic insights from human and animal research. *National Review of Neuroscience*, *11*(9), 651–659. https://doi.org/10.1038/nrn2897
Hanson, J., Chung, M. K., Avants, B. B., Rudolph, K. D., Shirtcliff, E. A., Gee, J. C., Davidson, R. J., & Pollak, S. D. (2012). Structural variations in prefrontal cortex mediate the relationship between early childhood stress and spatial working memory. *Journal of Neuroscience, 32*(23), 7917. https://doi.org/10.1523/jneurosci.0307-12.2012
Holmes, C. J., Barton, A. W., MacKillop, J., Galvan, A., Owens, M. M., McCormick, M. J., Yu, T., Beach, S. R. H., Brody, G. H., & Sweet, L. H. (2018). Parenting and salience network connectivity among African Americans: A protective pathway for health-risk behaviors. *Biological Psychiatry*. https://doi.org/10.1016/j.biopsych.2018.03.003
Hughes, D. A., & Baylin, J. (2012). *Brain-based parenting: The neuroscience of caregiving for healthy attachment*. W.W. Norton.
Kuhl, P. K. (2004). Early language acquisition: Cracking the speech code. *Nature Reviews Neuroscience, 5,* 831–843.
Kurth, S., Dean, D. C., Achermann, P., O'Muircheartaigh, J., Deoni, S. C. L., Huber, R., & LeBourgeois, M. K. (2016). Increased sleep depth in developing neural networks: New insights from sleep restriction in children. *Frontiers in Human Neuroscience, 10*. https://doi.org/10.3389/fnhum.2016.00456
Macvarish, J. (2016). *Neuroparenting: The expert invasion of family life*. Palgrave Macmillan.
Macvarish, J., & Lee, E. (2019). Constructions of parents in adverse childhood experiences discourse. *Journal of Social Policy and Society*, *18*, 467–477. https://api.semanticscholar.org/CorpusID:199174449
Macvarish, J., Lee, E., & Lowe, P. (2014). 'The "first three years" movement and the infant brain: A review of critiques. *Sociology Compass, 8*(6), 792–804.
Morgan, J. K., Eckstrand, K. L., Silk, J. S., Olino, T. M., Ladouceur, C. D., & Forbes, E. E. (2021). Maternal response to positive affect moderates the impact of familial risk for depression on ventral striatal response to winning reward in 6- to 8-year-old children. *Biological Psychiatry: Cognitive Neuroscience and Neuroimaging*. https://doi.org/10.1016/j.bpsc.2021.12.014
Narvaez, D. (2017). Evolution, child raising, and compassionate morality. In P. Gilbert (Ed.), *Compassion* (pp. 173–186). Routledge.
PACE: A brain-based parenting program. (n.d.). Retrieved April 20, 2023, from https://www.communityservices.act.gov.au/data/assets/pdf_file/0004/1549750/PACE-web.pdf
Patterson, G. (1971). *Families: Application of social learning theory to family life*. Research Press.
Rogers, C. (1961). *On becoming a person*. Houghton Mifflin.
Schore, A. N. (2000). Attachment and the regulation of the right brain. *Attachment & Human Development*, *2*(1), 23–47.
Schore, A. (2023). Dr. Allan Schore on attachment trauma and effects of neglect and abuse on brain development [video]. In *Psychalive*. https://www.psychalive.org/video-dr-allan-schore-attachment-trauma-effects-neglect-abuse-brain-development/

Schore, J. R., & Schore, A. (2007). Modern attachment theory: The central role of affect regulation in development and treatment. *Clinical Social Work Journal, 36*(1), 9–20.
Sheridan, M. A., Mukerji, C. E., Wade, M., Humphreys, K. L., Garrisi, K., Goel, S., Patel, K., Fox, N. A., Zeanah, C. H., & McLaughlin, K. A. (2022). Early deprivation alters structural brain development from middle childhood to adolescence. *Science Advances, 8*(40). https://doi.org/10.1126/sciadv.abn4316
Siegel, D. J. (2007). Mindfulness training and neural integration: Differentiation of distinct streams of awareness and the cultivation of well-being. *Social Cognitive and Affective Neuroscience, 2*(4), 259–263.
Siegel, D. J. (2010). *Mindsight: The new science of personal transformation*. W.W. Norton.
Snoek, A., & Horstkötter, D. (2021). Neuroparenting: The myths and the benefits, an ethical systematic review. *Neuroethics, 14,* 387–408.
Suffren, S., La Buissonnière-Ariza, V., Tucholka, A., Nassim, M., Séguin, J. R., Boivin, M., Singh, M. K., Folan-Ross, L. C., Lepore, F. R., Gotlib, I. H., Trembley, R. E., & Maheu, F. S. (2021). Prefrontal cortex and amygdala anatomy in youth with persistent levels of harsh parenting practices and subclinical anxiety symptoms over time during childhood. *Development and Psychopathology, 34*(3), 957–968. https://doi.org/10.1017/S0954579420001716
Sydnor, V. J., Larsen, B., Seidlitz, J., Adebimpe, A., Alexander-Bloch, A. F., Bassett, D. S., Bertolero, M. A., Cieslak, M., Covitz, S., Fan, Y., Gur, R. E., Gur, R. C., Mackey, A. P., Moore, T. M., Roalf, D. R., Shinohara, T. T., & Satterthwaite, T. D. (2023). Intrinsic activity development unfolds along a sensorimotor-association cortical axis in youth. *Nature Neuroscience, 26*(4), 638. https://doi.org/10.1038/s41593-023-01282-y
van de Werff, T. (2017). Being a good external frontal lobe: Parenting teenage brains. In J. Leefmann & E. Hildt (Eds.), *The human sciences after the decade of the brain* (pp. 214–231). Elsevier.
Winnicott, D. W. (1960). The theory of the parent–infant relationship. *International Journal of Psychoanalysis, 41,* 585–595.
Zeanah, C. H., Nelson, C. A., Fox, N. A., Smyke, A. T., Marshall, P., Parker, S. W., & Koga, S. (2003). Designing research to study the effects of institutionalization on brain and behavioral development: The Bucharest early intervention project. *Development and Psychopathology, 15,* 885–907.

PART II

Putting It All Together

6

ATTACHMENT, SYSTEMS THEORY, AND NEUROSCIENCE

Using Indirect, Implicit, and Paradoxical Methods

Parenting Policies

In contemporary societies, parenting is more complex and anxiety provoking than in times past. Much of this difference rests on the evolving of society into more economic, social, and political complexities. Over the course of these changes, there is concern that children are vulnerable and prone to dysfunction partly because parents fail to provide adequate parenting. To address the inadequacies in parenting, social agencies and governments developed ways to improve parenting skills through parent education and programs.

A major change in government policies was not trusting the instincts of mothers to provide a natural environment where the child can thrive. Consequently, good parenting comes from parents who have developed skills from expert training (Stearns, 2003). What evolved from a carefree natural expectation of parenting became, in the 19th century, the beginning of the modern period where inadequacies in parenting began to take center stage. Thus, parenting began to move toward a *scientific approach to parenting* and away from individualized natural instincts. This focus led to the belief that the children's behaviors could be understood from the application of scientific methods. In the United States during the late 19th century and early 20th century, academics began research into child studies that was meant to address parenting based on its research findings (Hulbert, 2004).

The role of the parent became less and less important as the role of experts who could teach parents new skills in parenting became more prominent (Hulbert, 2004). In both the United States and the United Kingdom, programs sprang up to help the most vulnerable and at-risk parents. Part of the concern of governments about child welfare was purely political in that the future of the country rested on the shoulders of the next generations. Most of this initial parenting focus was

DOI: 10.4324/9781003381679-8

aimed at poor families who had higher rates of divorce, job interruptions, and poor education (Romagnoli & Wall, 2012).

Not all child development theorists were on board with the belief that experts were needed to advise families and that mothers needed training to provide the best care for their children, such as Winnicott (1964) who believed that the intrusion of parenting experts into the family was detrimental. Other popular writers such as Benjamin Spock (1985) suggested that mothers' trusting their parenting instincts was sufficient without expert help. Spock's book went beyond simply trusting mothers' instincts, however, and was awash with "expert" advice. Spock's sentiments were shared by many other writers of the time who seemed, on the one hand, to acknowledge that mothers knew how to parent, but on the other hand, there existed an undercurrent of caution and concern that mothers might need expert help.

Over time, the shift from trusting mother's instincts to suggesting that mothers could still need help transformed the full-blown belief that experts were essential in advising and training parents (mothers) how to parent. The experts believed that mothers needed to be consistent in parenting, which necessitated skill development that they lacked (Reece, 2013). Believing that mothers lacked skills and needed training to be better parents instituted a new era in parent–child relationships. No longer were mothers trusted to optimally perform the role of parent. The behavior of mothers became the important pivot in understanding the developing child. This view was criticized by Furedi (2008) who stated that the new assemblage of various *parenting experts* believed that not only parents need help but that helping was also necessary else children would be at risk of developmental dysfunction.

Furedi (2008) further believes that when experts become necessary for parenting competence, the results are negative for parents who then lose confidence, which increases their stress level. Furedi cites the lack of research on this shift of authority in parenting from the parent to the expert as a concern that needs addressing. Furthermore, according to Furedi, the teaching of parenting skills by this collection of experts is an invasion into the privacy of families. While there are genuine experts on parenting who can be a valued resource for families, there is a need to distinguish legitimate from illegitimate experts.

For Furedi (2008), distinguishing legitimate experts from illegitimate experts is based on authority and knowledge. The parents' relationship with an expert is hierarchical since the expert's confidence is verifiable based on their scientific foundation. He believed this level of authority too often is missing in parenting experts in contemporary society.

According to Furedi (2008), no parenting skills approach can measure up to the years of relationship development and maintenance that exist between parents and their children. Furedi believed that the fundamental issue is not if parents can be taught skills, but how something is learned. Although Furedi did not use the term *unconscious learning*, he stated that learning does not have to be taught. In fact, he did not believe that parents can learn how to parent from reading books or gleaning advice from experts. Children learn how to behave from the relationship with parents and parents learn how to parent through their interactions with others.

In both the United Kingdom and the United States, contemporary parenting dominated by questionable parenting experts has been adopted by governmental and childcare agencies meant to both correct poor parenting and prevent later problems in adolescence and adulthood. The UK program *Sure Start* and the US program *Head Start* were aimed at poor uneducated parents (Clarke, 2006 as cited in Furedi, 2008). In the 1990s, the swing toward government intrusion into parenting ramped up and has continued regardless of which political party was in power. The implications of such policies are that families are fragile and that intervention into parenting practices of families can help all families. The justification for intervention in poor families is based on the view that these families are diverse, children are more stressed and lack resources, family disruption is high, and parents lack the skills necessary to raise functional children. Poverty was cast as the cause for poor parenting and for poor outcomes in children.

The US Head Start program began in the 1960s with the main goal of improving the school readiness for children of poverty. These intensive efforts were believed to be necessary to provide an equal playing field for children of poverty. This program and similar ones, such as the *Perry Preschool Project*, showed improvement in school readiness. Head Start programs produced a bump in cognitive development of children in the early grades that faded over time. Despite this lack of cognitive sustained improvement, Head Start continued to be supported by the government. Perry Preschool Project, a longitudinal study that followed participants into their 20s, provided an intensive preschool educational program for poverty-level children. The study found that follow-up of participants as young adults had lower poverty rates, less criminal involvement, and less unemployment of the participants (Phillips, 2017). Subsequent projects, however, have not replicated the success of the initial project.

These early intrusions into the family aimed at poverty-level families soon expanded to include single-parent mothers and even dual-career families that lacked time and energy to deal with raising their children properly. It was no leap of logic to continually expand the net of parents needing help to include other categories of parents (Furedi, 2008). Under the rubric of supporting families in the United Kingdom, it soon became common practice in family programs to give advice on several relevant topics, such as healthy eating, spending playtime with children, and using positive parenting strategies (Churchill & Clarke, 2009). According to Furedi (2008), due to several laws meant to make parents accountable for the antisocial behavior of their children, the focus of agency intervention expanded in both making parents responsible for the child's behavior and in the age for monitoring beyond the age of 3. As a result of expanding the age of child vulnerability into the teenage years, new avenues for intruding into family life opened.

In both the United Kingdom and the United States, it was only a short jump from this expanding of the concern of the causes of child problems to redefining what constituted good parenting and designing programs to train parents. While in the past, the major parenting concern was with poor families, the shift in viewing parents as responsible for child outcomes meant that all parents needed help to ensure the best result for children. Some scholars warned that families were too individualized and complex for governmental programs aimed at improving parenting of all families to work effectively (Furedi, 2008). Furedi viewed the relationship between parent and child to be too unique and personal for broad-based generic programs to be of help. Consequently, the generic approach would perhaps address problems that were nonexistent for some families and would mechanize parenting toward unrealistic and unattainable goals. It could be argued that family life was no longer seen as the creation of the family itself, but successful families were those that fit a mechanized view of relationships that distorted the reality of family relationships. According to Clarke (2006 as cited in Furedi, 2008), this generic focus on techniques may undermine the actual parent–child relationship because it was created from a false narrative.

Attachment Theory Redux

It should not be shocking that the critics of the government intruding into the family by blaming parents, especially mothers, for the poor outcomes of children would lead straight to the heart of the matter, attachment theory. As long as the focus was on intrusion into the privacy of the family, attachment theory escaped a full-frontal assault. This began to change in the mid- to late-1990s as researchers began to hone in on the theoretical base for government interventions.

One of the major voices to alter the concept of attachment was Judith Harris (1998). Her book, *The Nurture Assumption*, was met with a mixture of praise and scorn. The very act of challenging such a widespread accepted view that attachment to the mother had profound long-term consequences on the child was heresy. Harris did not deny that children learn and are influenced by their parents and primarily the mother, but she claimed that they learn more from their peers. While children are influenced by both genes and *nurturance* evenly, Harris opted for peers being more influential in nurturing than parents. Harris' insight points to understanding attachment devoid of preconceptions. For example, to presuppose that attachment is good or bad, depending on how the parents act toward the child, precludes an unbiased assessment and leads to a self-fulfilled prophesy.

Harris' (1998) main argument centers around a belief that *attachment theory is reductionistic*—that is, outcomes in children depend on how parents behave toward them. A problem with viewing parents in the pivotal role affecting development is that parents do not generally follow predetermined plans for how to interact with their children. Their parenting varies according to the personality and needs of each child and the present circumstances. This point is well taken because when parents behave the same way to all their children, they do not turn out the same way. Furthermore, Harris points to research findings that outcomes with most children are good regardless of whether the child was "abused" or treated with extravagant love. However, while there may be some research that shows no difference in outcomes between abused children and nonabused children, the preponderance of evidence would not support that claim.

According to Harris (1998), the attachment model of parent–child behavior has several serious flaws when one steps back and merely observes human relationships. For example, the view that parents socialize children does not fare well when unbiasedly observed. Children are different from their parents and take on the culture of their peers. The simple observation that children are not focused on being successful adults, but on being children, according to Harris, undermines the argument that parents are more important than peers.

Harris' critique of attachment theory cuts into the intensive parenting models that by doing certain things, parents will increase the cognitive ability of their children. Instead, Harris believes that the reason some children are smarter than others is their heredity, not from explicit acts by parents. She believes that parenting should be natural and easy. The contemporary practice of skills training to be better parents precludes parents from acting naturally with their children, which creates undue stress and guilt at not being the best parent, and reduces love and affection to artificial behaviors that are done at the suggestion of so-called parenting experts. Furthermore, she believes that one of the dangers of contemporary parenting is trying too hard. What parents should be concerned about, according to Harris, is to love their children, not trying to produce certain outcomes prescribed by parenting experts.

Harris (1998) debunks the belief that the family environment is responsible for the personality development of children by observing that in adoptive families, adopted children's personalities are not shaped by the family environment. Likewise, the type of family structure, two-parent, single-parent, and LGBTQ, does not determine personality development. Parents' influence on children appears to be momentary and geared toward specific times with the parent but does not carry over to when the child is alone or with their peers.

Although Harris (1998) raises legitimate concerns about the deterministic underpinnings of attachment theory, there are caveats that arise. For example, to conclude that there is no difference in the personalities of children who have been abused and those who have not may reflect the wrong choice of measure for child outcomes. Personality is a different measure than psychological or behavioral outcomes and there is a wealth of research that concludes that even corporal punishment that is not considered abusive has psychological effects on children (Kaltenbach et al., 2018). The welfare of children depends on much more than being friendly with them throughout their life course, as Harris suggests.

Perhaps the most critical mistake in Harris' (1998) views is that, while she criticizes the presumption of parental nurture as predetermining the outcomes of children, she is also guilty of presupposing. Her presumption is that genes are more important in child outcomes than environment which is the conduit for the rest of her arguments. Research and observation would not lead you to that conclusion. She is heavily steeped in evolutionary theory and ignores a plethora of research on environmental factors that address outcomes in children.

Other attachment theory critics have focused on is Ainsworth's stranger situation. Briefly, Ainsworth developed the stranger situation to determine the components of attachment to the mother during eight 20-minute segments (see Table 6.1).

The experimenter scores the stranger situation according to the following criteria: *Proximity-Seeking*, such as greeting and approaching, reaching toward, and crying; *Proximity-Avoiding*, measured when the stranger enters the room or attempts to interact with the infant and includes ignoring, not looking at, turning or moving away; *Contact-Maintaining*, upon reunion with mother, the infant may cling, embrace, hold on, and show displeasure if they lose contact; *Contact-Resisting*, includes angry behavior at mother who attempts to initiate contact; *Ambivalent* attempts to push away, hit, or kick the mother who tries to make contact; *Search behaviors* after mother leaves the room that include watching door, or orientation mother's empty chair. In addition, the infant is assessed on exploring in the presence or absence of mother and the degree of *stranger anxiety*. An analysis of these behaviors leads to identifying the infants in one of four styles of attachment—secure attachment, insecure attachment, insecure ambivalent attachment, and disorganized attachment.

Jerome Kagan (1998) made a forceable argument against parental determinism as implied by attachment theory. While not denying the importance of development during infancy, he believed that this period and later life events underemphasized personality traits. Furthermore, he believed that other factors such as poverty, lack of education, birth order, one's self-identity, and the historical context were more influential factors in outcomes of children than was the attachment period in infancy. For Kagan (2013), the infant's temperament cannot be attributed to the

TABLE 6.1 Stages in the Stranger Test

The Stranger Tests	
Segment 1	Mother and infant enter a playroom with experimenter
Segment 2	Mother and infant alone, with infant free to move about and explore
Segment 3	Stranger enters, converses with mother, interacts with child, and mother leaves the room (3 minutes)
Segment 4	Separation #1 from mother; stranger remains in room, interacts with infant as needed
Segment 5	Reunion with mother; mother appears at door, greets infant, stranger leaves
Segment 6	Separation #2, mother leaves, infant is alone for 3 minutes
Segment 7	Stranger reenters, interacts with infant when needed
Segment 8	Reunion; mother returns and stranger leaves

sensitive care of the mother. The deciding factor in outcomes with children, Kagan believed, was a combination of social class, experiences with peers, and later life events. Kagan's views are echoed in the writings of Plomin (2018), who stated that no differences in outcomes in children can be found after controlling for genetics.

Other critics have spoken out against attachment theory. For example, Granqvist et al. (2017) challenged the use of attachment styles to identify psychopathology and mental health treatment of children. It was also noted that attachment therapies, such as adoption, do not remove deficits attributed to attachment disorders (O'Connor & Zeanah, 2003). Neckoway et al. (2003) acknowledged the importance of attachment for understanding outcomes with children but believed that attachment has been applied across the board with little regard for cultural and parenting differences, which even Ainsworth noted (as cited in Neckoway et al., 2003). Breuer (1999) concluded that the styles of attachment given to infants are not consistent over time. It can be implied that attachment changes over time, but when the mother–child relationship remains unchanged, the infant's identified attachment style will remain constant across time.

The question of attachment theory changing over time has prompted critics of parental determinism to pay attention. Generally, researchers have viewed attachment styles as changing either due to individual's increased or decreased security as they mature from children to adolescents to adults. The turbulent teenage years are noted for less closeness with parents and greater closeness with peer groups (Buist et al., 2002), which has a direct effect on attachment style with parents. In a longitudinal study, Chopik et al. (2017) found that attachment anxiety decreased during middle age while attachment avoidance decreases sequentially as one ages. As a result of new experiences, one's *working model* of the world derived primarily from one's attachment style would be expected to be altered, and even Bowlby (1982) acknowledged that. The important challenge for attachment theorists is to articulate precisely the factors that are indicated with attachment style change.

While it would appear to be of major concern that attachment styles can change over time, there is a paucity of scholarly research on the topic. The existing research findings are contradictory in that some find attachment to parents consistent over time (Jones et al., 2018) and others have demonstrated that attachment styles can change over time (Fraley, 2019). Much of the literature comes from psychotherapists who provide techniques and remedies for insecure attachment. Attachment styles in adulthood are generally related to romantic partnerships that reflect one's internal working model (Hazan & Shaver, 1994). Recently, emerging research on attachment is labeled *global attachment*, the tendency to act with similar attachment styles with different persons (Allen et al., 2018). A limitation of global attachment research is that it does not focus on specific relationships and whether attachment to the same person can change over time.

The above point was the focus of a research project of Bohn et al. (2019). Subjects for this research considered emerging adults (late adolescence) and parents who were assessed over a one-year time frame. Results indicated that mutual attachment over time was stable but emerging adults showed changes due to accumulation of situational occurrences, but this was not true for adults. The researchers were able to distinguish between stable and changing attachment.

According to Fraley (2002), there are two types of research models in the literature—the internal working model, which states there is a basic prototype of stable attachment; and the revisionist model, which argues no underlying stable attachment exists. Fransburg (2015) investigated these models to delineate the nature of stability, change in attachment over time, and the factors associated with relationship experiences that lead to change more accurately. The results of the study found that a latent stable element existed over the life course, but a second element existed that changed over time in reference to negative and positive relationship experiences, and internalizing and externalizing emotional states.

Changing attachment styles is a popular topic in psychotherapy models. While some research as noted earlier supports that attachment styles can change over time, they do not typically address the decision and conscious efforts to change them as do therapeutic models. Some researchers have found that when persons want to change a personality trait, they are more likely to change than someone who does not want to change (Hudson et al., 2019). When a person's circumstance over a long-term time frame changes, different thoughts and feelings are produced and corresponding traits, such as attachment style, change accordingly (Roberts et al., 2017). Psychotherapy models emphasize that, with time and repeated patterns, the new response becomes habituated and can change the internal frame of reference.

The scenario for changing attachment follows from repeated conscious efforts to alter what was developed unconsciously. An assumption is that one must practice new behaviors until they become automatic. Another assumption is that the attachment style took time to development and, consequently, will take time to change. Recent research reveals that personality traits can change over the life course with or without conscious awareness and volition (Roberts et al., 2017). These changes are highly correlated to life events and may be either positive or negative.

The question should be raised that if attachment is difficult to change and can only change from repeated efforts, is it worth it? It could also be asked: Why try to change an implicit process through explicit means? If something is formed implicitly without conscious awareness, is it not better to change it implicitly? And how would an implicit change occur? To change a trait, such as attachment, implicitly, requires a complete addressing of how attachment develops. Some therapeutic models suggest that it is necessary to recreate the same environment in which the original attachment occurred (Cain, 2020). This requires recreating the atmosphere of dependence on the therapist in place of the parents. While this therapy intervention may seem strange and untenable, it does illustrate the mechanism by which change occurs implicitly.

It is not disputed by researchers on attachment theory that attachment develops from relationship interactions (Fraley & Shaver, 2008). What is disputed is that attachment forms a lasting determinism throughout the life course based on that first attachment bond. Life experiences, which are implicit emotional experiences that occur throughout one's life, change attachment far more effectively than direct conscious attempts. According to Fraley et al. (2021), life events can initiate both short-term and long-term changes in attachment. These life experiences, which have no explicit expression, change personality traits and attachment unconsciously.

The term that generally refers to the capacity to change the brain and, consequently, behaviors is plasticity. As stated before, the infant's brain develops through interactions and experiences, which form a basic pattern for how the infant views the world. As the child ages and gains life experiences outside the family, brain plasticity allows for altering of the original neural networks and, consequently, changes occur in the implicit internal working model. The internal working model is not determinism as was once believed. Brain researchers now report that the brain is alterable throughout the life course and even capable of making new neurons, although decidedly more so in the early years (Zhou et al., 2022). Learning from new experiences affects brain change by altering the structure of the brain. The interactions with others throughout the life course change attachment generally without conscious awareness. Relationships with significant others, romantic partners, children, work colleagues, therapists, and close friends, all have an influence on how the internal working model, including attachment, changes over time. Thus, neuroplasticity happens due to the emotional system's response to experiences, and less through intentional cognitive and verbal actions (de Zulueta, 2006).

Implications for Parent Education and Parenting Models

This section of the chapter will discuss how parent education and parenting in general can be enhanced by implicit techniques. Second order parenting, in contrast to first order parenting, uses intuitive, creative, paradoxical, and indirect interventions that do not require conscious awareness to produce change. Grounded in systems/dialectical perspective, second order parenting focuses on change of the structure of the parent–child relationship rather than changing individuals. Change occurs from new experiences that unbalance the structure and sets in motion reorganizing the parent–child relationship. The following discussion and summary of previous literature review will justify the thesis that indirect interventions that reflect neuroscience findings need further consideration in parent training and parenting.

Conscious and Unconscious Processes

One of the major beliefs about change is that it should be conscious and, to change, a person must use their rational thinking to understand their problem and make different decisions to change (Figure 6.1). This understanding of change as emanating from cognitive awareness permeates the helping professions, including parent

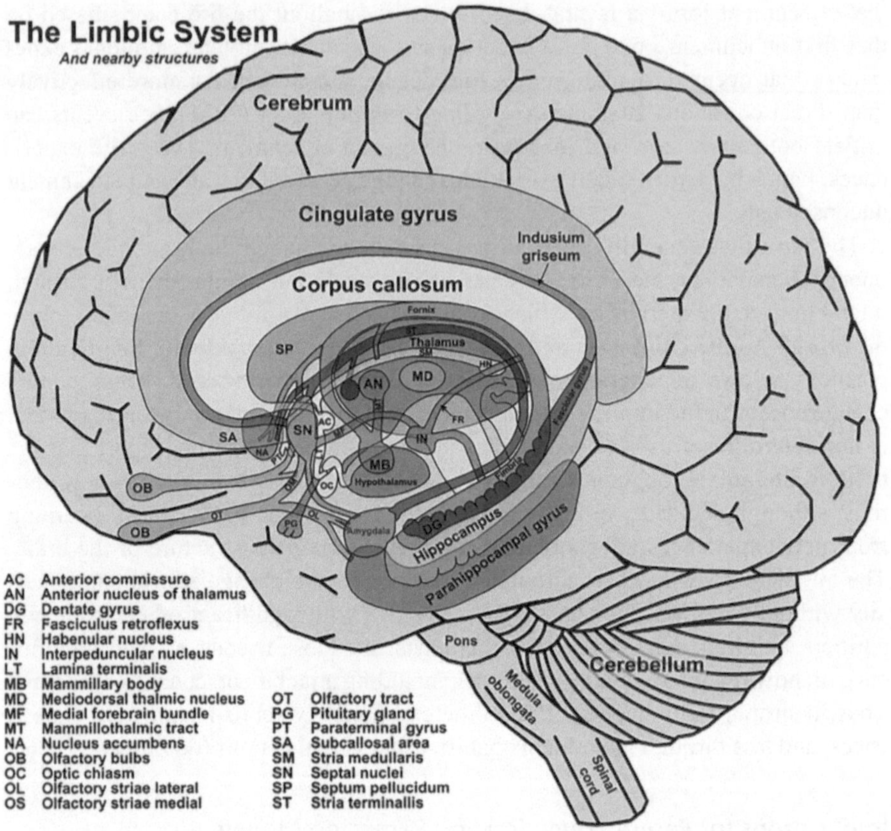

FIGURE 6.1 The brain's limbic system is involved in processing emotions, which aids in learning, decision making, and unconscious processes. (Taylor, 2013)

education. Recent neuroscience research, however, implies that conscious awareness is not necessary for change. For example, a recent development in neuroscience labeled predictive mind is based on evidence that the brain is geared toward predicting future personal and social outcomes (Carruthers, 2017). This brain process is automatic and outside of conscious awareness, but consciousness can break in when there is a disruption to the predicted outcome. The implication of Carruthers' research is that thoughts and mental processes are directed by implicit and automatic processes, not by the conscious brain.

Other neuroscience research tends to come to similar conclusions as Carruthers. For example, Kahneman (2011) noted that although the conscious and unconscious work together, the conscious mind is limited to the contents of the working memory, which means most mental processes come from the unconscious. Furthermore, Solms & Friston (2018) demonstrated that consciousness was tied to the emotional systems of the brain and not the rational centers.

In sum, recent neuroscience research on consciousness and unconsciousness supports the view that unconscious processes account for most of brain activity. Furthermore, the limbic or emotional center of the brain is the source of decision making and not the neocortex. Although this research would appear to support the view of determinism, it supports a view that the brain is experience-dependent, and as a systems/dialectical perspective would imply, changes occur because new experiences require the brain to change, which interrupts the automatic processes. In other words, plasticity occurs because the brain's automatic function is challenged in a dialectical manner and a new equilibrium ensues.

Another focus in neuroscience research that has relevant implications for conscious and unconscious processes is *epigenesis*, the investigation of how genes interact with environmental factors. Research in epigenesis supports the view that early experiences in childhood can have long-term effects on genes by turning genes on or off (Isles & Wilkinson, 2008). Early experiences, such as abuse, poverty, and exposure to environmental hazards, can alter gene expression. Although experiences can have long-term effects, new experiences over the life course can continue to turn genes on and off (Costa & Johannes, 2020).

It follows from the above research that early experiences do not determine later outcomes. In systems/dialectical terms, that which occurs before another occurrence is related in a circular manner, not a linear manner. Rather, one response will elicit a response in the other which repeats endlessly. Applied to parenting and parent education, there is no cause-and-effect relationship between the parent's behavior and the child's behavior. The parent does not cause the child's behavior or vice versa, but behavior in general reflects a circular pattern of interaction. Consequently, the change that happens is a change in the structure of the relationship rather than a change in either party. Because the focus of change is on the structure of the parent–child interactional patterns, the focus on skill development is largely ineffective.

Implicit and Explicit Actions and Decision Making

The involvement of the unconscious even in behaviors deemed to be cognitive moves the scales toward the importance of understanding implicit processes. Implicit processes mean that they take place outside of conscious, or explicit awareness. Much of what occurs in the parent–child relationship takes place outside of awareness, even though there is a cognitive bias that awareness is necessary for change. Examples of implicit communication include gestures, tone of voice, and intuition gleaned from the interaction (St Quinton & Brunton, 2017). While understanding implicit forms of communication is important, the inferences from implicit processes go far beyond communication theory and include changes in genes as noted earlier, indirect actions, and decision making.

Decision making is popularly framed as a conscious explicit behavior that is the purview of the rational center of the brain and the conscious mind. This popular view is in sharp contrast to a large body of evolving research that paints a different picture of decision making. Conscious or explicit processes reflect awareness of intent in decision making, but researchers have found little support for the view that explicit or conscious processes are involved in behavioral change (Schwarzer, 2008). Decision making processes seem to happen because of unconscious rather than conscious means. This means that they are part of the implicit memory system and operate outside of consciousness (Papies, 2016). Behavioral change prior to recent research came from identifying one's automatic responses and making conscious efforts to change them through practice. Recent research concludes that the unconscious is not suppressed, so there is no need to identify the unconscious or implicit processes to change them. Instead of the old view of the relationship of conscious explicit processes and unconscious implicit processes, the new view proclaims that they work together, and it is the implicit processes that inform the conscious mind what to decide (Kahneman, 2011).

Neuroscience research has focused on intentionality in behaviors, including change behavior. The old view was that intentionality in behaviors and decision making involved only conscious awareness. In this view, thoughts and behaviors outside of awareness were considered "dumb" in contrast to "smart" processes of the conscious mind (Bargh & Morsella, 2008). Believing that the unconscious was incapable of motivation or intentionality meant that persons lacked an understanding for much of their behaviors. Research began to accumulate that found that intentionality was also present in behaviors outside of awareness. Knowing that one does not have to be conscious to learn or to direct their own behaviors chips away at the popular view that the conscious mind oversees motivations.

Second Order Parenting and Learning New Skills

Parent education programs and interventions that parents use are typically understood to be learned. Parents learn how to parent from different input. For example, in books on parenting, a basic framework for how change in parenting behavior occurs helps guide the parent to desired outcomes. In parent education, parents are taught new skills that are believed to be necessary for optimum parenting. This framework has been described variously, but the "*conscious competency ladder*" model developed six decades ago is a good description of a generic approach to skill development (dePhillips et al., 1960). The model consists of four stages—*unconsciously unskilled, consciously unskilled, consciously skilled*, and *unconsciously skilled* (see Table 6.2).

The first step, unconsciously unskilled, states that, in general, persons are unskilled but do not have conscious awareness of it. People tend to evaluate their competency higher than it is and, therefore, lack a true understanding of how unskilled they are. A research study by Kruger and Dunning (1999), referred to as the *Dunning–Kruger Effect*, illustrated that people are unaware of and inflate their

TABLE 6.2 The Conscious–Competence Matrix Developed by dePhillips et al. (1960)

Consciousness	**Level 2:** Consciously unskilled	**Level 3:** Consciously skilled
	Level 1: Unconsciously unskilled	**Level 4:** Unconsciously skilled
	Competence	

perceived skill level. They showed that the lowest skill-level person rated themselves as being highly competent.

The second step, consciously unskilled, is becoming aware that a person's skills are underdeveloped. For example, at this stage there is a realization that communication skills are poor, and the level of empathy is low amid other poor skills. This stage is only the realization of a need for skills training. Optimally, this stage would be necessary for trainees in parent education to be motivated to change.

Consciously skilled is the third stage and the beginning of learning new skills. For example, in learning communication skills, one must change their automatic responses, send clear messages, and show understanding and empathy from listening to the other's messages. Much practice is required to become effective in using the skills.

The final stage, unconsciously skilled, comes after much practice when the skills become natural and automatic. Reaching this stage takes effort, time, and considerable practice. The old automatic responses are replaced with new automatic responses that are outside of awareness.

The above steps in skill acquisition are reflected in skill development exercises in parent education models. Generally, it is believed that parents referred to parent education classes lack skills in dealing with their children, particularly in showing love and using interventions to stop unwanted behaviors. The basic implication of this model is that skills that parents lack can be identified and then practiced until they become automatic. This model is cognitive in nature and the parent must have conscious awareness of what needs to change and make conscious efforts to change them. While change *can* occur this way, this book offers a perspective that is often ignored.

As stated before, this book integrates systems theory and dialectical theory that is grounded in new neuroscience research. The above discussion of the conscious competency model represents a generic model for skill development. This book takes a different view, namely, that conscious awareness is not needed for behavioral change. In place of skill development which generally reflects a conscious model, this book uses the broader term of second order or transformational change, because it lacks any connotation with the conscious linear model. The last section of the chapter will discuss how neuroscience informs the development of second order parent education and parenting.

Neuroscience-Informed Parent Education and Parenting Model: Systems/Dialectical Second Order Parenting

First, this model is based on the view that the unconscious is the primary force in behavioral change. A brief review of neuroscience findings made earlier in this chapter and previous chapters about the conscious and unconscious reveals that the unconscious is dominant in decision making, is capable of intentionality, works on finding solutions outside of consciousness, and breaks into consciousness when it has found a solution in the form of the aha experience. A systems/dialectical perspective supports this assessment of the relationship of the conscious and unconscious in that conscious awareness is not necessary for change to occur. Transformational or second order change happens because the system changes, not because of conscious insight into the problem. The focus of change is the relationship between parent and child rather than individual change in either parent or child.

Second, instead of an emphasis on skill development based on the belief that parents lack competency in parenting, a systems/dialectical perspective focuses on a structural change in the parent–child interactional system. This is not to conclude that parents do not come to new understandings and cognitive appraisals of their relationship with their child. Based on the view that brain plasticity is grounded in new experiences and novelty, the way parents gain a new understanding is through new and novel experiences that change the context of the problem, that is, the parameters in which the problem exists. Consequently, the training model needs to be a collaborative, experiential involvement that challenges the status quo.

Third, a systems/dialectical perspective believes that learning is enhanced by *circular causation* in contrast to linear causality, in which the trainer sets the content and procedures of the training. Training goals from this perspective are set bilaterally by the trainees and the trainer. A linear model means that the trainer is the source of the goals and the implementation of them in the training session. Trainees are not passive subjects who need skills that only the trainer can guide them in acquiring. Each trainee enters the training with goals and aspirations, which drive the motivation to participate and the willingness to change. When the contents of training programs are predetermined, the goals of the program may not mesh with the goals of the trainees. The contents of the training should reflect the goals of the trainees in addition to the goals of the trainer.

In contrast to the conscious cognitive ladder approach, parent education trainees may know more than their parenting actions show. Many factors other than competency or knowledge can affect the patterns that develop between parent and child, such as stress. The context in which the pattern occurred may be unique to that specific dynamic and requires an understanding of that context. The trainer is part of this dynamic and therefore must be considered part of the system. Consequently, the parent education training group is a system that operates in the same way as other systems, such as the family. Trainees and trainer form an interdependent system in which the action of any member affects the action of others. For change to the system to occur, all parties in the system must change (see Table 6.3).

Fourth, trainees have different styles of learning which will affect their participation and understanding of the didactic portions of the training and the interactions with other trainees. The system/dialectical perspective side steps, to some degree, the question of presenting style due to the focus on experiential and unconscious learning. If cognitive awareness is unnecessary for learning to take place, the learning styles of the trainees are not centrally important.

Fifth, a linear model of parent education training and parenting in general fixates on the problem as needing to change and developing new skills to eradicate the problem. That view contrasts with the systems/dialectical view where no single correct way exists for resolving the problem. The important consideration is how the problem is defined because it determines the interventions. In contrast to a linear model of training which uses a skill development approach, a systems/dialectical perspective would focus on a malfunctioning system that needs altering. Parent trainees are not viewed as lacking skills but are one component in a malfunctioning system. The lack of the parent's skill competency is conceived as the symptom of a malfunctioning system and not its cause.

Sixth, the point of intervention in a linear parent training model is always the parent, while the systems/dialectical perspective would intervene at the most beneficial point for change to occur. Unfortunately, while most parent education models have a goal of improving the family, the point of intervention is never the family, but always the parent. This raises the question: Should parent education training models include children and, therefore, be focused on family dynamics and not primarily on parenting strategies? Furthermore, interventions from a systems/dialectical perspective should be made within the context in which they occurred or within an environment that approximates the original context.

TABLE 6.3 Characteristics of Neuroscience Informed of a Second Order Systems/Dialectical Model of Parent Education

	Characteristics of an Implicit Model of Parenting
1	The unconscious is the primary focus in behavioral change
2	Structural change in parent–child relationship versus skills training
3	Learning is enhanced by circular causation
4	The context of the biobehavioral must be understood
5	The trainer is part of the system
6	Experiential and active learning emphasized
7	The system is viewed as malfunctioning
8	The point of intervention not limited parents
9	Trainees should understand how systems function

Seventh, a systems/dialectical perspective expects change to be a second order and not a first order change. Because the focus in parent training is on developing new skills in the parent, first order direct interventions are common. Even improving the current parenting skills of the parent is also first order change rather than second order change. A systems/dialectical perspective suggests, instead of emphasizing skill development in the parent, there should be an openness for changing the system. This is not to conclude that first order change is not helpful, but parenting models should be expanded to include second order change.

The training group is a system and operates under the same principles as the family system. Therefore, the training model should provide experiential modules for understanding and experiencing how a system functions. Instead of focusing on skill development, trainees could experience firsthand the nuances of the underpinnings of the system to maintain the problematic patterns. Such an approach would diminish the tendency to isolate small components of the problem and identify them as the problem, such as the parent using too harsh discipline interventions. In addition, it would curb the assumption that certain skills are needed by everyone. Parent education models have been criticized because the skills that are commonly taught represent the popular view of what constitutes a functional family, which is determined by what society values and does not represent individual families (Macvarish, 2016).

A Second Order Parent Education Model from a Systems/Dialectical Perspective

A circular causality model is applied to parent education and considered to be the same dynamic as the parent–child relationship within the family. Participants would include both partners in a two-parent family and anyone involved in parenting in a single-parent family. Groups should be formed based on the age of children. Forming groups in this way will facilitate group cohesion and sharing. Family measures will be used rather than individual measures to determine the change within the family.

The model consists of three stages. In stage one, trainers meet with each family member individually to ascertain individual and family goals. Stage two consists of 12 weekly meetings for 2.5 hours each. Stage three comprises the evaluation of the training which takes place at the end of the training, six months after completion, and one year after training (see Table 6.4 for description of training module sessions).

This model avoids the skills development approach and instead emphasizes that a child's misbehavior occurs within a specific context and both the parent and the child have used erroneous efforts to solve the problem. The goal of the training is for families to understand the components of a system and how the family operates as a system. Furthermore, the first six sessions of the training are meant to focus on normal development in the family according to a systems/dialectical view of family relationships. Family members affect each other in indirect and implicit ways,

TABLE 6.4 A Second Order Systems/Dialectical Model for Parent Education

Session	*Description*
1	This session introduces the idea of how families operate as a system. The concept of circular causality is explained. Exercises allow the family to experience circular causality
2	Focuses on physical and mental developmental throughout the life course
3	Moral development is emphasized, and exercises address how parents appropriately give reasons for their interventions consistent with the reasoning ability of the child
4	Improves understanding of both implicit and explicit communication. The marital or partner relationship will be emphasized
5	How systems work in family interactions. Triangles, boundaries, and differentiation will be the focus and exercises will illustrate how they work in families
6	Focuses on understanding how we learn unconsciously
7	Describes how parents and children affect each other through their actions. Parents model behavior and unconsciously influence how their children feel about many things
8	Storytelling is underdeveloped as a disciplinary intervention by most parents. Exercises will help the parents be able to see how storytelling can enhance their parenting interventions. The module will help parents learn how to use storytelling in disciplining misbehavior
9	Reframing is the ability to see actions in a different context. Exercises help parents understand that changing the context changes the problem
10	Humor is a trait that redefines the problem behavior. How to use humor effectively is discussed in this session through exercises
11	This session will describe how confusion, confrontation, and novelty can be used to change problem behavior. Distractions and opportunities for an "aha experience" be a significant part of this module and other modules as well
12	Paradox is a seemingly absurd statement that when analyzed can be truthful and have the opposite meaning. Parents are sometimes afraid to use paradox, but appropriate use can be a very effective implicit intervention

which are often underemphasized in parent education models. The last six sessions will detail how unconscious, implicit, and indirect interventions are constantly at work in families. These interactions include modeling, storytelling, reframing, humor, play, and paradox. Change component is embedded in the exercises in each session.

References

Allen, J. P., Grande, L., Tan, J., & Loeb, E. (2018). Parent and peer predictors of change in attachment security from adolescence to adulthood. *Child Development*, *89*, 1120–1132. https://doi.org/10.1111/cdev.12840

Bargh, J. A., & Morsella, E. (2008). The unconscious mind. *Perspectives on psychological science*, *3*(1), 73–79.

Bohn, J., Holtmann, J., Ulitzen, E., Koch, T., Luhmann, M., & Eid, M. (2019). Analyzing stability and change in dyadic attachment: The multi-rater latent state-trait model with autoregressive effects. *Frontiers in Psychology, 12,* 604526. https://doi.org/10.3389/fpsyg.2021.604526

Bowlby, J. (1982). Attachment and loss: Retrospect and prospect. *American Journal of Orthopsychiatry, 52*(4), 664–678. https://doi.org/10.1111/j.1939-0025.1982.tb01456.x

Breuer, J. T. (1999). *The myth of the first 3 years: A new understanding of brain development and lifelong learning*. Free Press.

Buist, K. L., Deković, M., Meeus, W., & van Aken, M. A. G. (2002). Developmental patterns in adolescent attachment to mother, father and sibling. *Journal of Youth and Adolescence, 31*(3), 167–176. https://doi.org/10.1023/A:1015074701280

Cain, C. S. (2020). *Attachment disorders: Treatment strategies for traumatized children.* Jason Aronson.

Carruthers, P. (2017). The illusion of conscious thought. *Journal of Consciousness Studies, 24*(910), 228–252.

Chopik, W. J., Edelstein, R. S., & Grimm, K. J. (2017). Longitudinal changes in attachment orientation over a 59-year period. *Journal of Personality and Social Psychology, 116*(4), 598–611. https://doi.org/10.1037/pspp0000167

Churchill, H., & Clarke, K. (2009). Investing in parenting education: A critical review of policy and provision in England. *Social Policy and Society, 9*(1), 39–53.

Clarke, K. (2006). Childhood, parenting, and early intervention: A critical examination of the Sure Start national programme. *Critical Social Policy, 26*(4), 699–721.

Costa, M.-C. D., & Johannes, F. (2020, December). Epigenesis: Switching genes on and off. *Frontiers for Young Minds*. https://kids.frontiersin.org/articles/10.3389/frym.2020.554136

de Zulueta, F. (2006). The treatment of psychological trauma from the perspective of attachment research. *Journal of Family Therapy, 28,* 334–351.

dePhillips, E. M., Berliner, W. M., & Cribbin, J. J. (1960). *Management of training programs*. Richard D. Irwin.

Fraley, R. C. (2002). Attachment stability from infancy to adulthood: Meta-analysis and dynamic modeling of developmental mechanisms. *Personality and Social Psychology Review, 6*(2), 123–151. https://doi.org/10.1207/S15327957PSPR0602_03

Fraley, R. C. (2019). Attachment in adulthood: Recent developments, emerging debates, and future directions. *Annual Review of Psychology, 70,* 401–422. https://doi.org/10.1146/annurev-psych-010418-102813

Fraley, R. C., Gillath, O., & Deboeck, P. R. (2021). Do life events lead to enduring changes in adult attachment styles? A naturalistic longitudinal investigation. *Journal of Personality and Social Psychology, 120*(6), 1567–1606. https://doi.org/10.1037/pspi0000326; Epub 2020 August 13

Fraley, R. C., & Shaver, P. R. (2008). Attachment theory and its place in contemporary personality theory and research. In O. John and R. W. Robins (Eds.), *Handbook of personality: Theory and research* (3rd ed., pp. 518–541). Guilford.

Fransburg, C. S. (2015). *Patterns and predictors of stability and change in representations of romantic relationships in adolescence and young adulthood* [Doctoral dissertation, University of Denver]. https://digitalcommons.du.edu/cgi/viewcontent.cgi?article=2022&context=etd

Furedi, F. (2008). *Paranoid parenting: Why ignoring the experts may be best for your child* (2nd ed.). Continuum.

Granqvist, P., Sroufe, L. A., Dozier, M., Hesse, E., Steele, M., van Ijzendoorn, M., Solomon, J., Schuengel, C., Fearon, P., Bakermans-Kranenburg, M., Steele, H., Cassidy, J., Carlson, E., Madigan, S., Jacobvitz, D., Foster, S., Behrens, K., Rifkin-Graboi, A., Gribneau, N., . . . & Duschinsky, R. (2017). Disorganized attachment in infancy: A review of the phenomenon and its implications for clinicians and policy-makers. *Attachment and Human Development, 19*(6), 534–558. https://doi.org/10.1080/14616734.2017.1354040; Epub 2017 July 26

Harris, J. R. (1998). *The nurture assumption: Why children turn out the way they do*. Free Press.
Hazan, C., & Shaver, P. R. (1994). Attachment as an organizational framework for research on close relationships. *Psychological Inquiry, 5*(1), 1–22.
Hudson, N. W., Fraley, R. C., Chopik, W. J., & Briley, D. A. (2019). Change goals robustly predict trait growth: A mega-analysis of a dozen Intensive longitudinal studies examining volitional change. *Social Psychological and Personality Science, 11*(6), 19485506198784. https://doi.org/10.1177/1948550619878423
Hulbert, A. (2004). *Raising America: Experts, parents, and a century of advice about children*. Vintage.
Isles, A. R., & Wilkinson, L. S. (2008). Epigenetics: What is it and why is it important to mental disease? *British Medical Bulletin, 85*(1), 35–45.
Jones, J. D., Fraley, R. C., Ehrlich, K. B., Stern, J. A., Lejuez, C. W., Shaver, P. R., & Cassidy, J. (2018). Stability of attachment style in adolescence: An empirical test of alternative developmental processes. *Child Development, 89,* 871–880. https://doi.org/10.1111/cdev.12775
Kagan, J. (1998). *Three seductive ideals*. Harvard University Press.
Kagan, J. (2013). *The human spark: The science of human development*. Basic Books.
Kahneman, D. (2011). *Thinking, fast and slow*. Farrar, Straus, and Giroux.
Kaltenbach, E., Hermenau, K., Nkuba, M., Goessmann, M., & Hecker, T. (2018). Improving interaction competencies with children: A pilot feasibility study to reduce school corporal punishment. *Journal of Aggression, Maltreatment & Trauma, 27*(1), 35–53. https://doi.org/10.1080/10926771.2017.1357060
Kruger, J., & Dunning, D. (1999). Unskilled and unaware of it: How difficulties in recognizing one's own incompetence lead to inflated self-assessments. *Journal of Personality and Social Psychology, 77*(6), 1121–1134. https://doi.org/10.1037/0022-3514.77.6.1121
Macvarish, J. (2016). *Neuroparenting: The expert invasion of family life*. Palgrave Macmillan.
Neckoway, R., Brownlee, K., Jourdain, K., Jourdain, L. W., & Miller, L. (2003). Rethinking the role of attachment theory in child welfare practice with Aboriginal people. *Canadian Social Work Review, 20*(1), 105–119.
O'Connor, T., & Zeanah, C. (2003). Attachment disorders assessment strategies. Treatment approach. *Attachment and Human Development, 5,* 223–244.
Papies, E. K. (2016). Health goal priming as a situated intervention tool: How to benefit from unconscious motivational routes to health behavior. *Health Psychology Review, 10,* 408–424.
Phillips, D. A. (2017). *Puzzling it out: The current state of scientific knowledge on prekindergarten effects*. https://www.brookings.edu/wp-content/uploads/2017/04/consensus-statement_final.pdf
Plomin, R. (2018). *Blueprint*. Allen Lane.
Reece, H. (2013). The pitfalls of positive parenting. *Ethics and Education, 8*(1), 42–54. https://doi.org/10.1080/17449642.2013.793961
Roberts, B. W., Luo, J., Briley, D. A., Chow, P. I., Su, R., & Hill, P. L. (2017, January 5). A systematic review of personality trait change through intervention. *Psychological Bulletin*. https://doi.org/10.1037/bul0000088
Romagnoli, A., & Wall, G. (2012). "I know I'm a good mom:" Young, low-income mothers' experiences with risk perception, intensive parenting ideology and parenting education programs. *Health, Risk and Society, 14*(3), 273–289.
Schwarzer, R. (2008). Modeling health behavior change: How to predict and modify the adoption and maintenance of health behaviors. *Journal of Applied Psychology, 57*, 1–29. https://doi.org/10.1111/j.1464-0597.2007.00325.x
Solms, M., & Friston, K. (2018). How and why consciousness arises: some considerations from physics and physiology. *Journal of Consciousness Studies, 25*(5–6), 202–238.

Spock, B. (1985). *Dr. Spock's baby and child care* (40th anniversary ed.). Pocket Books.

St Quinton, T., & Brunton, J. A. (2017). Implicit processes, self-regulation, and interventions for behavior change. *Frontiers in Psychology*, *8*, 1–7. https://doi.org/10.3389/fpsyg.2017.00001

Stearns, P. (2003). *Anxious parents: A history of modern childrearing in America*. New York University Press.

Taylor, J. (2013). *General science*. Taylor Electronics. Archived from the original on June 9, 2013.

Winnicott, D. W. (1964). *The child, the family, and the outside world*. Penguin.

Zhou, Y., Su, Y., Li, S., Kennedy, B. C., Zhang, D. Y., Bond, A. M., Sun, Y., Jacob, F., Lu, L., Hu, P., Viaene, A. N., Helbig, I., Kessler, S. K., Lucas, T., Salinas, R. D., Gu, X., Chen, H. I., Wu, H., Kleinman, J. E., . . . Song, H. (2022). Molecular landscapes of human hippocampal immature neurons across lifespan. *Nature*, *607*(7919), 527–533. https://doi.org/10.1038/s41586-022-04912-w

7
MODELING

Early Theories of Socialization

The study and research of the socialization of children primarily by parents and those in proximity has a long history. It is well documented in child development studies that children learn by *imitation* from observing parents and others in their sphere of influence (Figure 7.1) (Kail & Cavanaugh, 2007). The *social cognitive model* of Albert Bandura (1977) is based on the belief that learning occurs when children observe and imitate their parents and others around them. For learning to be complete according to Bandura, however, more is needed than mimicking others, which means that children tend to copy behavior that is reinforced or punished. Learning by imitation can take place without the parent's awareness and can have a positive or negative influence on the child's behavior. Behaviors that are more likely to occur from observation are labeled *disinhibition*, and behaviors less likely to be mimicked are labeled *inhibition*.

Social learning for most children takes place around 2 years of age and is a powerful influencer of behavior thereafter. To demonstrate that children learn from interaction patterns, Bandura initiated research referred to as the *Bobo Doll Experiment* (Bandura et al., 1961). The findings of this experiment confirmed that when children witness violent actions by an adult, the observing child would be more prone to commit violent actions. In a follow-up study, Bandra found that the child witnessing violence that was rewarded would be more likely to commit violence and less likely if the violence was punished.

Another perspective on learning by observation is the *sociocultural theory* of Vygotsky (1978), who believed that children learn by social interactions that can be outside of conscious awareness. The social interactions occur within a precise social and cultural setting (Bates, 2019). Cultural influences generally reflect the

DOI: 10.4324/9781003381679-9

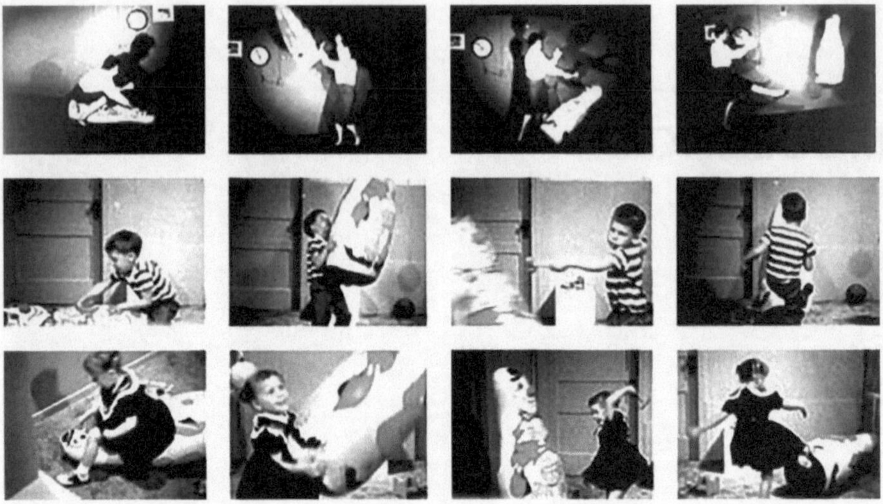

FIGURE 7.1 Children are heavily influenced to copy behaviors, including violent behavior, that they observe. (CC BY-SA 4.0)

context in which the family is immersed. *Internalization* of what a child observes reflects those in close contact and becomes the source for the child's memory and automatic behaviors.

Observational Learning

Studies demonstrated that children do not merely imitate indiscriminately what they observe but choose what to imitate from the vast input of behaviors in their social sphere of influence (Kuczynski et al., 1987). Children can be as affected by the tone and behavior of the parent as they are by the content of the interaction. Consequently, disruptions in the communication patterns may occur due to an ambiguous message.

New research on observational learning focuses on whether children need to actively engage in behaviors or whether observation learning can take place without active involvement. The findings in this area of research are rewriting what is known and widely held about observational learning versus active learning. It has been widely held that learning is enhanced by "doing" but requires reinforcement for observational learning to occur. A recent research project calls that conclusion into question (Cross et al., 2009). The study involved one group of subjects learning dance routines from physical practice and another group passively observing a screen. Researchers obtained fMRI recording of brain activity for both groups of subjects in the Action Observance Network (AON), neural network in the inferior parietal and premotor areas that are associated with motor skills and partial memory activity. Findings indicated that there were parallel processes in the AON in both groups of subjects. The researchers concluded that the same mental processes occurring in both groups indicate that learning from observation need not be practiced for learning to occur.

Hill et al. (2016) have identified specific brain cells that are involved in observational learning. They concluded that observational learning is the foundation for transformational change because a basic trait in humans is to learn from other people's mistakes. The experiment was conducted at UCLA Medical Center by implanting electrodes deep into the brain of ten epileptic patients, a procedure used to identify the roots of seizures prior to brain surgery. The electrodes noted specific brain activity, while the subjects played a card game. The electrodes recorded individual neurons deep in the anterior cingulate cortex of the frontal lobe, an area related to decision making and social interaction, that reacted in anticipation of whether their opponent would pick a winning card. The rate of neuron firing varied according to whether the patient expected a winning or a losing card and according to whether their prediction of the card was accurate. The researchers concluded that, in observing the other players to determine from which deck to pick a card, specific brain neurons were activated. Further, when a patient won or lost, cells in proximity activated strongly and diminished.

Other research on observational learning was conducted at the University of Washington and Temple University by Saby et al. (2013). Their findings are pertinent to how infants learn basic activities, like holding a ball, from watching others. The study was based on the *somatotopic map* of the brain, the outer portion of the brain in which different areas of the body are reflected in specific areas of the brain. The study demonstrated that areas in the brains of seventy 14-month-old babies lit up when the baby watched someone perform a physical movement or activity. As the baby observed an adult moving a particular body part such as a hand, a corresponding brain area in the baby lit up.

The research procedure included the infants wearing electroencephalogram (EEG) caps with sensors that could register brain activity in the regions of the cortex associated with body parts. The experiment was conducted with the baby sitting in the parent's lap and watching a researcher move a toy on a table in front of the baby. The toy was equipped with a clear plastic top that could be pushed by the experimenter's hand or foot, causing music to play and confetti to swirl in the cap. This action was repeated if the baby was observant. The researchers believe that infants learn how to distinguish the body part involved which facilitates the baby's ability to imitate and accomplish the same bodily action. Interestingly, infants learn the linking between action and body parts prior to language development. Imitation of others' actions occurs because the baby can distinguish the body part the other person used, which is the basis for being able to understand their own body. Consequently, when babies see others act, it allows them to experience themselves and is the basis for how imitation takes place.

The fact that infants can imitate body movements of caregivers very early has created an enormous interest in the role imitation plays in socialization

(Meltzoff, 1988). The ability to imitate caregivers implies a built-in or genetic process whereby offspring form an indelible connection. In addition, it initiates investigation into the neurobiology of human bonding and emotional connection. Furthermore, infant imitation has opened new doors in understanding the components of human thought.

Another outcome of the study of imitation is greater understanding of the memory system (Meltzoff & Williamson, 2013). One of the fascinating findings of infant imitation is that infants can recall past information without it having been formed through language. In other words, infants can recall preverbal memories of past events, a process referred to as *deferred imitation.* The implication is that infants' memory development is not restricted to habit formation but can execute actions that they have visually witnessed. Consequently, in addition to habit memory, infants already have in place declarative memory that is pre-language.

Mirror Neurons

The discovery of mirror neurons has debunked some of the theories about how observational learning takes place. The old belief was that to learn, one needed to experience an action themselves. Mirror neurons, discovered over 30 years ago in studies with macaque monkeys, have opened the door to a clearer understanding of how social learning takes place (di Pellegrino et al., 1992). It has enhanced knowledge about how one understands social interactions across the lifespan and particularly in the pre-language infancy stage of development. What distinguishes mirror neurons from other neurons is that they are activated by both doing an activity and observing an activity, while other motor neurons are activated only by motor action or observation. Most research of mirror neurons use monkeys instead of humans because current brain imaging techniques that rely on oxygenation of the blood to determine activity do not capture the activity of motor neurons. While mirror neurons have been reported in various areas of the macaque brain, including the lateral and ventral intraparietal areas of the inferior parietal lobule, the dorsal premotor and primary cortex, and the rostral division of the ventral premotor cortex (F5), the latter is more associated with it.

Hundreds of articles and research studies have been done seeking to understand the function of mirror neurons in human social interactions. These studies have described three types of mirror neurons—strictly congruent, broadly congruent, and logically related (di Pellegrino et al., 1992). Strictly congruent mirror neurons fire during motor actions and observation of that action. Broadly congruent mirror neurons fire during an action and an observation of a similar, but not identical action. Logically congruent mirror neurons fire during actions and observation of different events. Most research studies of children's socialization and imitation have been done with strictly congruent mirror images. For example, research findings indicate that young infants can imitate parents' actions that they observe

(Heimann et al., 2017), and the majority can imitate an action after the passage of time. The ability to use pre-language declarative memory is present by 14 months according to Meltzoff (1988), much earlier than believed by Piaget (1951/1962).

A recent study has expanded knowledge on imitation by focusing on infants' awareness of the parent's imitation of them (Sauciuc et al., 2020). This research raises questions about Meltzoff's conclusions regarding how and when children acquire the ability to imitate others. This study was based on providing more support for the belief that infants learn cultural norms and interactional patterns from recurrent experiences of being imitated. While the role of imitation has long been touted as present in early learning, the research support was missing. The experiment was conducted with 6-month-old infants and the researcher doing one of three behaviors: (1) imitating the infant's actual behaviors like a mirror image; (2) acting as a reverse mirror; (3) while making no facial expression, infant response to being imitated was also evident even when the researchers showed no facial expression (Figure 7.2).

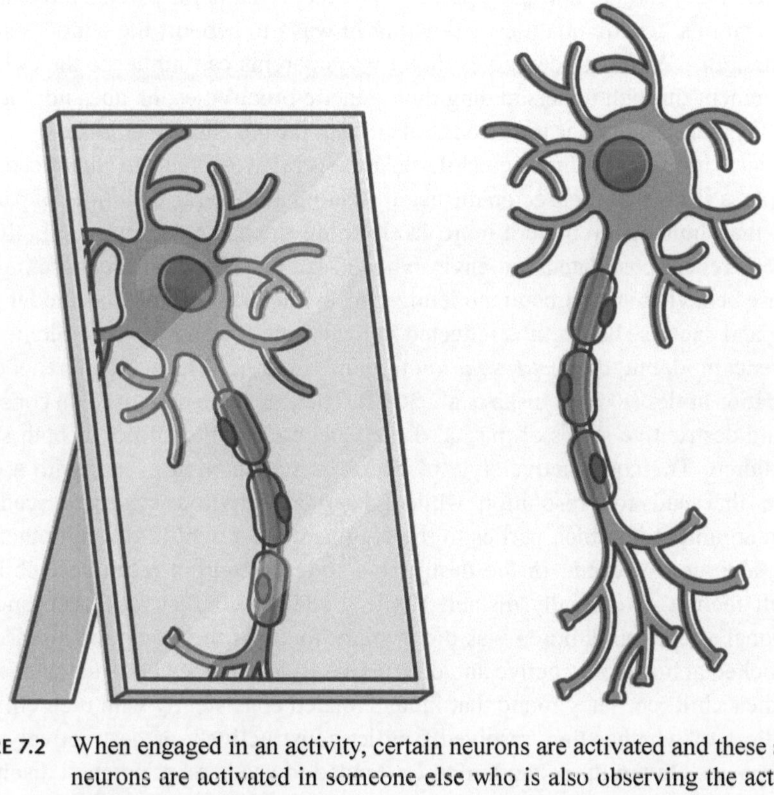

FIGURE 7.2 When engaged in an activity, certain neurons are activated and these same neurons are activated in someone else who is also observing the activity. These are mirror neurons.

Parental Modeling

How parents act, rather than what they say, can be very influential to their children. This type of influence may not be conscious by either the parent or the child. Parents influence career choices, level of education, stable relationships, religious affiliation, and so on. While parents can influence their children in positive ways, they can also influence them in negative ways. Smoking, drinking, philandering, irresponsible and criminal behavior, manipulation of others, and other negative parental behaviors can be seen in children. Clinicians and marriage and family therapists have long seen a connection between an acting-out teen and a parent who has a current problem or had a similar problem as a teenager (Haley, 1980). The child's behavior does not copy the parent's in all cases, but can be encrypted into their unconscious automatic responses.

Holden (2010) developed a new approach to the nature–nurture debate by concluding that the way children turn out is both nature and nurture and is mainly influenced by parental guidance. That conclusion is not unique in and of itself, but the way Holden expressed it gives a new nuance to the old debate. Good parenting considers nature in the nurturing process. His theory calls for parents understanding the child's genetic qualities and acting in ways to support the child's interest and strengths. While Holden gives direct ways parents can influence their child's development through understanding their genetic proclivities, he does not include how the parent's behavior is a strong role model for the child to emulate.

Parental modeling influences children in several ways that go unnoticed. For example, a study that focused on the healthy eating and exercise routines of parents found that their children were more likely to do the same (Østbye et al., 2013). The researchers postulated that environmental factors affect children's eating and exercise behavior, and parental modeling is a key factor. When parents model good eating and exercise habits, it is reflected in lower rates of obesity in children.

Parents modeling *conflict resolution* to their children influence children's communication styles (Kopystynska et al., 2017). The researchers focused on constructive and destructive styles of marital disagreements and the effects of both styles on children. The constructive style of couple argumentation occurs with a calm manner that leads to a resolution, while a destructive style was characterized as a heated argument in which parties to the argument are resentful of each other and resolutions do not occur. In the destructive style of conflict resolution, children are left feeling emotionally distant. While modeling conflict resolution and the emotional effects on children was the primary focus of the study, the researchers also looked at how constructive and destructive styles affected how they interacted with their children. They found that fathers related consistently with their children regardless of whether they resolved conflict constructively or destructively with their spouse. On the other hand, mothers tended to use harsher parental discipline when the conflict style used with the partner was destructive.

A similar study conducted by Brauner-Otto et al. (2020) focused on child outcomes and the quality of the parents' marital relationship. This study conducted by researchers at the University of Michigan and McGill University in Quebec with couples in Nepal found that when the couple showed love and affection for each other, there was a direct effect on children. The researchers interpreted the findings to describe how married couples who express love and affection to each other model positive components in a relationship and children are more likely to choose a partner where they are likely to have a similar experience.

Parents are role models for physical activity of children. Most parents do not realize that their lack of physical activity is a model for their children's activity level. Voss and Sandercock (2013) obtained data from 4,000 schoolchildren who completed a cardiorespiratory test and gave feedback on the activity level of parents. The children whose test placed them as physically unfit had inactive parents. Furthermore, the researchers found that fathers' activity levels were more predictive of children's fitness level than mothers. The research underscores the role parental modeling plays in influencing children's behavior.

It has been known that around 16 months of age, toddlers begin helping behavior, but what was not known was the mechanism for how the helping behavior developed. A recent study helps answer that question. Schuhmacher et al. (2018) found that imitation is the basic factor in why or how toddlers learn helping behavior, defined as reaching to give an object to their caregiver or picking up a sibling's fallen toy. The study was the first of its kind to show that imitation of prosocial behavior results from watching others behave in a prosocial manner (Figure 7.3).

The research consisted of two experiments, one of which consisted of the researchers needing help in stacking a cup. Toddlers who observed the researcher getting help were significantly more likely to help than toddlers who did not. The second experiment attempted to determine whether imitation was the important factor in the helping behavior. The same experiment was conducted, but this time the researcher didn't need help and the toddlers who had witnessed help in the first experiment were less likely to offer help. The researchers concluded that toddlers learned helping behavior as efficiently from imitation as from being instructed. In addition, they concluded that prosocial role modeling of parents is an important aspect of toddlers acquiring prosocial behaviors.

The parent's level of anxiety and how he/she handles stressful situations can be imitated by the child. The parent's poor stress management creates unconscious responses to the environment as a frightening place that needs to be avoided. Such fearful attitudes not only affect the child's implicit responses to the present environment but may also condition them to further anxiety disorders (Burstein & Ginsburg, 2010).

Studies have found that aggression in teens reflects parents who act out aggressively or have attitudes conducive to the acceptance of violence (American Academy of Pediatrics, 2012). Because of this major influence, clinicians working with

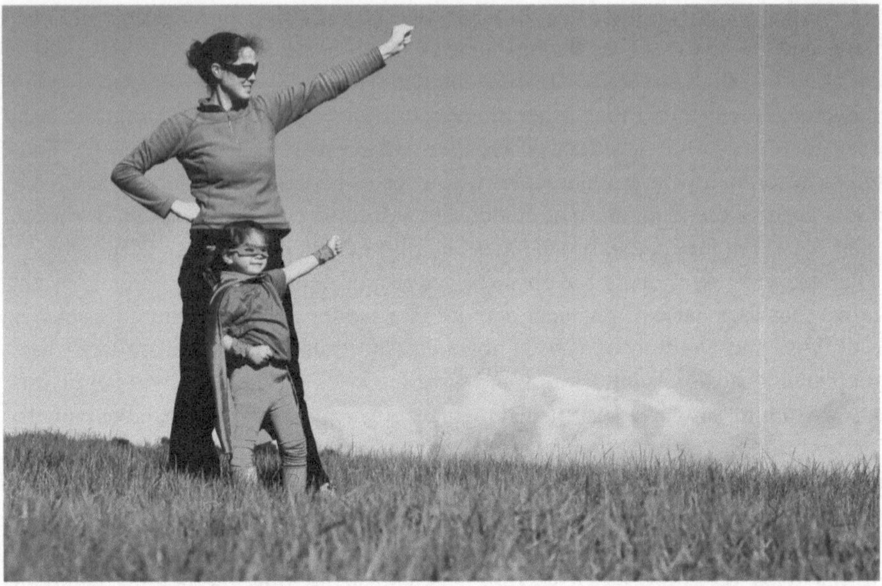

FIGURE 7.3 Children tend to behave according to what they observe others doing, particularly their caregivers.

aggressive teens believe that parents should be actively involved in treatment. Reasons for male teen fighting include defending themselves against other aggressive teens, gaining respect from others, and having a high level of anger that gets out of hand. Female fighting occurs more commonly due to gossip or jealousy. Parental models of conflict resolution were an essential influencer in whether teens engaged in aggressive behavior. Parents who used positive means of conflict resolution were more likely to have teens who walk away or ignore situations that could lead to fighting. Teens whose parents modeled aggressive behavior were unable to walk away and were cued to act aggressively.

Undesirable teen behaviors, such as smoking cigarettes, are related to several influencing factors such as peer relationships, poor academic school performance, parent–child problems, and parental modeling. Of these factors, parental smoking is a major significant influencer in whether children smoke (Vuolo & Staff, 2013). This finding is true even when parents who smoke lecture and prohibit their children from smoking.

Parents who have substance abuse issues tend to have difficulty in parenting and model behavior that negatively affects their children. The research on parent's use of drugs and the effects on children have focused mainly on alcohol consumption (Chassin et al., 2004). Early onset of adolescent use of drugs or alcohol has been frequently researched because of the association with lifetime drug and alcohol problems (Warner et al., 2007). Parents who drink or use drugs model that it is okay to use them regardless of what they verbalize about the harmful effects. When teens see their parents using any type of substance, it signals to them that using any form of drug is okay (Capaldi et al., 2016).

Research that examines both paternal and maternal substance abuse is little in the literature. Studies that have been done with both parents' substance use found that problematic substance use by both mothers and fathers predict alcohol use by their children (Hussong et al., 2012). Kerr et al. (2012) found that problematic substance use by either parent could predict alcohol use in their children.

While most research on drug, cigarette, and alcohol use focuses on fathers, there is clear evidence that mothers have a more profound effect on children's onset of alcohol use than fathers' use. Although a few factors may predict this occurrence, mothers spend more time with children and her use of cigarettes has a more powerful impact than fathers' use (Craig, 2006). Capaldi et al. (2016) conclude that it may be important to identify children of polysubstance-using parents for targeted prevention programs and to identify children of substance-using mothers regardless of father's use levels.

Several researchers have focused on children's intention to use alcohol in the future. The important connection of this type of research is when children have an intention to use drugs and alcohol, they are more likely as teens to do so (Andrews et al., 2003). Webb and Sheeran (2006) found the relationship between intention to use alcohol and the actual using of alcohol later was causal and not correlational.

Parents model an assortment of behaviors to their children, including their attitude about money and debt management. Concerns over college dropout rates due to financial concerns have spawned several studies. For example, Hancock et al. (2013) investigated the connection of college students' credit card debts and financial modeling of their parents. This study was one of the first to associate college students' financial behavior with their parents' mode of communication, work experience, and financial attitudes. Students were twice as likely to have multiple credit cards and financial distress if their parents argued about financial matters compared to students whose parents did not disagree about financial matters. In addition, students who had significant debt had parents who disagreed about financial matters. The researchers concluded that students are influenced indirectly by the mere attitude and disagreement over finances by their parents. The researchers suggested that any intervention for college students regarding their financial management should include their parents.

The other side of parental modeling addresses the positive effects of good role modeling by parents (Emamzadeh, 2018). Some of the benefits of good modeling reflect generational factors, such as members of the same family through the generations tend to have similar professional and employment histories. Self-esteem, which cannot be consciously taught, is modeled in the way that parents make decisions, react to disappointments, and present themselves socially, and their children tend to develop similar levels of self-esteem. Levels of education and stability in relationships generally are similar across generations in families. While genetics plays a role in child-rearing outcomes, along with direct instruction from parents, positive modeling plays an equally important role because it manifests itself in the implicit memory system.

An internet search reveals many websites and blogs focused on giving advice for how to be a good role model. For the most part, these sources for good modeling are aimed at making the parent more conscious of their modeling and how to make changes (Center for Parent Education, n.d.). For example, parents are encouraged to be consistent so that what they say matches what they do. Parents should support education and their child's unique gifts, have a positive attitude, be slow to anger, be flexible, show good judgment in making decisions, and be respectful of others' feelings. While these and similar suggestions are made on parental modeling websites and are helpful general suggestions for family living, they lack specific application and represent the kind of thinking that only the selected skills are good for all families.

A systems/dialectical perspective takes a different approach to parental modeling and will be addressed later. Parental modeling is a much more nuanced concept than can be reduced to offering a few suggestions for all families. The perspective offered later is not a cookie-cutter approach to families and believes that families are uniquely different. Functional parenting does not look alike in every family. Consequently, the overarching goal in systems/dialectical parent training is not to make all families look alike when they emerge from the training program, but to aid the family in claiming their uniqueness and undergo with them the changes they want to make.

A Systems/Dialectical Perspective of Parental Modeling and the Effects of Children

Resistive Parents

The literature on parent–child relationships in social work (Forrester et al., 2012) in addition to parent education and parenting is largely missing on the topic of parental resistance, which is perhaps the most important component of change. The underlying assumption is that parents lack skills and are allies with the trainer to bring about change in the family by improving or acquiring new parenting skills. The definition of *parental resistance* includes both parents who model bad behavior and refuse to see the connection of their behavior and the problems with their child, and parents who mean well but are limited in efforts to change. No doubt a fine line exists between blaming parents for the child's behavior and acknowledging that a bidirectional approach to family issues means that parents must change their behavior as well. This concern leads to a conundrum for trainers and, perhaps, the reason why parental resistance is marginally addressed in parent education programs.

Parental resistance to change is a formidable problem and much more is needed than for parents to simply complete the training; that is, parents must be collaborative in creating new structural alignments in the family (Jones et al., 2017). To begin with, the concept of resistance needs redefining. Typically, parental resistance referred to parents as noncooperative. This definition is linear in that it only represents the parents' behavior from the standpoint of the parent trainer. When parents are cooperative and accepting of training, they are viewed as collaborative, and when they fail to support the trainers' perspective or get with the program, they are labeled resistive. What this definition of resistance implies is a linear unidirectional approach in which the trainer determines what is to be learned by the trainee. In this sense, parent training is not only reductionistic, that is, reduced to the program of the trainer, but also non-collaborative because the trainee has no input into the training material.

The Family System and a Second Order Perspective

The goal in addressing role modeling with parents is not to create perfect role models and provide a rendition of various positive role modeling the parent should be doing. Rather, the goal is to acknowledge that some actions by the parents parallel the negative behaviors of the child. The parent may become aware of how their actions have cued similar actions in their child. For example, a parent who smokes but tells the child not to smoke and forbids certain privileges of the child due to their smoking has little clout in changing the child's behavior. What ensues from this type of parental response is a vicious circle that escalates.

It must be kept in mind that the family is a reciprocal interacting system that is governed by a set of rules (Crane et al., 2020). Rules are regular or redundant ways of doing things. They may be acknowledged verbally, or they may be implicit and non-acknowledged. Everyone has a sense of what the rules are and act accordingly. However, in the scenario where the rule is that the parent can do as they please but the child cannot do the same behavior (i.e., "do as I say, not as I do"), the parent has little authority to change the child's behavior. In terms of a systems/dialectical perspective, the child views this rule as unfair or unjust and this leads to resentment and a feeling of inequality.

Changing a rule in the family system can be difficult. It requires the family to view family relationships in a different light. Making explicit rules that exist implicitly can require much effort. A bidirectional understanding of relationships means that all members have equal standing in reference to outcomes. Rules can change when families have designated a rule for change, called a meta rule (Szkody & McKinney, 2021). A meta rule allows the presence of new input into the system, which is a prerequisite for change.

Any change in the system can be disruptive, scary, and overwhelming. Attention should be given to these feelings in the training model. When any change occurs, even a desired positive change, realignment in the systems must take place.

Even positive change can have negative consequences. Since family systems are rule-governed, a change initiates new rules, with the intention to have increased functionality.

Change in the system is the desired outcome of parent training. To think of any one part of the system causing the problem is reductionistic. Parents may not buy into the parenting program as outlined by the trainers. For this reason, input from each family is needed to determine how they perceive their problem and how they think it should be addressed. From this perspective, the more the trainers attempt to direct the change through preplanned interventions and skill-building, the more the things will stay the same. The belief is that major change occurs as the result of a series of small changes. As a small change takes place in part of the system, a ripple effect is felt throughout the system and, over time, more change occurs. On the other hand, when a major change, such as a total overhaul to the system, is attempted, homeostatic forces are activated to keep things the way they are.

The homeostatic function to maintain a balance allows for the family to make consistent predictions that make adjustments easier (Kim & Rose, 2014). The fear of loss of control runs deep in the family psyche and that fear can be exacerbated when family members feel marginalized even in a preplanned training session. These feelings of loss of control are further impacted by the Western cultural values of self-reliance and individualism. The training situation is a reminder that trainees need help and cannot solve their own problems, which contributes to the feelings of loss of predictability and fear of change.

Traditional models of parent–child relationships assume a unidirectional pattern where the parent affects the child, or the child affects the parent in a deterministic manner. Even in claiming bidirectionality, a unidirectional pattern of causality is reflected in the premise that each causes the behavior of the other. The bidirectional model emphasizes that parents and child change over time due to reciprocal interactional patterns. Observation of parental behaviors by the child creates a spoke in the wheel of the interaction with parents.

One of the central aspects of a systems/dialectical perspective is that change results from contradictions (see Table 7.1). Any interaction between parent and child contains a thesis and antitheses, or opposite points of a continuum, which are viewed as "both/and," rather than "either/or" (Overton, 2006). A both/and

TABLE 7.1 Hegel's Triad of Thesis, Antithesis, and Synthesis

	Contradictions	
1. Thesis	↔	2. Antithesis
When you have a need, you go		*Search for it, find it, and take it*
	↓Change↓	
	3. Synthesis	
	Then return, changed	

interactional pattern suggests a bilateral relationship in which one aspect of the interaction exists in chorus with an opposing aspect that will produce an innovative likeness of both aspects. According to Baxter and Montgomery (1996) who developed the *relational dialectical theory*, contradictions are necessary and successful relationships learn to manage them.

The parent–infant relationship is one that is endlessly changing. These changes can be explained by different theories but can be more clearly understood from the systems/dialectical perspective. A systems/dialectical perspective emphasizes that the forces of homeostasis and morphogenesis, or stability and change, work toward a functional interactional pattern between caregiver and infant. Riegel (1976), whose dialectical theory of development departed from Piaget (1951/1962) on the issue of change, believed that there were no periods of stability as such because contradictions continued to occur and were the force behind change.

While it has been noted that infants imitate selectively and at other times persistently, little research explains why this happens (Over & Carpenter, 2012). Over and Carpenter argue that the reason infants and toddlers imitate serves a social function and is relevant to the context of their social group, which reflects the systems view of the importance of the system of which one is a member. In human relationships there is the need to fit in, which means that infants selectively imitate those in proximity while not imitating more distant others.

The above view is reflected in the work of Grusec et al. (2000), who believe that the practice of parents using specific parenting techniques or styles to teach children values and acceptable social behaviors has emphasized appropriately the need for reciprocal parent–child relationships, but it has at the same time not emphasized the different forms of interaction. This practice has also highlighted how it is accepted that children internalize these parental directives without consideration for the specific needs of children. Instead, they recommend parents have a precise understanding of their child's unique features and situation rather than the use of specific generic strategies. Generally, missing in assessing parenting behaviors are larger goals that parents have for their children that surpass their goals for internalization of specific goals and behaviors. Finally, Grusec et al. (2000) suggest that a wide range of parenting strategies should be available to parents.

From a systems/dialectical position the interaction between parent and child forms a feedback system in which each provides input to the other. Any interaction or gesture can be an input of new information, which acts to stimulate a response in the other. This feedback system is constantly in motion and mirrors changes that occur in the relationship. The parent–child relationship has been characterized as different from adult relationships because of the various forms and content involved within the relationship (Maccoby, 2000). The dialectical aspect of this feedback system posits that when an input occurs, it may be in the form of a contradiction or challenge. In terms of dialectics, it represents a thesis that generates an antithesis. According to Riegel (1976), contradictions occur as *inner*—those within a person—or *outer*—contradictions associated with one's relationship with another person or involvement with the environment. The contradiction leads to a synthesis which holds both thesis and antithesis together rather than splitting in an either/or fashion.

Both inner and outer contradictions are constantly created in the parent–child relationship because each has conflicting needs, and opposing interests, values, and perceptions. The parent–child relationship is interdependent, and contradictions are entrenched within the relationship union. Contradictions caused by the different internal and external needs are the dynamic energy in development (Vygotsky, 1978). Contradictions in the parent–child relationship are present in parent modeling because the modeling behavior is inconsistent. Parents' behavior toward their child is a mixture of nurturance and control tactics that vary according to the current situation. *Ambivalence* can be a frequent state in the parent–child relationship due to parental inconsistent verbal and modeling behavior. For example, the child may hear warm and nurturing verbal comments from their parents, but simultaneously experience fear and rejection based on the parents modeling aggression and violence (Kuczynski & Parkin, 2009).

Managing contradiction from a systems/dialectical perspective takes a different route than the common assumptions about resolving them. As previously stated, a systems/dialectical perspective is based on the view that the dialectical process brings about transformational change. Contradictions create novel solutions that lead to transformational change, and the process continues because new contradictions occur. This is due to the interactive nature of communication that is circular rather than linear, which means that continuity is not the goal from a systems/dialectical perspective. Because of the contradiction in subparts of the system, the parent and the child, the system moves forward in a novel response.

The dialectical tension between two points, such as between verbal and nonverbal parental behavior, involves a synthesis. The circular or nonlinear concept of synthesis requires some analysis to determine its definition. A simple and inaccurate definition is that either the thesis or the antithesis dominates in the outcome (Valsiner, 2012). In addition, the synthesis cannot be considered a mixture of thesis and anthesis where neither dominates. According to Valsiner, synthesis emerges as a novel development that is unpredictable from what is known.

The outcome of any process in which confrontation exists leads to neither conformity nor similarity because both are grounded in linear causality. Rather, transformational change and the advent of novel syntheses from a systems/dialectical perspective emerge as outcomes. Parenting interventions taught by parenting experts often leads to conformity and an overemphasis on the control function of parenting, which is present in all forms of parent–child interaction, including the concept of parental modeling. The underlying assumption of parental modeling rests on the belief that there is a unidirectional cause of bad behavior when children imitate parents.

A bidirectional understanding of relationships is based on the view that in close emotional relationships, such as the parent–child relationship, meanings are created and reshaped through verbal and nonverbal elements (Sameroff, 2009). According to Sameroff, the interaction between parents occurs on two levels: (1) a macro level, or what is expressed externally, and (2) a micro level of how each interprets the interaction. The process of interpreting the interaction on a micro level may be different from what is expressed on a macro level. Children are influenced by interactional input from parents and their own past perceptions and experiences. Due to the two levels of interaction, no causal link can be established for any specific interaction. Consequently, a synthesis is never one-dimensional and what appears to be the outcome on one level may not present an outcome on another level.

Parental modeling of either prosocial or negative behavior is a good way to further illustrate this process. Modeling behavior may outwardly influence a child in one direction on a macro level and another way on a micro level. Parenting styles and behaviors (both direct and verbal, and indirect and nonverbal) can influence a child, but not determine the outcome (Kuczynski & De Mol, 2015). In terms of parental modeling, it seems plausible to suggest that a child witnessing good or bad parental behavior may be influenced in multiple ways, but not in a deterministic way. The child's response to a parental modeling incident may contain compliant, noncompliant, and novel elements. This process of synthesis is not deterministic and continues over the lifespan through the dialectical process of thesis, antithesis, and synthesis.

According to Kuczynski and De Mol (2015), much of parenting behavior is geared toward the future in terms of child outcomes. The future success of the child is assumed to be dependent on specific aspects of the parent–child relationship. For example, prosocial parental modeling can be viewed as the cause of children developing empathic and caring relationships. Kuczynski and De Mol show how this deterministic process fails through analyzing the dialectical concept of *equifinality*—many starting points in a sequence can have the same outcome, and one starting point can have many outcomes.

The principle of equifinality suggests that inflexible parenting that expects certain outcomes in their children may be harmful to children in the long run (Kuczynski & De Mol, 2015). When parents behave in particular ways to get a predetermined outcome in children, they deny the child's creative and novel response. For example, when parents attempt to instill specific beliefs in children and expect no deviation, they may be met with extreme rebellion or resistance. Instead of demanding complete compliance with their requests, parents tend to allow for flexibility in the child's response, which can lead to novel responses. The quality of the parent–child relationship in the long term seems more plausible than the short-term focus on fixing the noncompliance (Cavell & Elledge, 2007).

In sum, parental modeling is important to the overall parent–child relationship. When parents model prosocial behavior naturally, the influence on the child may not be coercive or inflexible but provides an opportunity for the child to respond naturally and creatively. In parent training, addressing the importance of modeling without prescribing specific modeling behaviors would allow for children to respond by accepting the model, rejecting the model, or creatively altering their response. The change element in this scenario is more than compliance and makes possible a change in the system, or transformational change.

New research on infant and child imitation challenges the older research that imitation is an internal trait active from birth, as espoused by Meltzoff (1988). The new research raises questions about Meltzoff's research design and concludes that imitation is a learned phenomenon rather than an internal trait. That is, the child learns to imitate from being imitated by the parent. This definition of imitation fits with a systems/dialectical perspective in that imitation is conceived of as developing from an interaction with the parent and is not deterministic and inflexible. Furthermore, the systems component of the interaction represents wholeness in which the whole is greater than the sum of the parts. The child is free to respond in a novel, creative, and nonlinear manner. The principle of equifinality is represented because the act of the parent imitating the child can lead to multiple outcomes. The child learning to imitate the parent also reflects a feedback loop where the child receives input that provides a catalysis for understanding one's own self-image.

References

American Academy of Pediatrics. (2012, April 29). Fight or flight: Violent teens may be following parents' lead. *ScienceDaily*. Retrieved June 11, 2023, from www.sciencedaily.com/releases/2012/04/120429085359.htm

Andrews, J. A., Tildesley, E., Hops, H., Duncan, S. C., & Severson, H. H. (2003). Elementary school age children's future intentions and use of substances. *Journal of Clinical Child and Adolescent Psychology, 32*, 556–567.

Bandura, A. (1977). *Social learning theory*. Prentice-Hall.

Bandura, A., Ross, D., & Ross, S. A. (1961). Transmission of aggression through imitation of aggressive models. *Journal of Abnormal and Social Psychology, 63*, 575–582. https://doi.org/10.1037/h0045925

Bates, B. (2019). *Learning theories simplified*. SAGE.

Baxter, L. A., & Montgomery, B. M. (1996). *Relating: Dialogues and dialectics*. Guilford.

Brauner-Otto, S. R., Axinn, W. G., & Ghimire, D. J. (2020). Parents' marital quality and children's transition to adulthood. *Demography, 57*(1), 195–220. https://doi.org/10.1007/s13524-019-00851-w.2020

Burstein, M., & Ginsburg, G. S. (2010). The effect of parental modeling of anxious behaviors and cognitions in school-aged children: An experimental pilot study. *Behavior Research and Therapy, 48*(6), 506–515. https://doi.org/10.1016/j.brat.2010.02.006; Epub 2010 February 25

Capaldi, D. M., Tiberio, S. S., Kerr, D. C. R., & Pears, K. C. (2016). The relationships of parental alcohol versus tobacco and marijuana use with early adolescent onset of alcohol use. *Journal of Studies on Alcohol and Drugs, 77*(1), 95–103. https://doi.org/10.15288/jsad.2016.77.95

Cavell, T. A., & Elledge, L. C. (2007). Working with parents of aggressive, high-risk children. In J. Briesmeister & C. Schaefer (Eds.), *Handbook of parent training* (pp. 379–423). Wiley.

Center for Parenting Education. (n.d.). *Being a role model—the promise and the peril.* https://centerforparentingeducation.org/library-of-articles/focus-parents/role-model-promise-peril/

Chassin, L., Flora, D. B., & King, K. M. (2004). Trajectories of alcohol and drug use and dependence from adolescence to adulthood: The effects of familial alcoholism and personality. *Journal of Abnormal Psychology, 13,* 483–498. https://doi.org/10.1037/0021-843X.113.4.483

Craig, L. (2006). Does father care mean fathers share? A comparison of how mothers and fathers in intact families spend time with children. *Gender & Society, 20,* 259–281. https://doi.org/10.1177/0891243205285212

Crane, J., Harper, J. M., Bean, R. A., & Holmes, E. (2020). Family implicit rules, shame, and adolescent prosocial and antisocial communication behaviors. *The Family Journal, 28*(1), 72–82. https://doi.org/10.1177/1066480719896563

Cross, E. S., Kraemer, D. J. M., Hamilton, A. F., Kelley, W. M., & Grafton, S. T. (2009). Sensitivity of the action observation network to physical and observational learning. *Cerebral Cortex, 19*(2), 315–326. https://doi.org/10.1093/cercor/bhn083

di Pellegrino, G., Fadiga, L., Fogassi, L., Gallese, V., & Rizzolatti, G. (1992). Understanding motor events, a neurophysiological study. *Experimental Brain Research, 91,* 176–180.

Emamzadeh, A. (2018). What factors are associated with positive parenting? *Psychology Today*. Retrieved December 13, 2023, from https://www.psychologytoday.com/us/blog/finding-new-home/201807/what-factors-are-associated-positive-parenting

Forrester, D., Westlake, D., & Glynn, G. (2012). Parental resistance and social worker skills: Towards a theory of motivational social work. *Child and Family Social Work, 17*(2), 118–129. https://doi.org/10.1111/j.1365-2206.2012.00837.x

Grusec, J. E., Goodnow, J. J., & Kuczynski, L. (2000). New directions in analyses of parenting contributions to children's acquisition of values. *Child Development, 71*(1), 205–211. https://doi.org/10.1111/1467-8624.00135

Haley, J. (1980). *Leaving home*. McGraw Hill.

Hancock, A., Jorgensen, B., & Swanson, M. (2013). College students and credit card use: The role of parents, work experience, financial knowledge, and credit card attitudes. *Journal of Family and Economic Issues, 34*(4), 369–381.

Heimann, M., Edorsson, A., Sundqvist, A., & Koch, F.-S. (2017). Thirteen- to sixteen-months old infants are able to imitate a novel act from memory in both unfamiliar and familiar settings but do not show evidence of rational inferential processes. *Frontiers in Psychology, 8*. https://doi.org/10.3389/fpsyg.2017.02186

Hill, M. R., Boorman, E. D., & Fried, I. (2016). Observational learning computations in neurons of the human anterior cingulate cortex. *Nature Communications, 7,* 12722. https://doi.org/10.1038/ncomms12722

Holden, G. W. (2010). Childrearing and developmental trajectories: Positive pathways, off-ramps, and dynamic processes. *Child Development Perspectives, 4*(3), 197. https://doi.org/10.1111/j.1750-8606.2010.00148.x

Hussong, A. M., Huang, W., Serrano, D., Curran, P. J., & Chassin, L. (2012). Testing whether and when parent alcoholism uniquely affects various forms of adolescent substance use. *Journal of Abnormal Child Psychology, 40,* 1265–1276. https://doi.org/10.1007/s10802-012-9662-3

Jones, H. A., Putt, G. E., Rabinovitch, A. E., Hubbard, R., & Snipes, D. (2017). Preventing stress, readiness, to change, and child externalizing behavior of clinically referred children. *Journal of Child and Family Studies, 26,* 215–233.

Kail, R. V., & Cavanaugh, J. C. (2007). *Human development: A life-span view* (4th ed.). Thomson Wadsworth.

Kerr, D. C. R., Capaldi, D. M., Pears, K. C., & Owen, L. D. (2012). Intergenerational influences on early alcohol use: Independence from the problem behavior pathway. *Development and Psychopathology, 24,* 889–906. https://doi.org/10.1017/S0954579412000430

Kim, H., & Rose, K. M. (2014). Concept analysis of family homeostasis. *Journal of Advanced Nursing, 70*(11), 2450–2468. https://doi.org/10.1111/jan.12496; Epub 2014 August 11; PMID: 25109705

Kopystynska, O., Paschall, K. W., Barnett, M. A., & Curran, M. A. (2017). Patterns of interparental conflict, parenting, and children's emotional insecurity: A person-centered approach. *Journal of Family Psychology, 31*(7), 922–932. https://doi.org/10.1037/fam0000343

Kuczynski, L., & De Mol, J. (2015). Dialectical models of socialization. In W. F. Overton & P. C. M. Molenaar (Eds.), *Theory and method: Vol. 1 of the handbook of child psychology and developmental science* (7th ed., pp. 323–368). Wiley.

Kuczynski, L., & Parkin, M. (2009). Pursuing a dialectical perspective on transaction: A social relational theory of micro family processes. In A. Sameroff (Ed.), *Transactional processes in development* (pp. 247–268). American Psychological Association.

Kuczynski, L., Zahn-Waxler, C., & Radke-Yarrow, M. (1987). Development and content of imitation in the second and third year of life: A socialization perspective. *Developmental Psychology, 23,* 276–282.

Maccoby, E. E. (2000). The uniqueness of the parent-child relationship. In W. A. Collins & B. Laursen (Eds.), *Relationships as developmental contexts* (pp. 157–175). Erlbaum.

Meltzoff, A. N. (1988). Infant imitation after a one-week delay: Long-term memory for novel acts and multiple stimuli. *Developmental Psychology, 24,* 4470–4476. https://doi.org/10.1037/0012-1649.24.4.470

Meltzoff, A. N., & Williamson, R. A. (2013). Imitation: Social, cognitive, and theoretical perspectives. In P. D. Zelazo (Ed.), *The Oxford handbook of developmental psychology: Vol. 1. Body and mind* (pp. 651–682). Oxford University Press.

Østbye, T., Malhotra, R., Stroo, M., Lovelady, C., Brouwer, R., Zucker, N., & Fuemmeler, B. (2013). The effect of the home environment on physical activity and dietary intake in preschool children. *International Journal of Obesity, 37*(10), 1314–1321. https://doi.org/10.1038/ijo.2013.76

Over, H., & Carpenter, M. (2012). The social side of imitation. *Child Development Perspectives, 7*(1), 6–11. https://doi.org/10.1111/cdep.12006

Overton, W. F. (2006). Developmental psychology: Philosophy, concepts, methodology. In W. Damon & R. M. Lerner (Series Eds.) and R. M. Lerner (Vol. Ed.), *Handbook of child psychology: Vol. 1. Theoretical models of human development* (pp. 18–88). Wiley.

Piaget, J. (1962). *Play, dreams, and imitation in childhood.* Routledge. (Original work published 1951)

Riegel, K. F. (1976). The dialectics of human development. *American Psychologist, 10,* 689–700.

Saby, J. N., Meltzoff, A. N., & Marshall, P. J. (2013). Infants' somatotopic neural responses to seeing human actions: I've got you under my skin. *Public Library of Science (PLoS), 8*(10). https://doi.org/10.1371/journal.pone.0077905

Sameroff, A. (2009). The transactional model. In A. Sameroff (Ed.), *Transactional processes in development* (pp. 3–22). American Psychological Association.

Sauciuc, G. A., Zlakowska, J., Persson, T., Lenninger, S., & Madsen, E. A. (2020). Imitation recognition and its prosocial effects in 6-month-old infants. *PLoS One, 15*(5), e0232717. https://doi.org/10.1371/journal.pone.0232717

Schuhmacher, N., Köster, M., & Kärtner, J. (2018). Modeling prosocial behavior increases helping in 16-month-olds. *Child Development, 90*(5), 1789–1801. https://doi.org/10.1111/cdev.13054

Szkody, E., & McKinney, C. (2021). Family communication patterns and relationship quality between emerging adults and their parents. *Journal of Social and Personal Relationships, 38*(11), 3177–3197. https://doi.org/10.1177/02654075211027217

Valsiner, J. (2012). *A guided science*. Transaction.

Voss, C., & Sandercock, G. R. H. (2013). Associations between perceived parental physical activity and aerobic fitness in schoolchildren. *Journal of Physical Activity and Health, 10*(3), 397–405. https://doi.org/10.1123/jpah.10.3.397

Vuolo, M., & Staff, J. (2013). Parent and child cigarette use: A longitudinal, multigenerational study. *Pediatrics, 132*(3), 568–577. https://doi.org/10.1542/peds.2013-0067
Vygotsky, L. S. (1978). *Mind in society: The development of higher psychological processes*. Harvard University Press.
Warner, L. A., White, H. R., & Johnson, V. (2007). Alcohol initiation experiences and family history of alcoholism as predictors of problem drinking trajectories. *Journal of Studies on Alcohol and Drugs, 68,* 56–65. https://doi.org/10.15288/jsad.2007.68.56.
Webb, T. L., & Sheeran, P. (2006). Does changing behavioral intentions engender behavior change? A meta-analysis of the experimental evidence. *Psychological Bulletin, 132,* 249–268.

8

STORYTELLING

Indirect Influence via Storytelling

One of the unique interactions of parents and children is storytelling. Young children are especially intrigued by stories and commit to memory the words they hear in the story. When parents mispronounce or leave out a word in their favorite story, the child quickly corrects them. Parents frequently read stories at bedtime as part of a regular bedtime routine. There are many great books that contain timeless motifs and become children's favorites, such as *The Velveteen Rabbit* (Williams, 1922). Stories that link to the child's experiences, such as getting a new babysitter, using the potty, going to school, making friends, having a new baby in the family, and being a small person in a big person's world are helpful for making transitions. Identifying with the characters in stories helps the child make transitions easier and less stressful. Stories can also introduce children to new behaviors and skills that encourage their willingness to learn them.

Stories in books and videos run the gamut of topics and can be helpful in learning and entertainment. Parents make available different media for their children that use a story format, but there is little application of stories in direct or indirect parenting strategies to control children's misbehavior. For example, parents' use of stories to discipline, increase compliance, or correct behavior is underdeveloped in the literature. Telling a child a story that connects creatively with what the child is experiencing can unconsciously influence the child's behavior more than using more direct means of influence, such as rewarding or punishing behavior or taking away privileges.

DOI: 10.4324/9781003381679-10

Storytelling as a Form of Child Therapy

While parents have been slow in using storytelling to influence children's misbehavior, therapists have long understood the positive effects of storytelling. One of the most renowned therapists to use stories and metaphors for all clients was Milton Erickson (1965, 1975). Erickson used hypnotherapy, storytelling, and metaphoric language to implicitly induce change rather than the more common practice of making explicit direct interventions. A *metaphor* is a figure of speech that is applied to an object or action that cannot be taken literally (Craiker, 2023). Metaphors are symbolic language that relates ideas and powerful influential messages indirectly. The implicit message in a metaphor enlarges one's understanding and perceptions in ways that are beneath consciousness. In children, metaphors are understood first on a conscious level in the narrative of the story. While the child may hear the words consciously, the impact of the story is on the unconscious. Fairy tales may be difficult to decipher consciously, but conscious awareness of the meaning of the fairy tale is not necessary.

The contents of storytelling tend to reflect the societal attitudes prevalent in contemporary society. Many parents and teachers alike prefer the telling of timeless fairy tales to more modern stories. The power of fairy tales may be in the implicit meaning and emotional development that not only is timeless but enacts a more effective emotional response than modern contemporary stories. According to Fleer and Hammer (2013), fairy tales should be an integral feature of early childhood education programs.

Hypnotherapy works in a similar fashion to storytelling. While hypnotherapy is not a widely used treatment for child problems, words and phrases in the form of suggestion on an unconscious level are frequently used to induce an altered state (Dolan, 1985). For example, for a child who has difficulty concentrating in school, a therapist might tell a seemingly unrelated story that contains an embedded message or suggestion, such as "YOU WILL NOTICE INCREASED ATTENTION when the pokey little puppy barks in the garden." The therapist creates a parallel story that has unrecognizable content but can embed a subliminal message. Stories can also be used to induce an altered state of consciousness that increases relaxation, reduces stress, and promotes good sleeping.

In the therapeutic techniques of storytelling, therapists create stories that have relevance to the child's problems. Instead of reading a pre-written story, the therapist comes up with a story and invites the child to engage in the creation of its narrative. Mutual storytelling provides a way for the child to unconsciously participate in a resolution to their problem (Gardner, 1971; Sommers-Flanagan, 2019). The mutual storytelling technique does not give the child conscious insight into their problems and is playful and fun in context. The child is told to begin an original story, not recount the plot of a story already written or told in other media such as TV. The therapist engages in the story to provide additional content. After the child's story comes to a resolution, the therapist retells the story to address the underlying psychological issues and create a more adaptive ending. Below is an example of the mutual storytelling technique:

Child:	Once there was a squirrel. He lived by the woods. He lived with his mom, dad, and sister. He didn't like his sister. He had to play with her all the time. He's a squirrel, so he might eat her. They were playing in the woods, playing hide and seek, and something bad happened. A bear came and chased the squirrel and his sister. They ran really fast. The bear almost got the squirrel, but he got away and got home in his tree. And the bear couldn't reach him. She got away too.
Therapist:	What's the moral of your story?
Child:	He could trip his sister, and the bear would get her, and he could get away.
Therapist:	OK, here's my story. Once upon a time there was a squirrel family, a boy, a girl, a mom, and a dad. And they lived in a tree by the woods. The boy and girl squirrel liked to play hide and seek in the woods, but it wasn't always safe because there was a bear that lived there. Sometimes the bear was really nice and played with the squirrels, and sometimes it was scary, and the squirrels wanted to get away. The scary bear mostly came out at night. The squirrels knew when the bear wasn't in a good mood, because it would harrumph and growl and complain and talk in a mean voice. So, they learned to stay away from the bear when it harrumphed, growled, and complained. They would go to their own holes in the tree, or sometimes they would just spend time with momma squirrel. They also learned that they could call Mr. Lion, who was the peace-keeper of the woods or tell Mr. Owl, their teacher, if the bear ever hurt them. So, the moral of the story is, stay away from bears when they are harrumphing and growling and talking in a mean voice! (My Play Therapy Page, 2011)

The retelling of the story is to add therapeutic value and influence the child sublimely. Gardner (1993) did not rush the attempt to be therapeutic and believed that multiple storytelling sessions might be needed for the child to divulge enough emotional content to create a therapeutic story intervention. It was primarily developed for children over 5 years old and is a technique that requires verbal skills and a thorough understanding of the child. Gardner's technique is helpful in a clinical setting but would not be recommended for parents. What is important for parents from Gardner's position is that storytelling can be an alternative means to punishment for influencing children's misbehavior. It can also be helpful for parents discovering hidden or unconscious feelings.

Learning through Storytelling

A brief history of storytelling reveals that it has been an effective means of passing on traditions and mores of society since the beginning of civilization and continues today with the explosion of technology (Yuan et al., 2018). Values and role expectations can be passed down from generation to generation through stories that influence unconscious thoughts and perceptions. Early story formation was oral, intended to make sense of existential concerns, and understood today as "mythology." With the advent of the printing press, advanced science, and technologies, storytelling has evolved with our progress as well, but serves the same basic function: It is a method to grasp at the ungraspable.

Storytelling can be in the form of written or verbal narrative, songs, poems, or chants, which provide connection and bonding of a group of people but may or may not contain factually accurate information. Storytelling can be replete with legends, mythical elements, moral implications, and spirituality. Native Americans had a rich culture of storytelling that passed on the traditions and values of the group (National Geographic, 2022). For example, the storytelling tradition of the Choctaw centered around migration to their present location and a creation story that was infused with values and expected morality. In Ireland, the itinerant *seanchaí* were storytellers who moved from one community to the next telling stories of honor and ageless knowledge. Telling stories of past heroes, such as kings, the seanchaí embellished historic myths and spawned national pride.

Storytelling may be the oldest form of teaching and is one of the best methods for illustrating some facts (Krause & Rucker, 2019). While the persuasive power of storytelling has been known by researchers for some time, exactly how and why that is true has been largely unexamined in the child and family research literature. According to Krause and Rucker, when facts are weak, stories can bolster the effect and when facts are strong and stand on their own, storytelling is not as influential or persuasive. Krause and Rucker speculated that this is true because stories can reduce the processing of information and therefore not be as effective when facts are in abundance.

Stories facilitate learning by placing the receiver of the story within the narrative, making abstract ideas easier to comprehend. Stories increase creative responses via mental images which facilitate higher order critical and dialectical thinking skills. As such, it can increase divergent thinking by encouraging people to think outside the box.

Perhaps the greatest effect in learning from storytelling is the use of *characters* because they allow for a human face to be put on facts or problems (Brown et al., 2014). The visualization of the character helps the learner associate a human form with material and increase recall of the information. From characters, children learn how to react to situations that help them adjust to unplanned events in their own lives. In addition, analyzing characters as they respond to situations and change is important in aiding the development of critical thinking.

Learning academic subjects is enhanced by storytelling (Padrón, 2018). Stories provide an emotional connection to academic subjects that are missing in the facts alone. Stories have the power to transport students into different dimensions of thinking that broadens the understanding of the world around them. Even principles of the hard sciences, such as physics and math, can be more easily remembered if stories are used to embellish the material.

Narrative science storytelling is a technique used in educational settings where the author uses suspense, tone of voice, character, and description to link different elements of the story together to create an in-depth story that facilitates learning of abstract ideas (Martinez-Conde et al., 2019). While emotional content in scientific writing is restrained, lay audiences are more open and reveal more acceptance of emotional links to science research and publications. Furthermore, researchers in scientific endeavors no doubt have experienced fascination and emotional excitement about the discoveries they have made and have found avenues through stories where this emotional reaction can be shared with others, which can be most rewarding.

Researchers have found that children are more focused and less distracted during *oral storytelling* than when material is presented without stories or when material is presented with written stories (Lenhart et al., 2020). The oral storytelling procedure has good outcomes with all types of students, including special needs children. Storytelling is a powerful technique to help students focus and comprehend difficult material. While there are many explanations as to why storytelling can be so powerful in conveying ideas, Turner (1996) summarized it as the thing that makes humans uniquely different from other creatures. Without it, there would be no thinking mind, no culture, no history, and no vision for the future. Even given this central role in thinking and learning, academics or those focused on human development have not universally touted its importance.

The importance of storytelling appears to be based on how the human brain functions. Researchers have demonstrated that even in utero, the fetus can hear and distinguish sounds, such as music and human voices and develop familiarity with such sounds after birth (Kuhl, 2010). Neuroscientists have discovered that the entire brain is involved in stories, which is described by the moniker of "*narrative brain*" to illustrate its prominence (Gonçalves et al., 2004).

Storytelling provides the child the opportunity to recognize emotions in themselves and others and to rehearse emotional responses (Bateman, 2020). Storytelling is an essential technique for *social–emotional development*, the ability to form meaningful relationships with parents and others. A technique developed to aid children in recognizing and comprehending emotion is the storytelling table. The storytelling table is a technique developed for kindergartners in which children can act out the story by using various props (Catala et al., 2023). Like the therapy technique mentioned earlier, the close supervision of an adult or a teacher in the classroom is needed because kindergarteners lack life experiences and insight into emotional expression. Guiding the child through the storytelling with questions and prompts is an important component for the child's recognition of emotional content.

The next section of the chapter will recount the association of brain activity and storytelling.

The Neuroscience of Storytelling

The fascination with storytelling as an area of academic research has gained in popularity due to the recognition of stories' effectiveness in changing behavior. To address why this is true, researchers and neuroscientists conducted in-depth investigations. An obvious assumption is that narrative stories affect the emotional system even though most stories in any form are fictional and not about real people or events. Nevertheless, the listener of the story reacts as if the events and characters are real. Stories open the listener to greater understanding of the human experience, which can lead to not only self-reflection but also fundamental new insights that can result in change (Carroll & Gibson, 2011). Not all emotional experiences in stories are for positive outcomes. Stories can cause negative emotions, which may have long-term effects on listeners, and some stories are structured to dampen or subdue emotional expressions (Aldama, 2015).

Brain imaging techniques are currently used to determine how stories affect the listener. There is evidence from neuroscience research that the meaning of words is based on visual and motor functions (Pulvermüller, 2005). For example, action words stimulate the same brain areas that are activated during physical movement, so the brain of the listener or reader produces the same response as if they were physically experiencing the situation. Therefore, the brain's response connects the listener or reader to a similar real experience, placing them in an active rather than a passive observational role. The implication of these findings is that there is a wide-ranging neural response, linked to how one experiences the real world and language in all forms, including stories (Speer et al., 2009).

Mapping the brain's response to emotional story content has been the focus of several research studies. For example, Vessel et al. (2013) attempted to map the neural responses to expressions of art that produced an emotional response. This research is based on the belief that a *default mode network* is activated when an emotional response to artistic expression occurs. Other researchers have found similar neural patterns from stories even for different languages and across cultures. Dehghani et al. (2017) found that subjects who speak English, Farsi, and Mandarin Chinese had similar brain responses to stories. The implication of this research is that storytelling can induce similar responses of self-awareness and understanding of others irrespective of native language. Furthermore, Suzuki et al. (2020) found that storytelling activates most of the cortical and subcortical regions of the brain across different languages, which means that storytelling creates the same neural responses in subjects who speak different languages.

According to Oatley (2019), storytelling involves creating a mental reality that exceeds the brain's localized language processing of the meaning of words. What is produced by stories is a *theory of mind*, and the more that younger children are exposed to stories, the more developed their theory of mind is. The theory of mind is enhanced by the impact of events on the characters and the choices they must make in the story. Effective decision making is grounded in these implicit processes that are based on exposure to stories.

Recent research on how the unconscious operates to make decisions has added a greater understanding to this process. For example, researchers have found that the decision making process is mainly unconscious rather than conscious; although appearing to be an *explicit conscious process*, the decision making process is, in fact, an *implicit unconscious process* (Creswell et al., 2013). This implies that the early maturing implicit brain is the rudimentary underpinning for decisions throughout life beginning in early childhood when stories are frequently consumed. What this means is that the unconscious never stops working. When one feels that they cannot find a clear path, the unconscious is still processing it and will come up with an answer. In addition, research of this nature clearly points to the importance of experiences in story form that activate the unconscious.

In other brain research, Bargh and Morsella (2008) posit that in early childhood the developing implicit brain is the foundation for values that make the world governable and predictable. While they do not link this directly to storytelling, the dots begin connecting. Stories form the basis for understanding actions that are processed unconsciously, with the conscious mind acting more as a concierge and becomes active only subsequently to the experience. Consequently, the unconscious mind works better to solve problems when the conscious mind is uninvolved. Thus, the conclusion can be drawn that stories told by elders are part of the foundation of the young individual's values and moral system, which develop unconsciously and later inform conscious thoughts and feelings regarding conceptualization of self, others, and the world.

While storytelling is viewed by scholars as important for a culture in the passing down of traditions and morality, there is little application to how storytelling is associated with healthy outcomes in culture. This much is known—culture plays a role in the brain's response to persons of the same culture, which tend to be more similar in response to stories than persons of different cultures. Researchers speculated that this similarity results from a shared understanding of the world (Suzuki et al., 2020). Consequently, a person constructs their beliefs and perspectives from those to whom they are connected. In a highly polarized culture, storytelling might be less effective in providing an experience of shared meaning. This means that, at the core, storytelling has both a personal and public function in providing meaning.

Storytelling, however, must not be viewed as linear and unchanging; every culture changes due to social and political events, impacting story creation. Individuals and families immigrating to a new culture go through a process of *acculturation* and stories aid in retaining the heritage and shared values of a subculture's original homeland. As acculturation takes place in the subgroup, stories can provide the dual purpose of maintaining the group's shared heritage while at the same time allowing for changes in the stories that promote acculturation. It is assumed that changes to these traditional stories would be cosmetic rather than surgical and maintain the latent messages that bind the subgroup together.

Yabe et al. (2018) used *near-infrared spectroscopy (NIRS)*, a common practice for studying the brains of young children, to measure the activity in the prefrontal lobe as children were read picture book stories by their mothers and were told stories. The researchers noted that past research was inconclusive and wanted to definitively address the extent to which picture book stories affected the prefrontal lobe. Using NIRS technique, Yabe et al. designed a study that measured brain activity in the prefrontal cortex during picture book reading and with storytelling, the degree of familiarity with the stories and the effect on the prefrontal cortex, and the effects of lateralization on storytelling and picture book reading. Findings indicate that picture book reading produced high prefrontal activity initially but decreased as familiarity with the book occurred. Overall, picture book reading produced less prefrontal activity. On the other hand, storytelling showed robust activation in the prefrontal cortex with no decrease with familiarization.

Yabe et al. (2018) assumed that the difference in prefrontal activity in picture book reading and storytelling was due to greater imagination of listeners when engaged in storytelling as compared to picture book reading. Storytelling requires visualizing happenings in the story, as well as predicting future happenings. The greater involvement of the child's imagination may provide more brain stimulation across regions of the brain. Consequently, picture book reading may not be as useful in helping children be creative because of the overabundance of visual images and the reduced fantasy imagination that occurs with picture book reading.

Children and Storytelling

Emotion Regulation

One of the main functions of early childhood is emotion regulation. As the child matures, emotion regulation moves from external control, the mother, to internal or self-regulation. Failure to regulate emotion is associated with a host of problems, especially in the turbulent teenage years. The brain regions associated with emotion regulation include the amygdala, dorsal anterior cingulate cortex, medial, lateral prefrontal cortices, left insula, inferior parietal cortices, and middle temporal and medial occipital gyri (Ochsner et al., 2004). Another brain process, attentional control, overlaps with the brain regions associated with emotion regulation (Wessing et al., 2013).

Emotion regulation and *pretend play* are two elements of successful maturing in children and have been viewed as opposing each other (Hoffmann & Russ, 2012). In other words, to develop emotion regulation, pretend play must be decreased and considered less important. This relation of pretend play and emotion regulation was challenged by Hoffmann and Russ. Pretend play is defined as play occurring in a narrative or story in which various objects represent other things. In pretend play, a child uses divergent thinking within a story narrative to create a fantasy where an object can symbolize other objects or characters. The content is fast moving and change in meaning occurs often. While the story may make perfect logic to a child, an adult might have problems following its contents. *Creativity* is enhanced by pretend play as the child uses divergent thinking to concoct various outcomes to the story using symbols to represent real-life scenarios. According to Hoffman and Russ, this process of creating a fantasy in pretend play improves both the problem-solving ability and affect regulation.

Pretend play aids in affect regulation because children can create specific emotional content and alter it as the story develops and changes (Hoffmann & Russ, 2012). Pretend play allows emotions to be expressed in symbolic ways that result in better emotional regulation. Even negative emotions appear to be expressed without harm to the child or playmates. Social interactions with other children during pretend play reflect a full range of content involving emotions, logical and divergent thinking, and problem-solving (see Table 8.1).

Conscious control of thoughts is one of the developmental accomplishments that comes with aging. As children age, they take turns and interact nonaggressively (Hoffmann & Russ, 2012). To determine the association between pretend play, creativity, emotion regulation, and conscious control, Hoffmann and Russ found that pretend play was associated with creativity and emotion regulation but not to conscious control of thought. A major limitation of this study is that the sample was highly restricted and may not apply to all children.

Educators are concerned about attention in the classroom and use various methods to increase it. A recent study found that storytelling results in increased visual attention in children, but the opposite is true when children read on-screen monitors, which has the same brain patterns as when children have attention deficits (Zivan et al., 2019). The brain response also differs in the same pattern as above when children read in print versus reading on a screen (Zivan et al., 2023).

Psychological and Behavioral Interventions

There is a paucity of research on biosocial markers of storytelling, which contribute to the underdevelopment of storytelling as a disciple intervention. Investigating the psychological and physiological impact of storytelling lays a foundation for expanding storytelling to behavioral interventions. In a recent study to determine the psychological and physiological properties of storytelling, Brockington et al.

TABLE 8.1 The Positive Effects of Storytelling on Children

Children and Storytelling	
1	Improves emotion regulation, pretend play, divergent thinking, and creativity
2	Increases visual attention
3	Increases oxytocin and prosocial behavior, decreases cortisol and stress
4	Affects children's emotional and cognitive experiences outside of awareness
5	Conveys ideas through metaphor and story that will increase bonding
6	Can be used to discipline, and implant cultural and societal values

(2021) emphasized two biomarkers, *oxytocin*, a hormone and neuropeptide, and *cortisol*, the stress hormone, associated with human psychological and physiological responses. Brockington and associates collected oxytocin and cortisol levels and pain readings from hospitalized children before and after storytelling, and compared them to a control group. Findings indicated that the storytelling group had a significant increase in oxytocin and decrease in cortisol when tested 30 minutes after the procedure. Pain levels were also significantly decreased. The research suggests that storytelling is an effective and cost-saving way of increasing positive biomarkers and decreasing negative ones.

Only a few studies illustrate how oxytocin levels are related to prosocial behavior during early development. For example, Simpson et al. (2014), using animal subjects, found that infant monkeys showed increased social behavior with elevated levels of oxytocin. Furthermore, in older children, increased oxytocin levels predict positive social behavior while lower levels of oxytocin were associated with mental and emotional disorders (Suzuki et al., 2020). Clinical studies show a clear relation between oxytocin levels and functional social interactions (Parker et al., 2017).

The above study addresses how storytelling can increase prosocial responses in children by increasing oxytocin levels and explains how children bond with others through storytelling. What remains to be developed is how biosocial factors, which are present in storytelling, can be utilized by parents and in parent training to change and redirect negative behavior. The power of storytelling is the implicit effect that is outside of consciousness. Stories that have an obvious, explicit message intended to influence the child can easily be rejected by the child in the same manner as a parent explicitly telling a child to do or not do something can be ignored. This is not to say that direct methods are ineffective or to be avoided at all costs, but rather to explore indirect methods that are often not used. To be effective in addressing children's behavior outside of their conscious awareness, the contents of a story and how it relates to the child should not be recognizable. Stories need to be tailor-made to fit the child situation, yet distinct enough to avoid conscious recognition of any underlying message.

As stated previously, control of behavior and providing nurturance are considered the two most important behaviors of parental interactions with their children. Both come into play as needing improvement when parents have difficulty in parenting. Chapter 1 of this book reviewed some parent education models that are used to improve parents' skills for both control behavior and nurturance. These models focus mainly on developing skills and using direct, explicit procedures and methods. Storytelling provides an alternative method that conveys ideas through metaphor and narrative that increases creativity, bonding, divergent and dialectical thinking, and problem-solving in children. Instead of telling them what to do, stories will invite them to use their imagination and use the story content to come to a resolution regarding problems they are experiencing.

Various parenting models attempt to create a positive and cooperative atmosphere in the parent–child relationship. For example, the Adlerian model, one of the most common parenting models, revolves around the principle that parents should control their anger and never discipline in anger (Dreikurs, 1990). Instead, the parent should remove themselves from the situation if necessary until they are no longer angry before addressing the situation. Faber and King (2017) float a similar idea in that listening carefully and addressing adequately what children are expressing, instead of rushing to assumptions, leads to more functional interactions with children.

While the focus on being positive is good, the techniques generally emphasize verbal interactions that are direct and appeal to the logical conscious mind. There is little focus on spontaneity, play, and storytelling. While typically not true in Western societies, storytelling in some cultures is used for discipline. Doucleff and Greenhalgh (2019) address the use of storytelling by investigating how the Inuits use it to discipline and implant cultural and societal values in their children. Doucleff and Greenhalgh recount how Jean Briggs, a Harvard graduate student at the time, lived for 17 months with an Inuit family inside the rigid arctic circle. Living conditions were extremely harsh, and the Inuit lived primitively as their ancestors had done. Briggs noted one glaring difference between herself and the Inuit family: She frequently showed anger and frustration at the challenges in living in the repressive and harsh climate, while the Inuit never reacted in anger at anything. Their response to any inconvenience or unexpected chaotic occurrence was to simply fix it without expressing anger or frustration. Exhibiting any degree of anger or frustration was considered a weakness of character and to be avoided.

How Inuit parents teach their children not to react in anger is fascinating. They do the opposite of what Western parents would do (Doucleff & Greenhalgh, 2019). For example, Briggs noted that an Inuit mother gave her child a rock and asked the child to throw it at her. After the child threw the rock, the mother reacted by displaying no anger but simply replying that it hurt. The cardinal rule is never to show anger or yell at small children. The Inuit believe that when children are acting out or misbehaving, they are doing so because they want or need something and, as a good parent, your job is to figure that out. Common parenting practices in Western societies, such as time-out or taking away a privilege, are considered inappropriate by the Inuit. Instead of teaching good behavior, the Inuit believe these common practices teach children how to be aggressive and resentful.

The method the Inuit use to teach children how to behave is storytelling (Doucleff & Greenhalgh, 2019). Their stories are oral and passed down from one generation to the next. In contrast to the Inuit, Western parents use print or screen stories that may be poor replicas of an oral tradition, based on ancestry and cultural knowledge. Disciplining children with the Inuit method can be fun and a nice respite from punitive or harsh discipline.

When Inuit children are aggressive or hitting other children, parents do not react with punishment (Doucleff & Greenhalgh, 2019). Instead, they create a story drama that reenacts the child's behavior. The parent dramatically acts out the child's behavior and the consequences of such behavior. The parent gives the option for the child to hit them which provides the opportunity for some playful teaching by simply saying that it hurts. Follow-up playful questions by the parent are meant to demonstrate to the child why hitting was not good. This procedure continues until the child stops hitting and the misbehavior stops. The purpose of the dramas is to teach that one must control their reaction and not be provoked by others. The parent must ask many questions and make sure the whole process is fun and playful. By creating these drama experiences, parents help their children learn how to control their anger implicitly. Neurologically, this approach significantly impacts the emotional system of the brain, such that, over time, this portion is more developed in the brains of Inuits. A more developed emotional system allows an individual to opt for more controlled emotional responses.

Disciplining children through stories provides an alternative to direct explicit methods. Typically, *discipline stories* in Western societies take the route of addressing common concerns and challenges of children and are generally print stories. Stories are adapted to be helpful for all age children, including teenagers where the narrative is more complex, although the main audience is preschool children. Discipline stories are different from fairy tales because the purpose is to change behavior in the present time frame. Stories to change behavior can be used by parents to address specific problems. While stories can be read from books or other media, adapting the mutual storytelling model and stories told by the therapist are the most effective model for parents to adapt for their own use. The personalized stories of the parent can be focused directly on the issues at hand, and the mutual storytelling procedure provides experiences in which both the child and the parent engage in a cooperative endeavor to address current problems and foster a closer bond.

Both stories by parents and mutual storytelling develop the story through characters that the child identifies with and knows (Figure 8.1). With young children, the characters may take the form of animals, or a lovable creature that has a special connection with the child. William Cook (1994) developed a technique for telling stories in therapy that can be easily adapted by parents. The procedure consisted of five steps; (1) The stage is set with the introduction of the main character, who is described as a great person with a single flaw; (2) The problem is acknowledged which may be similar but not exactly as experienced by the child; (3) Conversation occurs with a wise person about the problem who shows unconditional positive regard and acceptance; (4) Engaging in divergent approaches occurs, wherein the problem is addressed in a healthy manner; (5) Summarizing. This procedure with the focus on character development is based on the belief that stories are more effective in changing children's behavior during early childhood than logical conscious control methods because children think in visual images utilizing more prominently their emotional brain centers, not their neocortex, or logical thinking center. Only later, around 10 years of age, do they develop a more formal logical thinking ability (Piaget, 1969). Furthermore, young children lack the depth of

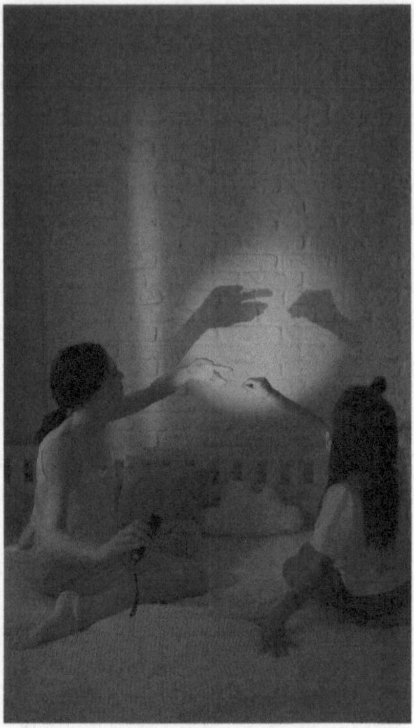

FIGURE 8.1 Pretend play improves cognitive, emotional, and social development. (Photo by Artem Podrez from Pexels)

recall of stories or comprehending metaphors to the degree that older children do (Carriedo et al., 2016). Their view of the world is limited because schemas for understanding relationships have not developed fully.

Storytelling as a Second Order Discipline Technique

Storytelling used for learning, cultural bonding, and fun can also be used in disciplining children. From the systems/dialectical position, too much emphasis is placed on control of children's behavior (Roberts, 1994). Although compliance is needed by children to parental directives, an overemphasis on control leads to punishment and negative and coercive parenting. An open interactive system that has a *nonlinear interactional pattern* in which parents do not express anger toward children can be effective in creating a healthy and functional system. A systems/dialectical model provides for an ongoing interactional system that is ever-changing. Stories become an integral part of the process of children incorporating metaphors in a story while, at the same time, disregarding some content.

No doubt, one of the concerns of parents in using stories to discipline children is the assumed skill that is required in constructing a story that can unconsciously affect children. While a structure for the content is needed, it must be remembered that storytelling with implicit and metaphorical meaning are present in fairy tales, religious allegories, and modern books and videos used by parents. To some extent, the art of storytelling permeates all human communication. Overtraining, or suggesting a right way to tell stories, would impede the parent's spontaneous and creative act of telling a story. The idea is not to make parents uptight in being creative, but to provide a simple structure that might also be subject to change (see Table 8.2).

Storytelling is not taken as the only or primary means of discipline and may be inappropriate for some types of misbehavior, such as repetitive, aggressive acting out, or when the child is in danger. The storytelling technique is appropriate for a wide range of adjustment issues and emotional concerns as children have experiences that they cannot understand. It is meant to suggest how parents can use a method steeped in metaphor and unconscious content to influence their child's behavior. It is a respite for parents and children from the overuse of controlling the child's behavior. It is also a cooperative approach that can be humorous and affirming of the child's individuality. In addition, it can improve the bonding between parent and child. Storytelling, as a discipline, is more effective with young children because stories and visual images are the way they understand their experiences. As children age, parents alter their storytelling to incorporate greater complexity and plot development.

Although the story needs to have a structure, it need not be too difficult for the parent to construct. Several steps are listed later as guidelines that can be altered depending on the situation and the parent's comfort level. First, of primary importance in constructing a discipline story, is to be very clear what the parents want to convey in the story. The story should be specific about the unwanted behavior but disguised in a way the child does not consciously recognize it. Not clearly

TABLE 8.2 Constructing Stories That Can Change a Child's Behavior

Storytelling as a Second Order Discipline Intervention
A nonlinear interactional pattern in which parents do not express anger toward children can be effective in creating a healthy and functional system
Storytelling does not need extensive instructions
In all types of stories, there are implicit and metaphorical meaning present
Overtraining or suggesting a "right" way to tell stories would impede the parent's spontaneous and creative act of telling a story
Storytelling may not be appropriate for kinds of discipline, such as aggressive behavior
The parents should be clear about the behavior they want to address
The background for the story should be something that the child understands and likes
The characters should be likable and relatable
The story should contain sufficient emotional content
The content of the story should be one that fixes the problem but is unrecognized by the child

identifying the problem the parent wants to change can lead to a subliminal message error on the part of the child and have little effect on the child's behavior.

Second, the background for the story is important because it must be one that is both familiar and of interest to the child. Young children have a great deal of interest in the setting for the story that may not interest their parents, such as garbage dumps or fighting, but parents must allow their child's interests to supersede their own. Knowing places and events that interest the child will help garner attention for the story.

Third, like setting, story characters should be likable and relatable. Most often these characters are fictional from literature or child movies. The characters should be positive in behaviors and attitude but have one problem that needs fixing. This problem or dilemma will need to be explained but should not be identifiable as the child's problem. While the problem should be different from the child's, the way to fix or change it should be similar. This is an important step because the message of the story should not be discernible, but the fix should be applicable.

Fourth, emotional content should not be avoided in the story. One concern with the Inuit storytelling tradition is that not expressing anger may also lead to not expressing other emotions. Humans are emotional and all learning, as has been previously noted, requires emotional input. The story should be constructed with emotional content, including anger, that is followed with an appropriate response to the emotion. In this way, the story can model functional and healthy responses to emotions.

Fifth, the story should contain humor and be fun for the child. Humor adds the human touch and provides a conduit for serious content. In addition, it adds a paradoxical layer of insight that can be missing from factual content.

Sixth, correcting the problem in the story is how the parent wants the child to behave and fixes the problem so that new and more adaptive behavior can develop. The danger here is also that the fix of the problem will be understood in conscious awareness. If the story content is well designed, the conscious decisions that the story carries will not be recognizable as pertaining to the child's situation.

Below is an example of how storytelling can be used as discipline. The story is only meant to be illustrative and not meant to be prescriptive for this or a similar problem. Stories told by parents should be constructed to meet the current challenges they face. Parents are free to be creative with only a few ideas to guide them.

Lisa is a 5-year-old girl and lives with her parents and 1-year-old brother, Ty. Over the past year since her brother was born, Lisa has developed problems both at home and in kindergarten. At home, she refuses to come to the table to eat, dawdles at bedtime, demands numerous stories to be read, or has a temper tantrum. Sometimes she interacts well with Ty and at other times takes toys from him and pushes him down. The parents are afraid to leave her unsupervised with Ty. Some days when she is not in kindergarten, her grandmother takes care of her. At kindergarten,

Lisa has been aggressive with other children, especially boys who are smaller than her. The following story was created by her parents:

> Piggie was a little girl who lived in the corner of the barnyard with her mother and father. She loved to play in the barnyard with other animals including other pigs, goats, geese, chickens, dogs, horses, squirrels, cottontail rabbits, birds, raccoons, and cats. She could not say which friend she liked the most. On the other side of the barnyard was Goose and Charley-Horse where she spent time playing with the toys there. One day when she went home from Goose's house, there was a present wrapped in a small blanket. The present was a very small little pig named Piglet. She loved Piglet but he was too small to play with and she thought they should give him back. Sometimes she just didn't want to be around Piglet. The wise owl sitting on the fence near the corner where she lived reminded her that she knew so much more compared to Piglet and one day, if she taught Piglet some of the things she could do, Piglet would become her favorite animal to play with. Just as Goose and her friends had helped her learn about the barnyard, she could pass on this knowledge to Piglet and this would help Piglet to become as knowledgeable in the barnyard as her.
>
> *(See another version of this story in Roberts, 1994, p. 200)*

References

Aldama, F. L. (2015). Storytelling: Perspectives from cognitive science, neuroscience, and the humanities. *Projections, 9*(1), 80–95. https://doi.org/10.3167/proj.2015.090106

Bargh, J. A., & Morsella, E. (2008). The unconscious mind. *Perspectives on Psychological Science, 3*(1), 73–79. https://doi.org/10.1111/j.1745-6916.2008.00064.x

Bateman, A. (2020). Young children's affective stance through embodied displays of emotion during storytelling. *Text & Talk, 40*(5), 643–668. https://doi.org/10.1515/text-2020-2077

Brockington, G., Moreira, A. P. G., Buso, M. S., da Silva, S. G., Altszyler, E., Fischer, R., & Mollh, J. (2021). Storytelling increases oxytocin and positive emotions and decreases cortisol and pain in hospitalized children. *Proceedings of the National Academy of Science USA, 118*(22), e2018409118. https://doi.org/10.1073/pnas.2018409118; Published online 2021 May 24.

Brown, P. C., Roediger, H. L., & McDaniel, M. A. (2014). *Make it stick.* Harvard University Press.

Carriedo, N., Corral, A., Montoro, P. R., Herrero, L., Ballestrino, P., & Sebastián, I. (2016). The development of metaphor comprehension and its relationship with relational verbal reasoning and executive function. *Public Library of Science, 11*(3), e0150289. https://doi.org/10.1371/journal.pone.0150289; Published online 2016 March 8.

Carroll, N., & Gibson, J. (Eds.). (2011). *Narrative, emotion, and insight.* Pennsylvania State University Press.

Catala, A., Gijlers, H., & Visser, I. (2023). Guidance in storytelling tables supports emotional development in kindergartners. *Multimedia Tools Applications, 82,* 12907–12937. https://doi.org/10.1007/s11042-022-14049-7

Cook, W. (1994). *The handbook of therapeutic storytelling* [Unpublished manuscript].

Craiker, K. (2023). What is a metaphor? Definition, meaning, and examples. *ProWritingAid.* Retrieved December 14, 2023, from https://prowritingaid.com/what-are-metaphors

Creswell, J. D., Bursley, J. K., & Satpute, A. B. (2013). Neural reactivation links unconscious thought to decision-making performance. *Social Cognitive and Affective Neuroscience, 8*(8), 863–869. https://doi.org/10.1093/scan/nst004
Dehghani, M., Boghrati, R., Man, K., Hoover, J., Gimbel, S. I., Vaswani, A., Zevin, J. D. Immordino, M. H., Gordon, A. S., Damasio, A., & Kaplan, J. T. (2017). Decoding the neural representation of story meanings across languages. *Human Brain Mapping,* 38(12), 6096–6106. https://doi.org/10.1002/hbm.23814
Dolan, Y. M. (1985). *The path with a heart: Ericksonian utilization with resistant and chronic clients*. Brunner/Mazel.
Doucleff, J., & Greenhalgh, J. (2019, March 13). How Inuit parents teach kids to control their anger. *NPR*. Retrieved July 24, 2023, from https://www.npr.org/sections/goatsandsoda/2019/03/13/685533353/a-playful-way-to-teach-kids-to-control-their-anger
Dreikurs, R. (1990). *Children the challenge*. Penguin.
Erickson, M. H. (1965). The use of symptoms as an integral part of therapy. *American Clinical Journal of Hypnosis, 18*, 143–155.
Erickson, M. H. (1975). The varieties of double bind. *American Clinical Journal of Hypnosis, 8*, 57–65.
Faber, J., & King, J. (2017). *How to talk so little kids will listen*. Scribner.
Fleer, M., & Hammer, M. (2013). Emotions in imaginative situations: The valued place of fairytales for supporting emotion regulation. *Mind, Culture, and Activity, 20*(3), 240–259. https://doi.org/10.1080/10749039.2013.781652
Gardner, R. A. (1971). *Therapeutic communication with children: The mutual storytelling technique*. Jason Aronson.
Gardner, R. A. (1993). *Storytelling in psychotherapy with children*. Jason Aronson.
Gonçalves, Ó. F., Henriques, M. R., & Machado, P. P. (2004). Nurturing nature, cognitive narrative strategies. In L. E. Angus, L. E. McLeoad, & J. McLeod (Eds.), *The handbook of narrative and psychotherapy: Practice, theory and research* (pp. 103–117). SAGE.
Hoffmann, J., & Russ, S. (2012). Pretend play, creativity, and emotion regulation in children. *Psychology of Aesthetics, Creativity, and the Arts, 6*(2), 175–184.
Krause, R. J., & Rucker, D. D. (2019). Strategic storytelling: When narratives help versus hurt the persuasive power of facts. *Personality and Social Psychology Bulletin, 46*(2), 216–227. https://doi.org/10.1177/0146167219853845
Kuhl, P. K. (2010). The linguistic genius of babies. *TedTalk*. Retrieved July 11, 2023, from https://www.ted.com/talks/patricia_kuhl_the_linguistic_genius_of_babies/transcript?language=en#t-598636
Lenhart, J., Lenhard, W., Vaahtoranta, E., & Suggate, S. (2020). More than words: Narrator engagement during storytelling increases children's word learning, story comprehension, and on-task behavior. *Early Childhood Research Quarterly, 51,* 338–351. https://doi.org/10.1016/j.ecresq.2019.12.009
Martinez-Conde, S., Alexander, R. G., Blum, D., Britton, N., Lipska, B. K., Quirk, G., Swiss, J. I., Willems, R. M., & Macknik, S. L. (2019). The storytelling brain: How neuroscience stories help bridge the gap between research and society. *The Journal of Neuroscience, 39*(42), 8285–8290.
My Play Therapy Page. (2011). *Storytelling*. https://myplaytherapypage.wordpress.com/2011/06/20/storytelling/
National Geographic. (2022). *Storytelling and cultural traditions*. Retrieved July 23, 2023, from https://education.nationalgeographic.org/resource/storytelling-and-cultural-traditions/
Oatley, K. (2019). The human unconscious in evolution. *Psychological Inquiry, 30,* 76–78.
Ochsner, K. N., Ray, R. D., Cooper, J. C., Robertson, E. R., Chopra, S., Gabrieli, J. D. E., & Gross, J. J. (2004). For better or for worse: Neural systems supporting the cognitive down- and up-regulation of negative emotion. *NeuroImage, 23*(2), 483–499.
Padrón, A. (2018). The importance of storytelling in learning. *Vista Higher Learning*. https://vhlblog.vistahigherlearning.com/the-importance-of-storytelling-in-the-learning-process.html

Parker, K. J., Oztan, O., Libove, R. A., & Hardan, A. Y. (2017). Intranasal oxytocin treatment for social deficits and biomarkers of response in children with autism. *Proceedings of the National Academy of Science, 114*(30), 8119–8124. https://doi.org/10.1073/pnas.1705521114

Piaget, J. (1969). *Psychology of the child.* Routledge/Kegan Paul.

Pulvermüller, F. (2005). Brain mechanisms linking language and action. *Nature Reviews Neuroscience, 6,* 576–582.

Roberts, T. W. (1994). *A systems perspective of parenting: The individual, the family, and the social network.* Brooks/Cole.

Simpson, E. A., Sclafani, V., Paukner, A., Hamel, A. F., Novak, M. A., Meyer, J. S., Suomi, S. T., & Ferrari, P. F. (2014). Inhaled oxytocin increases positive social behaviors in newborn macaques. *Proceedings of the National Academy of Science, 111,* 6922–6927. https://doi.org/10.1073/pnas.1402471111

Sommers-Flanagan, J. (2019). *Using therapeutic storytelling with children: Five easy steps.* https://johnsommersflanagan.com/2019/07/08/using-therapeutic-storytelling-with-children-five-easy-steps/

Speer, N. K., Reynolds, J. R., Swallow, K. M., & Zacks, J. M. (2009). Reading stories activates neural representations of visual and motor experiences. *Psychological Science, 20*(8), 989–999. https://doi.org/10.1111/j.1467-9280.2009.02397.x

Suzuki, S., Fujisawa, T. X., Sakakibara, N., Fujioka, T., Takiguchi, S., & Tomoda, A. (2020). Development of social attention and oxytocin levels in maltreated children. *Scientific Reports, 10*(1), 7407. https://doi.org/10.1038/s41598-020-64297-6

Turner, M. (1996). *The literary mind.* Oxford University Press.

Vessel, E., Starr, G. G., & Rubin, N. (2013). Art reaches within: Aesthetic experience, the self and the default mode network. *Frontiers in Neuroscience*, *7*(7), 258. https://doi.org/10.3389/fnins.2013.00258

Wessing, I., Rehbein, M. A., Postert, C., Fürniss, T., & Junghöfer, M. (2013). The neural basis of cognitive change: Reappraisal of emotional faces modulates neural source activity in a frontoparietal attention network. *NeuroImage, 81*(1), 15–25.

Williams, M. (1922). *The velveteen rabbit.* George H. Doran.

Yabe, M., Oshima, S., Eifuku, S., Taira, M., Kobayashi, K., Yabe, H., & Niwa, S. (2018). Effects of storytelling on the childhood brain: Near-infrared spectroscopic comparison with the effects of picture-book reading. *Fukushima Journal of Medical Science, 64*(3), 125–132. https://doi.org/10.5387/fms.2018-11

Yuan, Y., Major-Girardin, J., & Brown, S. (2018). Storytelling is intrinsically mentalistic: A functional magnetic resonance imaging study of narrative production across modalities. *Journal of Cognitive Neuroscience, 30*(9), 1298. https://doi.org/10.1162/jocn_a_01294

Zivan, M., Bar, S., Jing, X., Hutton, J., Farah, R., & Horowitz-Kraus, T. (2019). Screen-exposure and altered brain activation related to attention in preschool children: An EEG study. *Trends in Neuroscience and Education, 17,* 100117. https://doi.org/10.1016/j.tine.2019.100117

Zivan, M., Vaknin, S., Peleg, N., Ackerman, R., & Horowitz-Kraus, T. (2023, May 18). Higher theta-bata ratio during screen-based versus printed paper is related to lower attention in children: An EEG study. *PLoS One*. https://doi.org/10.1371/journal.pone.0283863

9

REFRAMING

Reframing as a Discipline Intervention

The chapter reviews the intervention of reframing that was developed by systemic psychotherapists and can be adapted as an intervention to disciplining children. *Reframing* is a therapeutic technique used to redefine a problem to develop a strategy to solve it. Systemic therapists use reframing as a major maneuver for change because the old definition of the problem was producing little change (Bowen, 1985; Haley, 1997; Minuchin, 1974). *Systemic therapy* is the application of general systems theory to individual and family problems. Individual problems are viewed as occurring within a larger social system that helps maintain the symptoms. Laypersons view mental problems in families as originating only within the mentally disturbed family member. They view the family as normal and want treatment for the mentally ill member. On the other hand, systemic therapists believe that the problem must be redefined from an individual to a family problem. Reframing the problem in family, rather than individual, terms helps create new behaviors that can break the repetitive cycle.

The rationale for reframing centers on the belief that the problem experienced by a family or an individual occurs within a particular context and the context must change to change the problem the individual is experiencing (Haley, 1997). For example, for a couple that constantly disagrees, affecting parenting and other dynamics within the family unit, the therapist could reframe their problem by identifying their heated disagreements, rather than as a negative such as arguing, as a form of communication expressing dynamic energy. This reframe would allow the couple to focus on their relationship in a new light, creating new interventions. Systemic therapists assume that many solutions have been tried resulting in the

DOI: 10.4324/9781003381679-11

solutions becoming the problem, which prevent change. The reframe changes the context and, therefore, allows for a solution.

Reframing by therapists is based on the belief that when individuals or persons have problems, they continue to do *more of the same* to solve them. Instead of trying something different, they continue trying to solve the problem the same way (Haley, 1997). Consequently, the definition of the problem must change. The automatic cycle produced by "doing more of the same" must be interrupted and when the therapist reframes the problem, even the exact opposite behavior can be suggested that would never have been a viable solution before the reframe. This intervention is referred to as "*doing less of the same*."

Haley (1973) described a process of systemic therapy with children that involved the parents. His assumption was the problem at the core was an overinvolved and an underinvolved parent. Simultaneously, the child was underinvolved with peers or other siblings because of the overinvolvement with one of the parents, usually the mother. The strategy in therapy was to reduce the bond with the overinvolved parent and strengthen the bond with the distant parent, peers, and/or siblings.

In strategic therapy with children, the focus moves from the child to the family context (Haley, 1997). In reframing the presenting symptom to a larger context, the intervention changes from the content of the problem to the *process of the problem*. The emphasis is on how the patterns develop that perpetuate the problem, rather than what the patterns are. From this perspective, the present time is more important than trying to change the past. Changes occur from enactments of the family system's dynamic within the therapy room (Minuchin, 1974). Instead of talking about their problems, the family is encouraged to enact them in the present. In this way, the systemic therapist can monitor the process of the interactions and, through reframes, can guide more adaptive responses.

Through reframing, the family can see the problem from a different perspective. The novelty of that alone can be of immense help to creating a more functional realignment in the family. Reframing continues throughout the treatment process and does not stop with reframing the symptoms. Reframing can change negative perceptions into more positive and functional ones. For example, when parents are very angry at a child for noncompliance, this anger can be reframed as love, caring, or wanting the best for their child. This reframe provides a different interactional pattern to emerge. In addition, a reframe of actions in the family interrupts the negative cycle that has engulfed the family. The therapist is constantly forging new directions that are adaptive and functional using reframes.

From the outset in systemic family therapy, the therapist assumes that the family is resistant to change due to the family being a self-regulating system that seeks to maintain balance or equilibrium. While the family may appear to be in chaotic imbalance, the prospect of change is far more disruptive to the family interactional patterns than remaining in chaotic imbalance. According to Minuchin (1974), the therapist is an outsider to the family and that position is weak in influence to change it. Joining means that the therapist is invited into the family and is better able to affect change. Entrance into the family is gained through the person who knows the most about the problem, typically the person who sought therapy for the family. In aligning with that person, the therapist gains credibility from inside the family and can make interventions that change the family structure.

Systemic family therapy is a unique form of therapy because it redefines the symptoms as reflecting the interactional patterns within the family and not the individual. Other forms of therapy generally believe or assume that if there is a presenting problem with a child, then the internal dynamics of the child need altering to address the problem. Although researchers have found both methods of reducing child problems effective, when the child is treated alone, family communication deteriorates (Robbins & Szapocznik, 2000). In addition, children who received treatment with the family unit improved significantly more than children who received group therapy.

In contemporary society, reframing is used in many disciplines, such as business and education (Desautel, 2023). The neuroscience of reframing has received attention in recent publications and training, but little attention exists in parenting literature. A purpose of this chapter is to discuss how reframing in parenting affects the developing brain of the child.

Reframing and Child Misbehavior

While *misbehavior* is generally defined as the child's willful actions in opposition to parental directives, it does not suggest an absolute classification of misbehavior. In essence, misbehavior is what the parent defines as misbehavior. One parent may define a temper tantrum as misbehaving, while another parent may define it as a cute display of emotional intensity. Even when parents define the same behavior as misbehaving, the broader meaning and behavioral significance attached to it may vary. Consequently, misbehavior in children is an arbitrary definition that belies attempts to categorize it into a specific label. This more nuanced meaning of misbehaving means that the general parenting practice of prescribing specific interventions for specific misbehaviors misses the mark and may result in more negative interactions between parent and child.

Not only is there an inconsistency in labeling misbehavior, but a significant number of parents also lack knowledge of normal development and mislabel normal expected behavior as misbehaving. These normal, *expected behaviors* of infants and toddlers include rolling over, beginning to crawl and later to stand and walk, and cognitive and verbal development, such as cooing and vocalizing sounds. Seeking self-identity, developing rational thinking, experiencing puberty, and striving for independence are other developmental sequences as the child develops into adolescence. Researchers have found that parents who are informed about child development milestones provide a healthier environment for children, and social and behavioral outcomes are enhanced (Rikhy et al., 2010). Pediatricians and childcare professionals often rely on the mother's knowledge of developmental milestones to tailor treatment plans, which may miss relevant information (Ertem et al., 2007). At best, parents uninformed about child development lack adequate attention to these behaviors and at worse mislabel normal behaviors as misbehaving. Their parenting practices may not correspond to the timeline of developmental sequences and place too much pressure on the child, resulting in greater problem behaviors. For example, a parent who begins potty training at six months, or one who punishes a child for wetting the bed at the same age, will invariably create a problem because the child is not developmentally ready for potty training and wetting the bed is a normal occurrence with a 6-month-old child.

As stated earlier, viewing the problem as the child's willful behavior may be a pejorative view that contributes to the parent's ineffectiveness in changing the behavior. The idea of misbehavior representing willful behavior has deep roots in parenting literature and contributed to the overemphasis on the control function of parenting. "*Breaking the will*" of a child or breaking the will without breaking the spirit (Dobson, 2017) so that the child submits to parental authority, no doubt, is associated with using harsh punishment if considered necessary and justified to change stubborn and resistive behavior. This perspective is part of the pop culture folklore of parenting interventions.

The question of whether the child is willfully disobeying is being raised in recent research by educators. Research shows that most teachers believe that children misbehaving in school is because of their choice to misbehave (Nash et al., 2015). Similarly, parents tend to perceive the child's misbehavior occurring due to their choice to misbehave. Reframing child misbehavior in school or at home as resulting from a stress response that ran amuck, rather than the willful conscious decision to respond defiantly, will change how teachers and parents respond to the behavior. This suggests that if parents view their child's behavior as stress-induced rather than defiance, a more reasoned response would occur. This view is consistent with a systems view that an individual's behavior reflects their interactional context within a system. For example, the child's misbehavior is more like a canary in a coal mine that reflects the conditions of the system, rather than occurring in a vacuum. The child alone is not the source of the problem. Thus, a child's misbehaving represents a dysfunctional system rather than a dysfunctional child.

The above redefinition is a reframe regarding the parent's perception of the problem and allows for different solutions to be tried. It means that the parent must make efforts to understand what is causing the defiant behavior rather than merely trying to control it. Parents must ask the "how" question and gain an understanding of how it is happening in the present. This shift in how the problem is perceived may not be easily accomplished by parents because it implies that the problem is not external to them but maintained and supported by their own beliefs and behaviors.

The underlying issue in highly stressed families is that stress is reflected in the child's misbehavior because parents tend to project the stress onto the child. The child responds with greater acting out and defiant behavior. The problem is greater than the parent or the child and implies that the family system should be the focus of interventions.

Stress is not the only aspect of child misbehavior. Other reasons for misbehavior stem from the child learning how to secure outcomes that give an advantage in their interactions with parents. For example, a child who dawdles at bedtime and demands more stories may not reflect stress, but rather a skill at knowing how to get what they want (Lerner, 2017). Like their parents, children want to get their way and use different ways of behaving to accomplish it. While these controlling child behaviors can be irritating to the parent, reacting to tighten control and demanding compliance may result in more resistance from the child.

Reframing in the parent–child relationship means one of two things: The parent relabels their own perception of the Child's behavior in a different way, or the parent relabels the child's behavior so that the child is not told they are misbehaving. Parents must realize that they are extremely limited in what they can make their child do, but they can change their perception of the child's behavior. That is, they reframe the meaning of the behavior into a different meaning.

The Neuroscience of Reframing

It is essential that parents know about the neurological underpinnings of their child's behavior. There is little research on the neuroscience of reframing, although there is research that can be applied from studies on negative and positive thoughts and emotions. Most research on the neuroscience of thoughts is on negative emotions. For example, Xie et al. (2023) found that negative emotions, among other things, reduce working memory. The emotional processing area of the brain is primarily the amygdala. One area of the brain, the basolateral, is associated with how the brain shifts emotions. Their preliminary findings indicate that the basolateral area of the amygdala is active in shifting from negative emotions. The findings indicate that alcohol is active in aiding these shifts and may explain how people can drink to excess to reduce negative emotions. Alcohol is a common method people use to self-medicate. Furthermore, the researchers located precise receptors consisting of GABA-A receptors in the basolateral amygdala that were responsible for the switch to positive emotions.

Other research that focused on basolateral amygdala found that if norepinephrine is blocked in this area of the amygdala, mice shift into a state of heightened anxiety. When the receptor α1A adrenoreceptor is disengaged, the fearful response is switched off. The researchers believe that knowing that this area of the brain can be shifted on and off can provide valuable insight into how to acquire equilibrium.

Neuroscientists argue that the brain is hardwired for negative thoughts (Hanson et al., 2021). This means that the brain has a negative bias. The focus on stress and threats to our safety, both psychologically and physically, continues today as seen in vast numbers of persons, including children, contributing to depression and forms of stress-related disorders. Even the smallest threats can set off the negative cycle in the brain, forming negative thoughts and emotions. For many people, this *negative brain bias* is debilitating, causing poor lifetime mental and physical health. Because of this negative bias, positive emotions and thoughts are minimized in neural activity. Negative emotions are quickly stockpiled in memory in the hippocampus, in contrast to positive emotions which require longer time and repeated presentations to store in memory (Table 9.1).

Researchers at Michigan State University have investigated how the brain may be hardwired for negative thoughts and emotions. Moser et al. (2014) showed graphic images to 71 female participants and asked them to think of positive outcomes. The researchers used a female sample because gender differences might affect the outcome of the study. The procedure included a pre-experiment to determine the degree of negative and positive thinking of the participants. For example, researchers showed an image of a man holding a knife against a woman's neck and explaining there were different possible outcomes. The researchers found that when asked to think of positive outcomes, the brain of the negative-thinking group reacted with greater negativity and was unable to put a positive spin on the image. The implication of this research is that telling someone, such as a child, who is worried about something, to think in a positive way will not help and could increase their negative thinking. It underscores the need to reframe the problem so that it changes the way the problem is perceived.

Negative thinking along with other types of thinking, such as deciding what to do in the afternoon, is considered by researchers to be a form of *mind-wandering* (Christoff et al., 2016). Christoff and associates believe that mind-wandering activity in the brain is related to the spontaneous brain function and they were interested in what takes place in the brain when it is at rest. They reviewed approximately 200 brain imaging studies when the brain was not engaged in a conscious activity, and found that the prefrontal cortex, the area of the brain associated with impulse

TABLE 9.1 The Neuroscience of Reframing

Neuroscience and Reframing
Researchers found that if norepinephrine is blocked in the basolateral the amygdala, there is a shift into a state of heightened anxiety, but when the receptor, α1A adrenoreceptor, is disengaged, the fearful response is switched off
Researchers believe that knowing that this area of the brain can be shifted on and off can provide valuable insight into how to acquire equilibrium
The reward center of the brain is activated by both positive and negative emotions
Negative thinking changes how information is processed in the brain
Positive thinking is associated with better physical health
Most of these popularized ways of changing negative thoughts are generic direct suggestions that may not be helpful to a specific person

control, was dominant. On the other hand, when the brain is experiencing a negative cycle, the emotional center of the brain is in control as it was in other forms of spontaneous thought. They hypothesized that the brain at rest vacillates between spontaneous and controlled thoughts. Other researchers have noted that depression is associated with an unbroken cycle of negative emotions (Rantamäki & Kohtala, 2020). The depression cycle strengthens the brain network connections associated with depression and weakens other connections associated with non-depressed thinking.

Recent neuroscience research on the *reward network* in the brain has found that negative emotions can activate the reward network similarly to positive emotions (Wang & Tsien, 2011). Using mice subjects, Wang and Tsien observed dopamine production in the ventral tegmental area and found increased activity in the reward network for both positive and negative experiences. The brain appears to be wired to allow both positive and negative experiences to generate an increase in dopamine.

Negative thoughts and decisions have recently been identified in the caudate nucleus, a region of the brain associated with emotional expressions, by scientists studying the brains of mice (Amemori et al., 2018). Scientists noted that when the caudate nucleus was stimulated, the mice made more negative decisions. The researchers believe that the atypical pattern in the caudate nucleus changes dopamine production.

Childhood stress or trauma, which alters brain chemistry, can continue to affect persons into adulthood and produce negative thinking cycles. Negative thinking changes how information is processed in the brain (Stuart et al., 2019). In investigating how depressed persons process information about faces and language, researchers found that when the subjects learned a particular negative reaction, they remembered it more than a positive reaction. According to Márquez et al. (2013), the brain is altered by early trauma. Using male rat subjects, Márquez et al. found that in teenage traumatized rats, the orbitofrontal cortex, which functions to decrease negative and aggressive impulses, was underdeveloped and the activity in the amygdala, the emotional center of the brain, was increased. In addition, the researchers investigated if the MAOA gene expression, which is related to aggressive attitude in the brain, was altered by the early trauma. The findings confirmed that the level of MAOA gene expression was increased in the prefrontal cortex, which continued into full development.

While there exists much research on negative thinking and the consequences thereof, research on positive thinking is limited and incomplete. *Positive thinking* is defined as an attitude of general optimism that one develops from a focus on thoughts that are conducive to healthy outcomes in mind and body (McGrath, 2004). As with negative thinking, the general attitude and thought patterns of positive thinking can be understood as a chicken-and-egg situation—it is less important which came first, and more important to realize the reciprocal feedback cycle, which serves to further entrench either the positive or negative thinking. In recent literature, mindfulness and other forms of positive thinking have become commonplace in research on moods and attitudes. A recent study sought to determine the effects of mindfulness and positive thinking on emotion regulation and defense mechanisms of borderline patients (Ebrahimi, 2022). The study concluded that training positive thinking skills and mindfulness improved emotion regulation in borderline patients.

Research on positive thinking is based on the premise that stress is not so much the culprit that prevents positive thinking as is the appraisal one makes about the stress. This means that negative thinkers do not necessarily encounter more stress than positive thinkers, but the way each assesses the stressful event accounts for the difference (Jamieson et al., 2018). The experience itself is neutral and can be viewed in multiple ways.

Researchers have found that positive thinking is associated with better physical health. A recent study by Kubzansky et al. (2018) found that cardiovascular health is improved through intervention strategies that enhance social relationships and psychological well-being in cardiac patients. Research indicates that the more optimistic a person was, the more they engaged in healthy eating habits and the less they consumed alcohol or smoked. Overall, optimistic patients had healthier diets, exercised more, and did not smoke. Further, to manage stress, optimistic thinkers planned and used problem-solving skills to combat difficult situations. The researchers felt the focus on healthy diet and exercise was directly related to good heart practices and contrasted with poor problem-solving skills and poor diet of non-optimistic patients. In addition, the social network of optimistic patients was another factor in creating the atmosphere of psychological well-being.

According to recent research, positive thinking is associated with increasing creativity (Nadler et al., 2010). Nadler and associates manipulated the mood of subjects using both happy and sad videos and music before giving them a learning task. The subjects who received the happy video and music performed far better on the learning task than did the subject receiving the sad input. The researchers suggested that a reason people prefer happy music and videos is due to how susceptible people are regarding this stimulus, enhancing a positive mood.

Positive thinking or changing negative into positive thoughts has generated several studies. Reframes generally change what is perceived to be not only negative but unsolvable as well into something that is not perceived as negative and may be considered positive. In contrast to negative feelings of unsolvable problems, a positive frame of mind is related to resilience and emotional health (Silton et al., 2020). Persons who experience positive emotions have increased prosocial behavior and lower levels of cortisol.

Researchers have determined that positive and negative feedback help children at different ages (Figure 9.1) (van Duijvenvoorde et al., 2008). For example, 8-year-old children learn better from positive feedback, while 12-year-old children learn better from negative feedback. Brain imaging shows that the cerebral cortex is the brain region most involved in learning at both ages. Although researchers

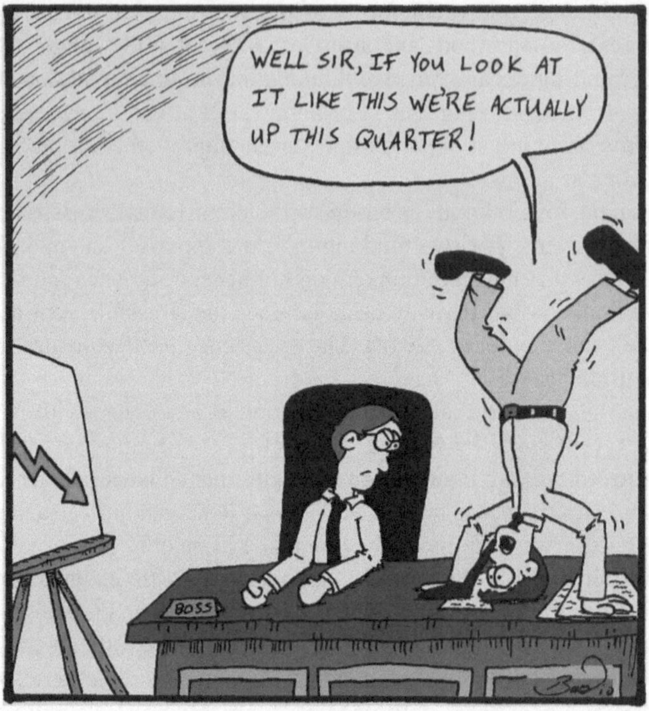

FIGURE 9.1 Reframing a problem can provide solutions that were not apparent before. (www.CartoonStock.com)

are unsure if this difference is due to the brain maturing or greater social experiences, the implication of this finding for teaching children and for disciplining misbehavior speaks for itself. It would say that children younger than 12 are much more amenable, compliant, and cooperative when parents use positive methods of discipline.

Researchers at the Stanford University School of Medicine studied 240 children aged 7–10 and found that being positive improved their ability to answer math problems, increased their memories, and enhanced their problem-solving abilities (Chen et al., 2018). They also used MRI brain scans to map the neurological effects of positivity. The hippocampus, the brain area closely associated with memory, showed improved functions. The impact of positivity on learning was found to be as important as overall IQ. The researchers concluded that although positivity is important and vastly underrated by teachers, it does not work in a vacuum and needs other factors to be successful. Positivity can improve one's ability to see multiple outcomes and, therefore, aid in decision making.

A major focus in the clinical literature on positive thinking is how to turn negative thinking into positive thinking. Researchers have not found a single definitive way to change thinking patterns from negative to positive. Rather, there is a smorgasbord of methods used by psychotherapists (Cuncic, 2023). Self-help websites and blogs are replete with suggestions for dealing with negative thinking and how to change them into positives (Awaken Potential, n.d.). Most of these popularized ways of changing negative thoughts are generic direct suggestions that may not be helpful to a specific person. Relying on oneself through the *self-help approach* popularized by these methods circumvent traditional approaches to therapy that have demonstrated a track record of successful outcomes

Cultural differences exist in conceptualizing positive and negative thinking. While it is not a major difference in Western and Eastern cultures, Westerners tend to prefer positive thinking and Easterners are more varied in preference (You et al., 2009). This difference may rest on the cultural expectations which focus on slightly different premises. For example, in Western culture, the emphasis tends to be on self-enhancement and, in Eastern culture, the emphasis is on self-improvement (Gierlach et al., 2010). While self-enhancement is focused on external goals, such as achieving success or gaining an advantage over others, self-improvement is more concerned with internal goals, such as personal growth and development. Some researchers have challenged this fixed cultural view of positive thinking by adopting a more situational perspective (Malouff & Schutte, 2017).

While noting that positive thinking has many benefits, some researchers have critiqued the popularized version of positive thinking in all forms of literature. For example, researchers have found that when optimistic people are faced with overwhelming negative circumstances, they adopt the worst-case thinking mode that prepares them for the eventual outcome (Shepperd et al., 1996). As optimists face the reality of a negative outcome, they change from being optimistic to being pessimistic. Furthermore, McNulty (2010), in studying newlyweds, found having one's partner in a positive frame may, over time, be detrimental because it dampens repair work that is needed in a long-term marriage. In similar fashion, Gruber et al. (2011) found that optimistic individuals have difficulty empathizing with friends who are, or become, pessimistic.

The cultural differences may reflect underlying philosophical and communication differences. For example, in Eastern cultures, the dialectical perspective permeates much of their view of reality, which allows for a more varied belief about positive and negative thinking (Spencer-Rodgers et al., 2010). This dialectical view is based on the belief that things are always changing and that positive and negative events will merge into each other. Consequently, both positive and negative thinking will converge and overlap. From the perspective of the dialectic, positive thinking is viewed more negatively, and negative thinking is viewed more positively. A recent study found that the differences in positive thinking across cultures are relative in contrast to the view that differences are fixed and distinct (Ji et al., 2021).

In Eastern thought, the dialectic is best understood as the yin and the yang, opposites are bound together in unity. This means that anything that exists carries with it the opposite so that one will lead into the other as day leads into night, which forms a cyclical, repeating pattern. Consequently, the yin and the yang do not occur as separate entities. Dialectical thinking is the antidote to separating negative and positive thinking into distinct camps where one is encouraged to always choose the positive and eliminate the negative (Beers, 2017). It is a reminder that a balance in negative and positive thinking is necessary to be happy and successful and that even positive thinking to the exclusion of the negative can lead to dysfunction. Norem and Chang (2002) come to a similar conclusion and stress that research on positive and negative thinking reflect varied ways in which persons adapt to outcomes or situations. They assert that there is no one condition humans are seeking to attain and one should not be blinded to the belief that one way of thinking is the only path to take. How this decision is related to reframing child misbehavior will be addressed in the following section.

Reframing Child Misbehavior

Reframing child misbehavior refers to changing the definition of the problem, which allows for new strategies to be enacted to solve the problem. In short, it is not about changing negative thoughts and actions into positive thoughts and actions. This use of reframing differs from the popularized version of changing negative thinking into positive thinking because the focus is on process and not outcome. This means that when the problem definition changes, the whole content that supports the problem and helps maintain it also changes. What seemed unsolvable, now has new options for solving the problem. For example, the situation in which a child who dawdles coming to the table at dinner time could be relabeled from misbehaving to having too many things happening at the same time. This simple reframe would change the meaning of the problem from willful defiance to inability to decide among different choices.

Reframing the problem behavior requires that the social system of the child is thoroughly investigated and understood (Haley, 1973). A problem with the child does not develop because the child is bad. Rather, it develops within a context in which a circular feedback loop occurs that provides direction of both present and future behavior. While this conceptualization of the problem may not account for or explain all child misbehavior, it does provide a useful guideline for understanding how child problems are intertwined and maintained within a social environment. This necessary first step is needed in any parent education model and without it, the parenting interventions are, at best, hit or miss.

From a systems/dialectical perspective, the assessment of the family would uncover how the family is organized according to triangles, wholeness, boundaries, hierarchy, roles, rules, among other aspects (Minuchin, 1974). Wholeness refers to behavior that reflects how the parents' behaviors overlap with the child's behavior leading to intervention that is based on the relationship between them, rather than focused solely on individual behavior. Boundaries refer to rules that determine how interactions occur and who is involved in the interaction. In families in which the child is the symptomatic member, one area of concern is *boundary alignment* between parent and child. Symptomatic behavior in the child can result from inappropriate boundaries between parent and child. Firm generational boundaries between parent and child are essential to having functional relationships.

Hierarchy refers to the status of members in the family. Parents should be in the first position of leadership and children should have a second or lower position (Minuchin, 1974). When children have more power than parents, the child is given the ability to control parents' behavior, encouraging symptomatic behavior to occur in the child. A parent who forms a coalition with a child elevates the child in influence and power within the system, which can also demote the other parent to a lower status or child position.

Triangles are interesting because they appear to be supportive and helpful. For example, when one parent is lenient in discipline and undermines the other parent's authority, who is stricter in discipline, initially a child may feel supported by one parent. As this dynamic continues, the close parent becomes ineffective in parenting because they are too close, and the distant parent is ineffective because of being too distant. Symptoms worsen because neither parent is effective (Minuchin, 1974).

One of the main concerns from a systems/dialectical perspective is that the child's symptoms can be a projection of the parents' problems onto the child (Madanes, 1980). As a projection onto the child, the parent is freed from repair work on their issues. This *protective function of the child's symptoms* for the parent is not addressed in parent education models and may be one of the reasons that many families are not changed in participating in parent education programs.

A Systems/Dialectical Perspective of Reframing Child Problems

James and Erica Bentley have been married for 20 years and have three children, Jack 12, Kaleb 10, and Marian 5. James and Erica waited for six years to start their family because they wanted to enjoy their relationship and get established in careers before adding children. They enjoyed outdoor activities together, such as overnight hiking and camping, and weekend ski trips to the mountains in winter. Eventually, they decided that it was time to start their family but it took almost a year before Erica became pregnant with Jack. They wanted their children close in age so, two years after Jack's birth, Kaleb was born. Marian was not planned for, but they were both delighted to have a girl.

After their children were born, many of the things they enjoyed as a couple ceased but they enjoyed parenting and being involved with their children in their activities. Some tensions began to develop in their relationship as the stress of two careers and raising three children begin to weigh on them. Conflict grew in their relationship over the past year and there were rumors that James was having an affair with a coworker, though he denied it and there was no evidence to support it.

To ease tensions, James moved out for a while, and they saw a marriage therapist. After a few months they reconciled, and James moved back home. James continued to deny that he was romantically involved with a coworker and there was no evidence that an affair had occurred.

Over the past year, Jack's behavior became very disruptive in the family, and his academic performance dropped, and social problems occurred at school. James and Erica frequently unfavorably compared Jack's behavior to his siblings, which tended to increase his negative behavior. They believed they had two perfect children and one bad child. Both James and Erica felt that Jack's behavior was out of control, and they had no idea what to do to stop it. They worried he will get with the wrong peer group and be influenced to use drugs or engage in delinquent behavior. James had a period of rebellion in his own teenage and early adulthood years that could have negatively affected his adult life, but after meeting Erica, he got back on the right path. Jack's disruptive behavior occurs at times when stress between James and Erica is intense. Jack's misbehavior evokes stronger reactions from Erica than from James and she accuses James of undermining her discipline of Jack.

At school, Jack's behavior is problematic in that he performs below his abilities and resists teachers' instructions in the classroom. He fails to complete assignments, talks inappropriately, and frequently engages other students in being disruptive. The teacher who complained about Jack's behavior is currently having family difficulty in her own life. She is divorced from her husband and in a custody battle for their 6-year-old son. A conference with the school counselor and the teacher was of little help as James refused to go because he sensed that he would be blamed for Jack's problems.

From a systems/dialectical perspective, a parent educator would be interested in the whole story, not just narrowly focused on Jack's behavior and how the parents are responding to it. The parents obviously need better parenting skills, but much more is needed to bring about second order change in this family. Of primary interest is the marital relationship, which would not be a focal point in most models of parent education. The escalation of Jack's symptoms coinciding with the upheaval in the marriage with James moving out of the home is not accidental; making Jack's behavior the cornerstone of interventions would do little to change the family environment pertinent to his misbehavior. In fact, his behavior is not misbehavior and is an appropriate response to the situation. The first reframe that is needed is to redefine Jack's disruptive behavior from an individual focus that Jack "is bad" to a group focus where the family is understood to crave chaos. The two "perfect children" might be encouraged to participate in the chaos because they have been missing out. While this suggestion for an intervention may sound like therapy, it illustrates that addressing child misbehavior is more nuanced than simply addressing parenting skills or narrowly focusing on improving family functioning through improving communication skills.

A systems/dialectical approach would assume that the marital difficulty and separation of the parents had an adverse effect on Jack, who is on the verge of his teenage years. His misbehaving and school problems brought the parents together to discuss how to deal with him. If they could focus on his problems, they could minimize their own. This protective function of child misbehavior is ignored in all parent education models.

A second reframe is needed to change the perception that Jack's behavior is harmful to the family to the belief that his behavior is necessary. Jack could be encouraged to try other behaviors that bring his parents together. For example, Jack could be encouraged to take his parents to a movie they want to see or an activity that increases positive interactions between the parents.

The neuroscience of this family suggests that Jack experienced trauma in the form of his parents' marital issues and separation. This traumatic experience changed his neuropathways and were repeatedly activated (Zhu et al., 2022). His behavior, mood, and goal-oriented focus were disrupted by the repetition of neural pathways associated with the trauma. The trauma caused Jack to have an overactive amygdala that seeks out and identifies threats in his social environment. The cortisol level, the stress hormone, would be elevated in all family members, but Jack is the family member with acute stress response. The consequence of an overactive amygdala affects the hippocampus by killing cells which affects motivation and memory retention. As a result, Jack continues in a threat mode even when no threat exists and experiences less ability to self-regulate mental and physical symptoms.

According to researchers Zhu et al. (2022), much has been learned about how the brain changes because of experiencing trauma or depression. Changes occur in the salience network, the brain area that is responsible for learning and survival, when an individual has been exposed to depression or trauma. In addition, the researchers found that the group of subjects who were exposed to trauma without psychopathologies, that is not experiencing depression, PTSD, or anxiety, were compensating for the changes in brain functioning by activating their executive control network. This means that individuals who do not develop symptoms are still affected but the response is dampened by the activation of the executive control network. These individuals are categorized as *resilient* and not recognized as having negative consequences from their negative experiences. Furthermore, the negative effects are exacerbated by the presence of negative emotion.

Jack's school problems could be reframed from being disruptive to being over-energized. This reframe would provide new options for changing his behavior. The more positive reframe would reduce his resistance to more appropriate behavior. Another reframe for Jack is that his behavior over the past years has been an unconscious response trying to help his parents stay together. This reframe takes his disruptive behavior out of a negative frame and allows for other behaviors that would be helpful to his parents. The more reframes that Jack experiences, the less likely he will experience negative emotions and the more likely he will experience psychological health (John & Gross, 2004).

Reframes with James and Erica might include reframing how they view their children's behavior, such as their belief that they have two perfect children and one bad child. Jack's behavior could be reframed as their "free-spirited" child. This reframe could dampen the activity in their amygdales which no doubt is stimulated in dealing with Jack's behavior (Buhle et al., 2014). It would also change their interventions from attempting to control his behavior to more positive goal-focused interventions. Researchers have found that persistent relabeling of a negative behavior to a positive behavior can have healthy long-lasting effects (Denny et al., 2015).

James' similar problems as a teenager make his parenting interventions with Jack ineffective because his projection onto Jack is a misplaced way of dealing with his own personal issues. His worry about Jack getting with the wrong crowd and using drugs would increase the likelihood that it will happen. This reframe could be that the future is unknown and that multiple outcomes are possible. James could be helped in envisioning different possible scenarios to Jack's problems.

Reframes could be used in both group and individual parent education models but are better-suited for individual sessions. Research shows that parents prefer individual parent education sessions to group sessions and expect to receive help with their specific problems. When their specific problems are not addressed, this serves as an explanation for why many parents fail to complete the program (Chacko et al., 2012). Researchers have found that parents' expectation for parent educators' interventions can lead to failed treatment and high attrition rates when expectations are not met (Nock & Kazdin, 2005).

The theory behind these reframes is, once the problem is viewed differently, the neural pathways and behaviors that maintain them will be interrupted and new patterns can emerge. This does not suggest that all parent educators need to do is to reframe a problem and solutions will occur. Rather, the implication is that when dysfunctional patterns are interrupted, different patterns will emerge. The use of reframes helps define the underlying dynamics and moves the family in a different direction. Once positive change occurs, the effect is magnified due to a cascading of new behaviors.

References

Amemori, K., Amemori, S., Gibson, D. J., & Graybiel, A. M. (2018). Striatal microsimulation induces persistent and repetitive negative decision-making predicted by striatal beta-band oscillation. *Neuron*. https://doi.org/10.1016/j.neuron.2018.07.022

Awaken Potential. (n.d.). *The power of positive affirmation for success and happiness*. https://awakenpotential.org/positive-affirmations/?utm_source=adw&utm_campaign=Free+books&utm_agid=151479160315&gclid=CjwKCAjw_uGmBhBREiwAeOfsdt4U8Fr1_iHXptlH5XgLMA0bFd1bmeCjs4_xFHXAXjSRSiPpBoAsxoCS1MQAvD_BwE

Beers, H. (2017, January). *The yin-yang of positive thinking*. https://www.linkedin.com/pulse/yin-yang-positive-thinking-helen-beers/

Bowen, M. (1985). *Family therapy in clinical practice*. Jason Aronson.
Buhle, J. T., Silvers, J. A., Wager, T. D., Lopez, R., Onyemekwu, C., Kober, H., Weber, J., & Ochsner, K. N. (2014). Cognitive reappraisal of emotion: A meta-analysis of human neuroimaging studies. *Cerebral Cortex, 24,* 2981–2990. https://doi.org/10.1093/cercor/bht154
Chacko, A., Wymbs, B., Chimiklis, A., Wymbs, F., & Pelham, W. (2012). Evaluating a comprehensive strategy to improve engagement to group-based behavioral parent training for high-risk families of children with ADHD. *Journal of Abnormal Child Psychology, 40,* 1351–1362.
Chen, L., Bae, S. R., & Menon, V. (2018). Positive attitude towards math supports early academic success: Behavioral evidence and neurocognitive mechanism. *Psychological Sciences, 29*(3), 390–402. https://doi.org/10.1177/0956797617735528
Christoff, K., Irving, Z. C., Fox, K., Spreng, R. N., & Andrews-Hanna, J. R. (2016). Mind-wandering as spontaneous thought: A dynamic framework. *Nature Reviews Neuroscience, 17*(11), 718. https://doi.org/10.1038/nrn.2016.113
Cuncic, A. (2023, April). How to stop negative thoughts. *Verywell Mind.* https://www.verywellmind.com/how-to-change-negative-thinking-3024843
Denny, B. T., Inhoff, M. C., Zerubavel, N., Davachi, L., & Ochsner, K. N. (2015). Getting over it: Long-lasting effects of emotion regulation on amygdala response. *Psychological Science, 26,* 1377–1388. https://doi.org/10.1177/0956797615578863
Desautels, L. (2023). The power of reframing to 'rewire' students' brains. *George Lucas Educational Foundation.* Retrieved August 1, 2023, from edutopia.org/article/reframing-rewire-student-brains/
Dobson, J. C. (2017). *The new strong-willed child.* Tyndale Momentum.
Ebrahimi, S. S. A. A. (2022). The effectiveness of mindfulness-based therapy and positive thinking on emotion regulation and defense mechanisms in people with borderline personality disorder in improving post-traumatic brain injury. *Journal of Assessment and Research in Applied Counseling, 4*(1), 6–10. https://doi.org/10.52547/jarac.4.2.13
Ertem, I. O., Atay, G., Dogan, D. G., Bayhan, A., Bingoler, B. E., Gok, C. G., Ozbas, S., Haznedaroglu, D., & Isikli, S. (2007). Mothers' knowledge of young child development in a developing country. *Child Care, Health and Development, 33*(6), 728–737.
Gierlach, E., Belsher, B. E., & Beutler, L. E. (2010). Cross-cultural differences in risk perceptions of disasters. *Risk Analysis: An International Journal, 30*(10), 1539–1549.
Gruber, J., Mauss, I. B., & Tamir, M. (2011). A dark side of happiness? How, when, and why happiness is not always good. *Perspectives on Psychological Science, 6,* 222–233.
Haley, J. (1973). Strategic therapy when a child is presented as the problem. *Journal of the American Academy of Child Psychiatry, 12*(4), 641–659. https://doi.org/10.1016/S0002-7138(09)61273-5
Haley, J. (1997). *Leaving home: The therapy of disturbed young people*. Brunner/Mazel.
Hanson, R., Shapiro, S., Hutton-Thamm, E., Hagerty, M. R., & Sullivan, K. P. (2021). Learning to learn from positive experiences. *The Journal of Positive Psychology, 18*(3), 1–12. https://doi.org/10.1080/17439760.2021.2006759
Jamieson, J. P., Hangen, E. J., Lee, H. Y., & Yeager, D. S. (2018). Capitalizing on appraisal processes to improve affective responses to social stress. *Emotion Review, 10*(1), 30–39.
Ji, L.-J., Vaughan-Johnston, T. I., Zhang, Z., Jacobson, J. A., Zhang, N., & Huang, X. (2021). Contextual and cultural differences in positive thinking. *Journal of Cross-Cultural Psychology, 52*(5), 449–467.
John, O. P., & Gross, J. J. (2004). Healthy and unhealthy emotion regulation: Personality processes, individual differences, and life span development. *Journal of Personality, 72,* 1301–1333. https://doi.org/10.1111/j.1467-6494.2004.00298.x
Kubzansky, L. D., Huffman, J. C., Boehm, J. K., Hernandez, R., Kim, E. S., Koga, H. K., Feig, E. H., Lloyd, D. M., Seligman, M. E. P., & Labarthe, D. R. (2018). Positive psychological well-being and cardiovascular disease. *Journal of the American College of Cardiology, 72*(12), 1382. https://doi.org/10.1016/j.jacc.2018.07.042

Lerner, C. (2017). Reframing “misbehavior”: Lessons from the toddler years. *PBC SoCal*. Retrieved August 4, 2023, from https://www.pbs.org/parents/thrive/reframing-misbehavior-lessons-from-the-toddler-yearsc

Madanes, C. (1980). Protection, paradox, and pretending. *Family Process, 19,* 73–85.

Malouff, J. M., & Schutte, N. S. (2017). Can psychological interventions increase optimism? A metaanalysis. *The Journal of Positive Psychology, 12*(6), 594–604.

Márquez, C., Poirier, G. L., Cordero, M. I., Larsen, M. H., Groner, A., Marquis, J., Magistretti, P. J., Trono, D., & Sandi, C. (2013). Peripuberty stress leads to abnormal aggression, altered amygdala and orbitofrontal reactivity and increased prefrontal MAOA gene expression. *Translational Psychiatry, 3*(1), e216. https://doi.org/10.1038/tp.2012.144

McGrath, P. (2004). The burden of RA RA positive: Survivors’ and hospice patients’ reflection on maintaining a positive attitude to serious illness. *Support Care Cancer, 12,* 25–33.

McNulty, J. K. (2010). When positive processes hurt relationships. *Current Directions in Psychological Science, 19,* 167–171.

Minuchin, S. (1974). *Families and family therapy*. Harvard University Press.

Nadler, R. T., Rabi, R., & Minda, J. P. (2010). Better mood and better performance: Learning rule described categories is enhanced by positive mood. *Psychological Science, 21,* 1770–1776. https://doi.org/10.1177/0956797610387441

Nash, P., Schlösser, A., & Scarr, T. (2015). Teachers’ perceptions of disruptive behavior in schools: A psychological perspective. *Emotional and Behavioral Difficulties, 21*(2), 167–180. https://doi.org/10.10802796015.2012.12087517

Nock, M. K., & Kazdin, A. E. (2005). Randomized controlled trial of a brief intervention for increasing participation in parent management training. *Consulting Clinical Psychologist, 73*(5), 872–879. https://doi.org/10.1037/0022-006X.73.5.872

Norem, J. K., & Chang, E. C. (2002). The positive psychology of negative thinking. *Journal of Clinical Psychology, 58*(9), 993–1001.

Rantamäki, T., & Kohtala, S. (2020). Encoding, consolidation, and renormalization in depression: Synaptic homeostasis, plasticity, and sleep integrate rapid antidepressant effects. *Pharmacological Reviews, 72*(2), 439. https://doi.org/10.1124/pr.119.018697

Rikhy, S., Tough, S., Trute, B., Benzies, K., Kehler, H., & Johnston, D. W. (2010). Gauging knowledge of developmental milestones among Albertan adults: A cross-sectional survey. *BMC Public Health, 10*(1). https://doi.org/10.1186/1471-2458-10-183

Robbins, M. S., & Szapocznik, J. (2000, April). Brief strategic family therapy. *Juvenile Justice Bulletin. U.S. Department of Justice*. https://citeseerx.ist.psu.edu/document?repid=rep1&type=pdf&doi=441fcaa5f973126df72fdcc5ffb9e74a0d54d9f5

Shepperd, J. A., Ouellette, J. A., & Fernandez, J. K. (1996). Abandoning unrealistic optimism: Performance estimates and the temporal proximity of self-relevant feedback. *Journal of Personality and Social Psychology, 70,* 844–855.

Silton, R. L., Kahrilas, I. J., Skymba, H. V., Smith, J., Bryant, F. B., & Heller, W. (2020). Regulating positive emotions: Implications for promoting well-being in individuals with depression. *Emotion, 20*(1), 93–97. https://doi.org/10.1037/emo0000675

Spencer-Rodgers, J., Peng, K., & Wang, L. (2010). Dialecticism and the co-occurrence of positive and negative emotions across cultures. *Journal of Cross-Cultural Psychology, 41*(1), 109–115.

Stuart, S. A., Hinchcliffe, J. K., & Robinson, E. S. J. (2019). Evidence that neuropsychological deficits following early life adversity may underlie vulnerability to depression. *Neuropsychopharmacology*. https://doi.org/10.1038/s41386-019-0388-6

van Duijvenvoorde, A. C. K., Zanolie, K., Rombouts, S. A. R. B., Raijmakers, M. E. J., & Crone, E. A. (2008). Evaluating the negative or valuing the positive? Neural mechanisms supporting feedback-based learning across development. *The Journal of Neuroscience, 28*(38), 9495–9503. https://doi.org/10.1523/JNEUROSCI.1485-08.2008

Wang, D. V., & Tsien, J. Z. (2011). Convergent processing of both positive and negative motivational signals by the VTA dopamine neuronal populations. *Public Library of Science (PLoS One)*, *6*(2), e17047. https://doi.org/10.1371/journal.pone.0017047

Xie, W., Ye, C., & Zhang, W. (2023). Negative emotion reduces visual working memory recall variability: A meta-analytical review. *Emotion, 23*(3), 859–871. https://doi.org/10.1037/emo0001139

You, J., Fung, H. H., & Isaacowitz, D. M. (2009). Age differences in dispositional optimism: A cross-cultural study. *European Journal of Ageing*, *6*(4), 247–252.

Zhu, X., Suarez-Jimenez, B., Lazarov, A., Such, S., Marohasy, C., Small, S. S., Wager, T. D., Lindquist, M. A., Lissek, S., & Neria, Y. (2022). Sequential fear generalization and network connectivity in trauma exposed humans with and without psychopathology. *Communications Biology*, *5,* 1275. https://doi.org/10.1038/s42003-022-04228-5

10

HUMOR

Theories of Humor

There are several theories about humor and how humor affects human mental states and interactions with others. *Relief theory*, the first theory of humor, was first popularized by Spencer (1911), over 100 years ago. He was interested in understanding the implicit meaning in the physiology of laughter, rather than the content of the joke. He concluded laughter was the release of pent-up emotions and subsequent increase of energy. Humor allows a release of tension and therefore provides a healthy alternative to being overwhelmed with emotional pressure. Humor allows for a healthier release of emotion and return to a state of equilibrium. There are some obvious weaknesses to this theory. For example, laughter is a spontaneous activity that often occurs in response to others in a social setting. Furthermore, the more stressed a person is, the less likely laughter will be engaged in, which would contradict the main tenant of this theory. If a stressed-out person does engage in laughter, it tends to be minimal and of short duration.

Another theory of humor is the *incongruity resolution theory*, which is based on the process involved in resolving an inconsistent experience (Couder, 2019). The human brain can entertain incongruities when they are framed within a logical context. What is set in motion by the incongruity is a type of problem-solving. When the joke is understood, the resolution brings a feeling of satisfaction like solving a problem. Incongruity theory is broad and can be described as an umbrella theory, which reduces explanatory significance. Said another way, incongruity theory does not specifically identify the difference between incongruity caused by humor and other incidences of incongruity. Furthermore, incongruity theory fails at the basic understanding of what constitutes humor in that it does not explain why some things are funny and other things are not funny.

DOI: 10.4324/9781003381679-12

The third theory of humor is the *superiority theory* (Wilson, 2017). There is an element in humor that delights in making fun of others who are perceived to be different or inferior. It also involves self-deprecating humor in which one can laugh at their former or present ignorance or limitations. Choosing certain people to make fun of is the use of humor to control interactions and keep some people in a submissive posture. This theory has detractors, such as Solomon (2002), who called for an "inferiority theory of humor." Instead of viewing oneself as superior, one uses self-deprecating humor and laughs at oneself as a way to not take a situation or oneself so seriously. Slapstick humor and laughing at one's physical foibles is a central element of cartoons and stand-up comedy and movie entertainment. Consequently, the feeling of superiority is not necessary to experience humor. It is also clearly obvious that feeling superior is unrelated to many things that a person could find humorous. For example, many people have pets that they feel superior to, but the pet is not necessarily a source of humor. While feelings of superiority might be a source of some humor, it cannot explain all humor and, therefore, is only a partial explanation.

These three theories of humor are only the tip of the iceberg in understanding the meaning and application of humor. While each specifies a unique understanding of humor, they are not in competition and should be viewed as different aspects of the same concept. Each theory answers different questions about humor and, therefore, work better as a group than as individual stand-alone, fully explanatory theories.

Humor is a human state of mind that is present in all societies of the world and reflected in a variety of human interactions, including disciplining children. Unfortunately, humor is underutilized in parenting, particularly in discipline strategies. Perhaps a reason for the reticence of using humor is an overemphasis on the control function of parenting and the belief that controlling the child's behavior requires a serious demeanor. Humor may not be appropriate for all parental disciplining behaviors, but for parents to resist using humor in all incidences of discipline is equivalent to throwing the baby out with the bath water.

Successful parenting requires a plethora of knowledge and techniques which are used in specific situations. It is a matter of knowing a lot of ways to intervene and then allowing the situation at hand to guide how the parent responds. Consequently, there is no need to prescribe what the responses would be to a situation that has not yet occurred. Parents must trust their instincts and allow themselves the flexibility of a spontaneous response. While this approach might seem to increase the anxiety of parenting, it serves as a freeing experience from having to follow certain set-in-stone intervention guidelines.

The use of humor in discipline creates novelty and is an abrupt change to what is expected. Humor is a surprise experience for the child and may increase the desire to cooperate. It can promote bonding and a sense of shared reality. Young children are prone to temper tantrums, which are not only disruptive but also can cause parents to negatively respond, resulting ultimately in a cycle of parental overcontrol and the child's resistance. Although there are other ways to increase bonding with one's child, the use of humor may have a profound influence on how the child responds to adversity throughout their lifetime.

According to Lawrence Cohen (2002), parenting should be playful and fun. It is done best when the parent joins the child's world with all the struggles in the process of maturing. Play and make-believe comprise the child's world. Entering that world with the child makes it possible for the parent to grow in their understanding of the child's behaviors. By partaking in the child's world, a new perspective on the child's emotions and motivations can be gained. This playful attitude need not be done as a last resort when the parent–child relationship has been damaged, but as an ongoing pattern which can help buffer this relationship from stress and dysfunction. Playfulness and humor in parenting can be a distinctive and authentic parenting technique in addition to being an intervention method to bond with the child. A review of the literature on humor summarized in the following section can reveal how essential humor is to a child's well-being.

The Benefits of Humor

Ample research over the past 40 years has demonstrated the importance of humor for positive outcomes in children (McGhee, 1989; Rutter, 1990; Tannenbaum, 1983). For Rutter (1990), humor is a way to increase resilience in children because it acts as an antidote to stress-related problems. Tannenbaum's investigation of gifted children revealed that they were more creative and innovative in seeing things from different perspectives and, therefore, more instrumental in constructing humor. Humor allows for the suspension of one's perceptions of reality and permits other alternative realities to be entertained simultaneously, which provides a benefit for dealing with difficulties. This means that one is not stuck in a single view of perceiving events and experiences (Figure 10.1).

The benefits of humor have been demonstrated through research in medicine, psychology, religion, and biology, to name a few areas. William Fry (1994) was one of the first and most noted researchers on humor and coined the phrase *gelotology*, the study of laughter. Fry's research was a forerunner for other research that established the relation between laughter and physiological changes within the human body. *Humor* is characterized by researchers as an emotion that has profound influence on heart rate, blood pressure, and other bodily functions, especially affecting the immune system (McGhee, 1999). Emotional responses, including humor, are consistent among humans regardless of culture.

According to research, humor reduces the stress hormone cortisol while simultaneously increasing antibodies that enhance the immune system (Bennett & Lengacher, 2007). Social interactions are more collaborative and cooperative when humor is an essential part to the interaction (Chadwick & Platt, 2018). The classroom experience can be one of reduced stress when subject matter is presented in a humorous way (Penberg, 2023). Additionally, humor is an essential element to the holistic approach to treating persons' mental and physical illnesses.

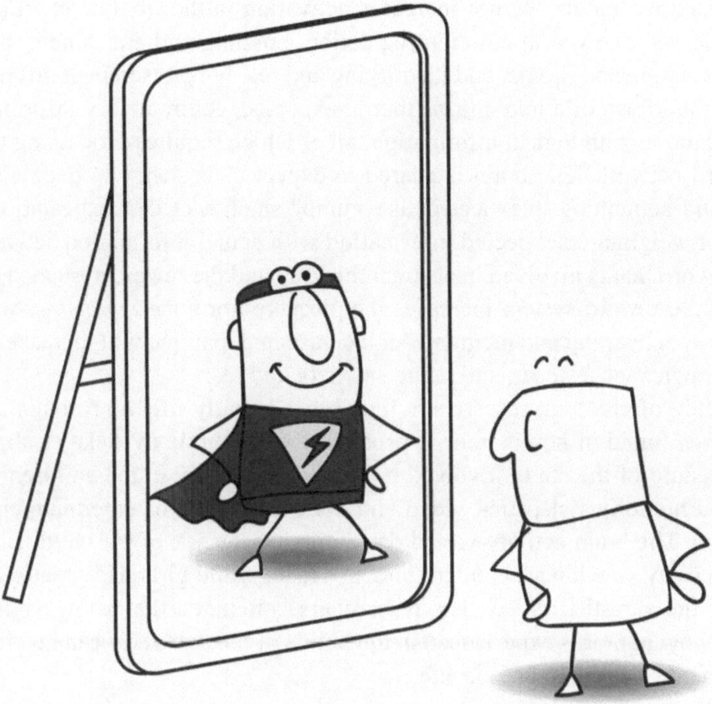

FIGURE 10.1 Humor allows us to see ourselves and others differently.

While much research has demonstrated that humor has many positive outcomes, some research has focused on the effects of an inability to experience humor in some mental disorders, such as in *schizophrenia* and depression (Berger et al., 2021). Childhood disorders that show reduced ability to engage in and/or appreciate humor have received much attention in the extant literature on childhood disorders. Research reveals that children 3–7 years of age with autism express less interest in telling humorous stories and respond less to others using humor (Reddy et al., 2002). The lack of humor responses is indicative of marked social and interpersonal skills among autistic children. On the other hand, teaching humor and using humorous stories with autistic children can improve their social skills and interpersonal relationships (Martin & Yip, 2006). Teaching autistic children the nuance of a joke is necessary since they may have difficulty processing the incongruence inherent in humor.

Humor and Brain Neuroplasticity

Humor enhances the learning experience because it affects brain plasticity (Cozolino, 2013). There is no "humor center" in the brain per se, but several brain networks are activated by humor. Humor increases activation in the frontal network of the brain which is involved in emotion regulation, bonding and attachment, processing contradiction and illogic, and identifying and resolving discrepant information. Humor in the form of a joke means that unexpected, contradictory information is presented along with logical information, all of which requires processing through the reward network. The brain is geared to expect consistency in people's experiences and something unexpected like humor sidetracks that expectation. This process of weighing unexpected information with actual information activates the brain network that is involved in abstract thinking and the reward system. The activation of the reward system increases the pleasure hormone *dopamine,* which in turn improves learning and memory. An increase in dopamine will increase energy, promote higher self-esteem, and reduce anxiety and fear.

In a study of children, researchers found that in early life, a profound sex difference was found in how humor is processed in the brain (Vrticka et al., 2013). The procedure of the study involved noting brain activity in the children as they watched a humorous slapstick video and a different type of entertainment, such as dancing. The brain activity varied depending on the sex of the child: Boys had greater activity watching the entertainment video, while girls had greater activity watching the slapstick video. The researchers concluded that knowing the processes of how humor is experienced in the brains of the two sexes can be important for treatment of children later in life.

In another study of children diagnosed with cancer who experienced significant physical pain, researchers found that, when viewing humorous videos, there was significantly more tolerance of, but not a decrease in the pain as compared to when watching other non-humorous videos (Stuber et al., 2009). The researchers concluded that the study should be taken with the caveat that other forms of pain tolerance were not studied, and humor may be one of many distractions that increase tolerance to pain.

Researchers have found that merely anticipating a humorous event can produce amazing results in the brain (American Physiological Society, 2008, April 10). For example, beta-endorphins, chemicals that reduce depression, increased by 27%, and *human growth hormone*, which improves immunity, increased by 87% from anticipating watching a humorous movie. In a follow-up study, the same researchers found that, using the same procedure, anticipating laughter reduced cortisol levels by 39%, *adrenaline* by 70%, and a chemical used to produce *epinephrine* by 38%. These chemicals, which produce epinephrine, are typically related to stress and anxiety.

Studies have demonstrated the efficacy of humor in adjusting to small failures (Stoeber & Janssen, 2011). Researchers conducted a study of college students using recordings of a daily diary of their experiences and how they felt about them, including what they did to alleviate them. Common strategies to dealing with their failures included seeking emotional support, religion, venting, denial, substance abuse, and disengagement. These strategies did not produce satisfaction at the end of the day and the more the students practiced these strategies, the less satisfied they were. On the other hand, when students used strategies that included positive reframes, humor, and acceptance, they were more satisfied at the end of the day. This study concludes that regardless of the experience of failure, the more the humor, acceptance, and reframing used, the better the adjustment.

Overall, research finds that when teachers use humor with their students, the students will rate them more positively than teachers who do not use humor. Researchers have concluded that curriculum-specific humor has an enormous impact on retention of material and positive rates for teacher performance (Garner, 2006). Humor in a learning situation increases attention and arousal that sparks greater interest in learning and retention of information (Cozolino, 2013). Humor also stimulates the right hemisphere of the brain, which connects to the right hemisphere of others, creating an intersubjective experience that facilitates bonding. As a result, social relationships are reinforced, and interactions are less stressful. The stimulations of numerous brain regions act to increase neural integration across the brain.

One of the key elements in learning is the social component: Children typically learn in a social or group setting. While humor has been touted as conducive to learning, some researchers have found that not all humor improves learning (Wanzer et al., 2010). Wanzer et al. concluded that not all forms of humor enhance learning and some types of humor may be met with considerable alarm. This may be due to lack of appropriate ways to evaluate how humor is perceived. Wanzer et al. state that teachers typically think that laughter at their humor means it is received well, but this may not be the best way to evaluate the effectiveness of humor as a learning tool. For learning to be enhanced by humor, Wanzer et al. conclude that the ability to process information is essential. The theory of processing, they propose, is *Instructional Humor Processing Theory* (IHPT), which posits that students must first cognitively process and judge the appropriateness of the humor and determine if the humor enhances the recall of information.

Brain injury can result in an inability to appreciate humor (Keegan et al., 2021). When the right brain, the network related to experiencing wholeness, has sustained injury, the inability to experience humor follows. The ability to shift between one's expectations of an interaction and the actual incongruity of the joke is damage resulting from a literal interpretation that fails to understand the joke.

Recent research on humor has identified that some forms of humor can have negative consequences (Plessen et al., 2020). Researchers differ on the number of styles of humor and reach different heuristic definitions. While different definitions of humor exist in the literature, a common aspect is that humor represents a stable personality trait. The most used research instrument for determining the style of humor is the *Humor Styles Questionnaire (HSQ)* (Martin et al., 2003), which identifies four styles of humor. Two of the styles, *self-enhancing humor* and *affiliative humor*, are related to positive outcomes (Greengross, 2019, December 6). The other two styles, *self-defeating humor* and *aggressive humor*, are related to negative outcomes. Affiliative and self-enhancing humor, both associated with positive interactions with others, reflect an outgoing, cooperative, or extroverted personality. In addition, positive styles of humor are related to being more conscientious and a desire to have positive and helpful relationships. On the other hand, the two negative styles of humor, self-defeating and aggressive, are associated with neuroticism and a more severe mental condition of psychopathology, in which persons have more pronounced symptomatology.

Although humor has been applied to coping and improving life experiences, it has only recently been advanced as an intervention in psychotherapy (Gremigni, 2012). In the marriage and family therapy literature, the use of humor was a central foundation in the writings of authors, such as Watzlawick et al. (2011) and Carl Whitaker (1975). Most notably was Whitaker's development of play therapy for the whole family. His therapy was based on the principle of families being stuck in rigid patterns and playfulness in therapy was one to break through this rigidity.

The use of humor in marriage and family therapy is based on the view that severe problems, in which clients resist change, require implicit and paradoxical interventions (Whitaker, 1975). In such cases, direct, cognitive interventions fail to create change because family members are stuck in patterns of interactions that are reinforced by explicit means. In general, systemic therapies embrace the use of humor as a spontaneous intervention that can help the family view things differently. Therefore, systemic therapists view humor to be present with the client or family and intervene strategically which goes beyond the comedic effect of viewing humor as laughter. Humor is a communication intervention that builds rapport and a sense of unity. Humor binds persons together, increases trust, and improves cooperation.

The benefits of humor in psychotherapy include improving self-reflection and processing one's beliefs and actions (Figure 10.2) (Gelkopf, 2011). Taking oneself less seriously can act to increase the likelihood of an aha experience and change the dynamic surrounding the problem formation and maintenance. Changing the perspective from viewing oneself as having problems or being deficient to having more acceptance and understanding of oneself is essential in reducing symptomatology. While all therapy models attempt to reduce symptomatology primarily through verbal means, humor cuts through the verbal content to make changes implicitly.

Increasingly, humor is popular in family therapy and other forms of group psychotherapy. In groups, there is an advantage of using humor due to the "*social contagion*" nature of humor (Gelkopf, 2011). Humor expressed in a group setting has social effects that are not present in individual expressions of humor. Humor promotes a feeling of well-being within the group and increases relaxation and acceptance among others.

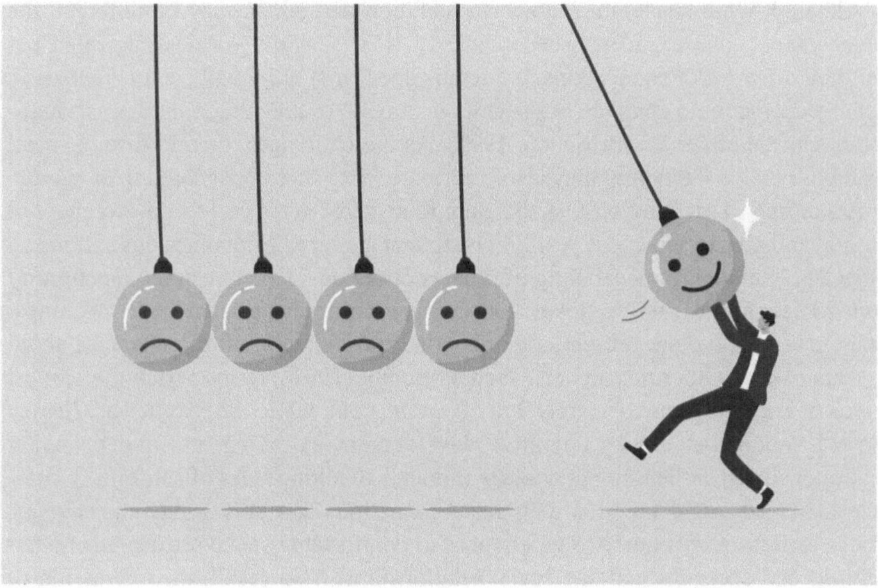

FIGURE 10.2 Humor can be used as a method to disrupt a chain of negative events; to shake up the brain's negative bias, lead to positive input, and affect change; and to impact others in a socially contagious manner.

How Humor Can Be Used in Parenting

Humor may be especially helpful when children are overwhelmed with too many demands on them and retreat into their own safe space. They may also act out with angry outbursts at parents for what they perceive to be parental intrusion into their sacred space. A typical reaction from parents is to identify the child as having an attitude problem or withdrawing from expected activities and begin a regimen of imperatives to get the child back on track. The parents' maneuvers can easily be misinterpreted as punishment and the child may commonly resist their efforts to amend the problem. A vicious cycle can ensue with the child feeling more isolated and resistive and the parent increasing control efforts.

Instead of increasing the parental control default response, parents could engage in a more spontaneous and free expression of humor. Humorous interactions, which occur spontaneously and mostly unconsciously, are important for both children and adults to adjust to stressful situations. No one must consciously think that they will use humor to reduce their stress level. Rather, humor is the common antidote to reducing stress and anxiety naturally. While humor is a spontaneous activity, parents can also plan and devise humorous response interventions to their children's behaviors.

Although what constitutes humor for children and adults may be different, the engagement in humor can have beneficial effects. The child's world is magical in that children often make connections to circumstances that are unique and paradoxical, which become more complex as the child matures. For this reason, humor is a natural circumstance for them (Mahon, 1992). As the child ages, the increase in social relations outside the family may also contribute to a better understanding of humor.

According to McGhee (1999), there are four stages in the child's development of humor, and all can supersede reality. The four stages are (1) incongruous actions on objects; (2) incongruous labeling of objects or actions; (3) conceptual incongruity and riddles; and (4) telling jokes that involve ambiguity and multiple meanings. Stage one and two are present beginning at approximately 18 months until about 3 years of age. Other researchers, such as Reddy (1991), pushed back the earliest forms of humor to approximately 9 or 10 months old, while others, such as Chaney (1993), found that child's cognitive development in telling and understanding humor occurred earlier than previously thought. Breaking rules of conformity characterize these stages coupled with slapstick actions and silly songs and rhymes. These expressions of humor happen more in comfortable social settings than other settings and serve to facilitate social relationships. As a result, the expression of humor from the earliest ages coincides with other developmental milestones that aid in emotional development. Stage three begins at about age 4 and stage four begins at about 6 years of age. These stages occur from the child's maturing brain, resulting in greater cognitive complexity and language development, which allows for increased appreciation for ambiguity and multiple meanings.

Understanding incongruity is an essential element in a child's appreciation and use of humor. Along with learning expected behaviors, children delight in upending the expected for novel or different outcomes. Children have a penchant for memes, impersonations, knock-knock jokes, and riddles and use any opportunity to express them. Other things that make children laugh are flatulate noises, swear words, wedgies, dressing pets to look like humans, cartoons, and many other things too numerous to mention (Bongiorno, 2019).

Childhood humor tells us a great deal about child development because their appreciation and use of humor corresponds to their developmental level. Specific developmental issues are highly present in children's humor. For example, a toddler struggling with toilet training may find jokes about the bathroom funny, while a child 10 years or older may not. Interactive games with parents reflect developmental issues as well. For example, the game of peekaboo is loved by 1-year-old infants but not paid attention to by older children. Likewise, 2-year-olds find an object of clothing placed differently on the body as very humorous because there is some recognition that it is out of the normal order of things, such as putting underwear on one's head.

Older children around 6 years of age will find more abstract and cognitively challenging actions to be funny. For example, a joke that makes them process the information is both funny and challenging. Asking a question like, "How do you turn soup into gold?" can be funny and cognitively stimulating. The answer requires cognitive processing and knowing the relation between the elements of the joke. If they can solve it by saying, "All you do is add 24 carrots," it is both funny and they feel satisfied in their thinking ability. If they cannot answer it, their thinking ability is strengthened by being told how the elements are unified.

As children enter adolescence and experience a new wave of developmental changes, their taste in humor shifts again (Fox et al., 2016). For example, the jokes they laughed at as younger children are not funny now and there is a clear gender difference to humor. Boys enjoy jokes about aggression and sexual content, while girls are more likely to laugh at situations that are embarrassing or socially awkward.

Researchers have identified three styles of humor related to developmental issues for adolescents. One type that is prevalent in adolescents is *disparaging humor* associated with aggressive media (Martins & Riddle, 2021). Martins and Riddle found that entertainment and movies that targeted adolescents was more aggressive than movies and entertainment geared to adult audiences, and tended to glamorize violence. This type of humor makes adolescents laugh and is associated with imitation of aggressive acts. Another type of adolescent humor is termed *coping humor* (McCullars et al., 2021), which aids in adjusting to stressful events. For example, seeing humor in looking unkempt in a social setting that otherwise would cause embarrassment.

Knowing how to appreciate and respond to humor that reflects developmental issues is necessary for parents to use humor in the most effective way. As in other forms of discipline, the use of humor must be appropriate to the circumstances. For instance, singing humor with an adolescent that fits with a toddler would not be very effective. As children grow and develop, their needs and interactions with their parents change (Duffy, 2014). For example, a boy can be very close with parents in the early years, and distant and uncommunicative in the middle school and high school years. Such a change in parent–child closeness can be problematic to some parents who fail to connect the change to the developmental changes with their son who is struggling with peer pressure and identity concerns. It is not uncommon that this withdrawal from the parent can be misinterpreted as depression, causing the parent to become intrusive, resulting in greater emotional distance from the son. Shifting the focus from verbal interaction to more physical activity is more in line with this developmental stage for boys. Too much verbiage at this time can be emotionally overwhelming.

The caveat for parents, however, is that some forms of withdrawal by their children can represent a serious mental or emotional condition that needs immediate attention. When teens are isolated from peers, and also express other behaviors, such as poor academic efforts, illegal drug or alcohol use, or feeling hopeless, there is a need for parents to take more direct interventions (Groth, 2013). The major concern when boys go silent during the teen years coupled with depression and hopelessness is the high rate of suicide. Girls are more verbal and expressive of their problems and suicide is not as common. Developmentally appropriate humor can be a tool for parents in all phases of development, including periods of more severe issues. The next section of the chapter will discuss the specific application of humor as a discipline tool.

Humor and Child Discipline

As stated earlier, humor is rarely taught as a discipline technique in parenting or parent education training. Yet it involves novel parent–child interactions that can be very effective in changing the child's behavior.

To use humor in discipline effectively, the parent needs to understand developmental periods and match humor to the developmental stage of the child. While all parenting behavior to some extent is deliberate in terms of outcomes, humor offers a chance to be less deliberate and more spontaneous. Humor appeals more to the emotional side of the child rather than the logical side. It is implicit and can change the child's misbehaving without focusing on the behavior in question. In sidestepping the misbehavior, the parent avoids a power struggle with the child by shifting from a confrontation to a more cooperative mode (see Tables 10.1 and 10.2).

Humor with Infants and Toddlers

Humor is very natural with infants and toddlers and most parents seem to intuitively know how to have fun with them. That being said, it is still true that spanking

TABLE 10.1 Understanding Humor to Discipline Children

Humor as a Discipline Technique
Not commonly used as a discipline intervention
Developmentally appropriate humor can be a tool for parents in all phases of development
Humor offers a chance to be less deliberate and more spontaneous
To label the humorous behavior of a toddler as misbehaving is a misnomer
Humor can be an antidote to depression when used in a developmentally appropriate manner

TABLE 10.2 Using Humor through Development

Age	*How to Use Humor*
Infants and toddlers	In contrast to engaging in power struggles with a toddler, distracting and redirecting through humor can produce positive effects
5–11-year old	5–11-year-old children react well to forms of humor not appropriate for toddlers, such as teasing
Adolescents	Humor can reduce mental health issues for adolescents

is one of the most frequent forms of punishment for toddlers (Anderson, 2021). No professional parenting expert recommends spanking a toddler, yet in popular culture there remains the fear that unless toddlers are submissive to parents, they will be spoiled. While approximately 50% of parents use some form of spanking to discipline a toddler, there is no known benefit. What is known is that toddlers do not have the cognitive connections to understand why they are being spanked and the trauma they experience from being spanked can have lifelong negative consequences.

The underlying issue in parenting toddlers is: Do they, in fact, misbehave? The answer to that question depends on how misbehavior is defined. If misbehavior is defined as willful and knowing resistance to parents, aggression toward parents or other acting out behavior, toddlers are incapable of misbehaving. Willful behavior is part of the developmental stage in toddlerhood and is different from older children's willful behavior. The best frame for understanding toddler behavior is learning that they are a separate entity and are learning how to emotionally regulate themselves, which requires guidance from the parent, not punishment.

Distracting and redirecting through humor can produce positive effects rather than set in motion a cyclical power struggle. For example, a parent and child are walking through a large parking lot with many rows of cars and the child breaks away from the parent's grip and begins running between cars. The parent is frantic with fear, worrying that the child will run in front of a moving car. The parent's first thought is to run after the child, yelling or screaming for them to stop. While humor is not always a good move for a dangerous situation, in this case the parent might employ humorous singing or dancing to get the child's attention to distract and redirect them, which might keep them from running away from the parent in the future.

Another example with toddlers is to prevent meltdowns, such as temper tantrums. Toddlers push limits and create power struggles with parents in a variety of situations, ranging from getting dressed to eating. For example, a parent is trying to dress a toddler who is squirming, kicking, and fighting the parent's effort to dress them. Such behavior can cause anger and a rush of adrenaline in the parent to stop the child's behavior. Instead of hastily acting in anger, the parent could resort to humor by putting a piece of the garment on their head and asking the child to help find where it goes. The parent could keep this up until the toddler reacts positively and joins in the fun. This example is not meant to be prescriptive, but to offer a way that humor could be used to get cooperation from the child.

A common behavior of toddlers is to create *power struggles* to get what they want. Eating at the prescribed times is difficult to structure for toddlers and can easily become chaotic with the parent forcing food on the toddler. Making this time fun instead of a confrontation over food can reduce the frustration of begging or bribing the child to eat. For example, instead of saying, "You will not leave the table until you clean your plate," a parent might say, "Hey, I'm so hungry that as soon as I eat my food, I will eat yours too if you haven't eaten it." Parents who keep things humorous around food will be less frustrated when the child goes through periods when all they will eat is a few grapes.

Humor with 5–11-Year-Old Children

One of the behaviors that are annoying to a lot of parents is their child using bad language, such as swearing. Like adults, preteens commonly express anger and disappointment by using swear words they learn from friends. The explanation that some parents give to children for using swear words—"I'm an adult, you are a child, and these words are not appropriate for you"—carries no credibility for the child. In addition, children can think swear words are cool and help them fit in with a peer group. Children who have a poor relationship with their parents may swear to provoke a negative reaction from their parents.

Some forms of expressing humor to children have been criticized for being inappropriate, or at the least, ineffective. These include derogatory, critical, or bullying statements that are meant to embarrass or intimidate the child. Most parenting experts couple teasing with bullying, encourage parents to not use teasing with their child, and encourage the parents to protect their child from others teasing them. On the other hand, a few researchers on humor have identified *teasing* as a type of humor discipline that acts as social control (Tholander & Aronsson, 2002) because teasing focuses on a desired social skill within groups. In social interactions, teasing and the ability to retort the tease are viewed as desirable traits. In fact, boys view teasing to create comradery with other boys and to position oneself within a social group (Evaldsson, 2005). Not accepting teasing can result in not being considered a member of the social group.

Like all forms of humor, teasing could be an effective parenting behavior under specific circumstances. While teasing is linked to bullying in contemporary literature, there are differences (Mills & Carwile, 2009). Teasing has historical underpinnings and can promote positive functionality in communicating. Teasing can be a playful way to challenge a child's behavior without causing anger. Teasing requires a playful and warm demeanor by the teaser and a willing reaction by the receiver. This exchange needs to be balanced in this way. If the receiver does not perceive the playful intent, teasing may be perceived as hurtful. There is research evidence that shows that children are better able to discern antisocial teasing better than prosocial teasing based on how their parents used teasing (Jones et al., 2017). If parents used teasing in a prosocial manner congruent with positive gestures and tone of voice, children are better able to discriminate between antisocial and prosocial teasing in social settings.

For example, Ben, a 10-year-old child, is getting all zeros on his schoolwork because the teacher cannot read his writing. The teacher knows that Ben is doing the work correctly from conversations with him about his writing but takes the position that if she cannot read it, she cannot be sure that he has completed it correctly. Ben is very bright and is bored in school. His position is that if he knows what he wrote and can read it, why does it matter if others cannot read it? Instead of making perfect letters and numbers, he prefers to write very fast so he can do other things. The parent has a real dilemma with the direction to take with Ben. The teacher is intractable in her position about Ben's handwriting and the parents fear that Ben could become more resistant to doing any homework. They do not believe that punishment would be of any value and would create a power struggle. The parents resort to humor and lightheartedness to address this problem. They suggest that Ben write with his feet because they are sure that his feet would be a better writer than his hands. The novelty of the idea impressed Ben who had a vivid imagination and he immediately removed his shoes and socks. He placed a pencil between his big toe and the second toe and tried to write. This proved to be very difficult, and he admitted that not even he could read it. He resorted back to writing with his hands and his writing became more legible.

Humor and Adolescents

Adolescence is a time of exploring and trying out new identities and behaviors. The experimentations with dress and appearance and searching for identities are impermanent and may not have any relevance to their adult lives (Figure 10.3). It is a particularly hard time for parents because they can overreact to their adolescent's behavior and further alienate them. Adolescents also begin the process of determining educational and career goals (Faber & Mazlish, 2006), which at times may seem like a poor fit for them. Adolescents expect to be granted more decision making opportunities about their personal and social lives and resist parenting authority over them (Lee, 2006).

Adolescence, in recent years, is associated with increased depression and increased suicide rates. The COVID-19 pandemic increased adolescents' feelings of isolation and loneliness, and contributed to increased suicides and clinical depression (Kuhlman et al., 2021). Researchers have found that humor can be an antidote to depression when used in a developmentally appropriate manner. Parents who discipline adolescents with humor have greater success in maintaining a positive relationship through this stressful time.

For adolescent girls, stress-reducing humor tends to be about certain developmental tasks, such as change in body, crushes on boys, or frustration with parental relationships. This humor was characterized by giggling and laughter. Humor is used to reduce the impact of frightening words and stories, but humor did not work if the content was too adult, such as fantasy of actual sexual content or sexual penetration (Ransohoff, 1975).

For both genders, the mental health of adolescents has been of considerable alarm in the past several years. A recent report by the CDC (February, 2023) found that as much as 60% of teen girls had felt hopeless in the last year and 13% had attempted suicide. For LGBTQ+ teens, 66% had felt hopeless and 22% had attempted suicide. Parents respond to adolescent angst in ways that may not be

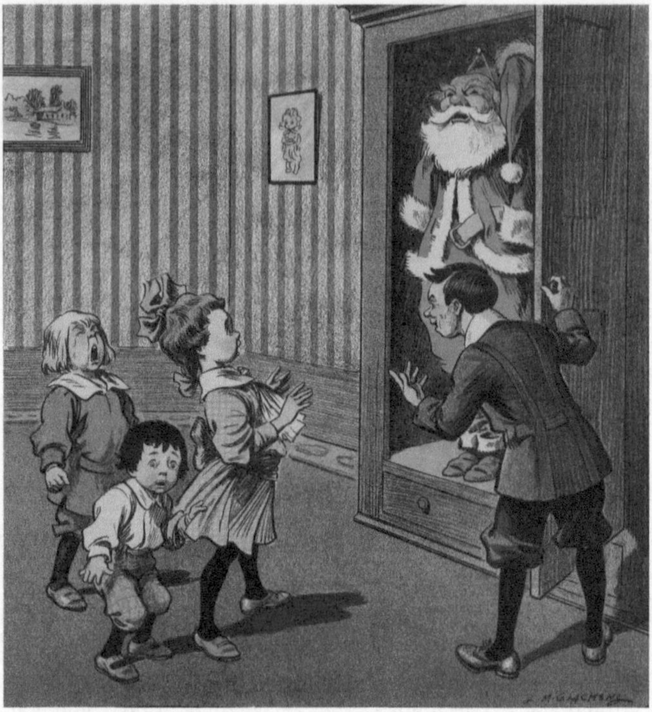

FIGURE 10.3 As children's brains mature, they possess an increasing ability to understand multiple meanings of situations (or to think divergently) and, thus, to utilize humor to come to terms with otherwise confusing situations. (J. Ottman Lithographic Company. Original from Library of Congress)

helpful, such as in anger, yelling, and making demands. These ineffective parenting behaviors make things worse for teenagers and reduce a cooperative and mutually satisfying relationship.

Using Humor to Discipline an Adolescent

Sam and Annabel have a 16-year-old daughter named Marianna. On a Friday night, she was supposed to be home by 11:00 p.m., as per the agreed-upon curfew. When the clock struck 11:30 p.m. and Marianna had not returned home, her parents were concerned and upset, but wanted to address the situation while maintaining a strong parent–child bond. Marianna walked through the door at 11:45 p.m. with both parents sitting in the living room impatiently waiting for her return. They resisted the urge to yell in anger or to unleash a lecture on rules and responsibility. Instead, they waited for the right moment to engage her. They noticed that she looked a bit flustered, so they broke the tension with humor.

With a playful grin, Sarah said, "Marianna, I thought you were auditioning for the role of Cinderella at the ball tonight, but the slipper hasn't dropped yet!" Marianna raised an eyebrow, surprised by her mother's humorous comment because it was not what she expected, and it immediately lightened the mood. Annabel continued, "Seriously, Mari, I was worried about you. Our agreement was to be home by 11:00 p.m. Can you tell me what happened tonight?" Marianna explained how she lost track of the time. Sarah responded to the explanation: "I understand that sometimes things don't go as planned, but it's crucial that we communicate when you'll be late. Let's work on that together." Marianna nodded, appreciating the way her mother approached it. Sarah followed up with a hug, saying "I love you and I'm always here for you."

In this case example, humor was used as an effective tool to address a curfew violation without resorting to anger or confrontation. By choosing the right moment, using a light-hearted approach, and balancing humor with seriousness, the mother was able to convey the importance of communication and safety while preserving the parent–child relationship. This approach fosters trust and open communication, ensuring that Marianna understands the rules while feeling supported and loved.

In sum, the use of humor in disciplining children's misbehavior is an underdeveloped technique that has potential to be transformational. This second order parenting style could enhance parent education training and supplement the explicit skill-building techniques that are widely used. Humor can help parents connect with their children on a more personal level. By sharing a laugh, parents create a positive atmosphere that makes it easier for children to accept discipline. It shifts the focus from blame to understanding, making children more receptive to the message being conveyed.

Humor often arises from incongruities or violations of expectations in a situation or statement. These incongruities prompt the brain to engage in problem-solving, and the process of resolving them contributes to humor's cognitive appeal. This mental exercise occurs predominantly at the unconscious level, as the brain automatically seeks to reconcile the disparity between what is expected and what is presented.

Humor is a potent tool for regulating emotions. Humor causes the brain to release endorphins and reduces the activity of the *amygdala*, which is responsible for processing emotions like fear and stress. This emotional regulation occurs both consciously and unconsciously, helping to alleviate negative emotions and create a more positive mental state. Neuroimaging studies reveal that humor engages various brain regions, including the prefrontal cortex (associated with higher-level thinking and decision making), the ventromedial prefrontal cortex (linked to emotional processing and reward), and the anterior cingulate cortex (involved in resolving cognitive conflicts). These findings illustrate that humor is a complex cognitive process that involves both conscious and unconscious brain activity.

Inappropriate Use of Humor

Some forms of humor have the opposite effects. Instead of helping children cope, increasing the bonding with parents, or changing behavior, they increase negative thinking, and cause anger, resentment, and hurt feelings. Parents should understand the forms of humor that are detrimental to their children. One type of humor that adults engage in often is *sarcasm*, which is caustic and can increase the emotional pain a child is feeling about a certain circumstance (Glenwright et al., 2013). While even playful use of sarcasm that pokes fun at a child may appear humorous to the parent, a sensitive child may feel attacked or put down and remember it long-term. When parents model sarcasm, children learn to use it in retorts to parents that parents interpret as disrespectful.

The extant literature labels inappropriate humor "aggressive humor," which includes sarcasm, and certain forms of teasing and jokes (Halfpenny & James, 2020). Aggressive humor is used to enhance oneself at the expense of the other person's feelings. It is a way to feel superior and has an overall negative effect on prosocial behavior in that it results in hostility, depression, lower self-esteem, and lack of social support.

References

American Physiological Society. (2008, April 10). Anticipating a laugh reduces our stress hormones, study shows. *ScienceDaily*. Retrieved September 5, 2023, from www.sciencedaily.com/releases/2008/04/080407114617.htm

Anderson, J. (2021, April 13). The effects of spanking on the brain. *Harvard Graduate School of Education*. Retrieved March 28, 2024, from https://www.gse.harvard.edu/ideas/usable-knowledge/21/04/effect-spanking-brain

Bennett, M. P., & Lengacher, C. (2007). Humor and laughter may influence health IV: Humor and immune function. *Evidence-Based Complementary and Alternative Medicine, 6*(2), 159–164. https://doi.org/10.1093/ecam/nem149

Berger, P., Bitsch, F., & Falkenberg, I. (2021, May 28). Humor in psychiatry: Lessons from neuroscience, psychopathology, and treatment research. *Frontiers in Psychiatry, 12*. https://doi.org/10.3389/fpsyt.2021.68190

Bongiorno, K. (2019). 21 things kids will always find funny. *Momtasic*. Retrieved September 13, 2023, from https://www.momtastic.com/parenting/756487-21-things-kids-will-always-find-funny/

Center for Disease Control and Prevention. (2023, February). *U.S. teen girls experiencing increased sadness and violence*. Retrieved September 29, 2023, from https://www.cdc.gov/media/releases/2023/p0213-yrbs.html

Chadwick, D. D., & Platt, T. (2018). Investigating humor in social interaction in people with intellectual disabilities: A systematic review of the literature. *Frontiers in Psychology, 9*. https://doi.org/10.3389/fpsyg.2018.01745

Chaney, C. (1993, February 14). *Young children's jokes: A cognitive developmental perspective*. Paper presented at an Annual Meeting of the Western States Communication Association, Albuquerque, NM.

Cohen, L. J. (2002). *Playful parenting: An exciting new approach to raising children that will help you nurture close connections, solve behavior problems, and encourage confidence*. Ballentine.

Couder, O. (2019). Problem solved? Absurdist humor and incongruity-resolution. *Journal of Literary Semantics, 48*(1), 1–21. https://doi.org/10.1515/jls-2019-2005

Cozolino, L. (2013). *The social neuroscience of education: Optimizing attachment and learning in the classroom*. W. W. Norton.

Duffy, J. (2014). *The available parent: Expert advice for raising successful, resilient, and connected teens and tweens*. Viva Editions.

Evaldsson, A. C. (2005). Staging insults and mobilizing categorizations in a multiethnic peer group. *Discourse & Society, 16*(6), 763–786.
Faber, A., & Mazlish, E. (2006). *How to talk so teens will listen and listen so teens will talk.* HarperCollins.
Fox, C. L., Hunter, S. C., & Jones, S. E. (2016). Longitudinal associations between humor styles and psychosocial adjustment in adolescence. *Europe's Journal of Psychology, 12*(3), 377–389. https://doi.org/10.5964/ejop.v12i3.1065
Fry, W. F. (1994). The biology of humor. *Humor*, *7*, 111–126. https://doi.org/10.1515/humr.1994.7.2.111
Garner, R. L. (2006). Humor in pedagogy: How ha-ha can lead to aha! *College Teaching, 54*(1), 177–180. https://doi.org/10.3200/CTCH.54.1.177-180
Gelkopf, M. (2011). The use of humor in serious mental illness: A review. *Evidence-Based Complementary and Alternative Medicine, 2011,* 342837. https://doi.org/10.1093/ecam/nep106
Glenwright, M., Parackel, J. M., Cheung, K., & Nilsen, E. (2013). Intonation influences how children and adults interpret sarcasm. *Journal of Child Language*, *41*(2), 1–13. https://doi.org/10.1017/S0305000912000773
Greengross, G. (2019, December 6). *The relationship between humor styles and personality; how healthy and unhealthy humor styles relate to your personality.* Retrieved September 9, 2023, from https://www.psychologytoday.com/us/blog/humor-sapiens/201912/the-relationship-between-humor-styles-and-personality
Gremigni, P. (2012). *Humor and health promotion.* Nova.
Groth, M. (2013, December 18). Silencing boys. *Psychology Today*. Retrieved September 15, 2023, from https://www.psychologytoday.com/us/blog/boys-men/201312/silencing-boys
Halfpenny, C. C., & James, L. A. (2020). Humor styles and empathy in junior-school children. *European Journal of Psychology, 16*(1), 148–166. https://doi.org/10.5964/ejop.v16i1.1934
Jones, T. L., Wadian, T. W., Barnett, M. A., Hellmer, M. K., & Pino, L. N. (2017). Young children's ability to discriminate between antisocial and prosocial teases. *The Journal of Genetic Psychology, 179*(1), 1–8. https://doi.org/10.1080/00221325.2017.1392280
Keegan, L. C., Suger, C., & Togher, L. (2021). Discourse analysis of humor after traumatic brain injury. *American Journal of Speech-Language Pathology, 30*(2S), 949–961. https://doi.org/10.1044/2020_AJSLP-20-00059
Kuhlman, K. R., Straka, K., Mousavi, Z., Tran, M. L., & Rodgers, E. (2021). Predictors of adolescent resilience during the COVID-19 pandemic: Cognitive reappraisal and humor. *Journal of Adolescent Health, 69*(5), 729–736. https://doi.org/10.1016/j.jadohealth.2021.07.006
Lee, T. Y. (2006). Resilience as a positive youth development construct: Conceptual bases and implications for curricular development. *International Journal of Adolescent Medicine and Health, 18,* 475–482.
Mahon, E. J. (1992). The function of humor in a four-year-old. *Psychoanalytic Study of the Child, 47,* 321–328.
Martin, R. A., Puhlik-Doris, P., Larsen, G., Gray, J., & Weir, K. (2003). Individual differences in uses of humor and their relation to psychological well-being: Development of the humor styles questionnaire. *Journal of Research in Personality, 37*(1), 48–75. https://doi.org/10.1016/S0092-6566(02)00534-2
Martin, R. A., & Yip, J. A. (2006). Sense of humor, emotional intelligence, and social competence. *Journal of Research in Personality*, *40*(6), 1202–1208.
Martins, N., & Riddle, K. (2021). Reassessing the risks: An updated content analysis of violence on U.S. children's primetime television. *Journal of Children and Media, 16*(5), 1–19. https://doi.org/10.1080/17482798.2021.1985548
McCullars, A., Richie, F. J., Klibert, J. J., & Langhinrichsen-Rohling, J. (2021). What's so funny? Adaptive versus maladaptive humor styles as mediators between early

maladaptive schemas and resilience. *Humor, 34*(1), 93–111. https://doi.org/10.1515/humor-2019-0082

McGhee, P. E. (1989). The role of humor in enhancing children's development and adjustment. In P. E. McGhee (Ed.), *Humor and children's development* (pp. 249–274). Haworth.

McGhee, P. E. (1999). *Health, healing and the amuse system: Humor as survival training.* Kendall/Hunt.

Mills, C. B., & Carwile, A. M. (2009). The good, the bad, and the borderline: Separating teasing from bullying. *Communication Education, 58*(2), 276–301. https://doi.org/10.1080/03634520902783666

Penberg, D. (2023). Learning and laughter. *Education Reimaged.* https://education-reimagined.org/laughter-and-learning/

Plessen, C. Y., Franken, F. R., Ster, C., Schmid, R. R., Wolfmayr, C., Mayer, A. M., Sobisch, M., Kathofer, M., Rattner, K., Elona, K., Maierwieser, R. J., & Tran, U. S. (2020). Humor styles and personality: A systematic review and meta-analysis on the relations between humor styles and the big five personality traits. *Personality and Individual Differences, 154*. https://doi.org/10.1016/j.paid.2019.109676

Ransohoff, R. (1975). Some observations on humor and laughter in young adolescent girls. *Journal of Youth Adolescence, 4,* 155–170. https://doi.org/10.1007/BF01537439

Reddy, V. (1991). Playing with others' expectations: Teasing and mucking about in the first year. In A. Whiten (Ed.), *Natural theories of mind* (pp. 143–158). Blackwell.

Reddy, V., Williams, E., & Vaughan, A. (2002). Sharing humor and laughter in autism and down's syndrome. *British Journal of Psychology, 93*(2), 219–242.

Rutter, M. (1990). *Helping troubled children.* Plenum.

Solomon, R. (2002). Are the three stooges funny? Soitainly? (Or when is it ok to laugh?). In J. Rudinow & A. Graybosch (Eds.), *Ethics and values in the information age* (pp. 179–185). Wadsworth.

Spencer, H. (1911). *On the physiology of laughter: Essays on education, etc.* Dent.

Stoeber, J., & Janssen, D. P. (2011). Perfectionism and coping with daily failures: Positive reframing helps achieve satisfaction at the end of the day. *Anxiety, Stress, & Coping, 24*(5), 477–497. https://doi.org/10.1080/10615806.2011.562977

Stuber, M., Hilber, S. D., Mintzer, L. L., Castaneda, M., Glover, D., & Zeltzer, L. (2009). Laughter, humor and pain perception in children: A pilot study. *Evidence-Based Complementary and Alternative Medicine, 6*(2), 271–276. https://doi.org/10.1093/ecam/nem097

Tannenbaum, A. (1983). *Gifted children: Psychological and educational perspectives.* Macmillan.

Tholander, M., & Aronsson, K. (2002). Teasing as serious business: Collaborative staging and response work. *Text, 22*, 559–595.

Vrticka, P., Black, J. M., & Reiss, A. L. (2013). The neural basis of humor processing. *Nature Reviews Neuroscience, 14*(12), 860–868. https://doi.org/10.1038/nrn3566

Wanzer, M. B., Frymier, A. B., & Irwin, J. (2010). An explanation of the relationship between instructor humor and student learning: Instructional humor processing theory. *Communication Education, 59*(1), 1–18.

Watzlawick, P., Weakland, J. H., & Fisch, R. (2011). *Change: Principles of problem formation and problem resolution.* W.W. Norton.

Whitaker, C. A. (1975). Psychotherapy of the absurd: With a special emphasis on the psychotherapy of aggression. *Family Process, 14*(1), 1–16.

Wilson, N. (2017). Superiority theory. *The Critical Comic.* Retrieved September 9, 2013, from https://thecriticalcomic.com/superiority-theory/

11

CONFUSION/ROPE-A-DOPE

Effective Parental Withdrawal

The use of confusion by a parent may be inappropriate at first glance or appear to reduce parental authority, but can be a powerful technique when the parent wants the child to take more initiative. This is a difficult technique but may be especially helpful for children who are performing below their capacity, are oppositional, or are defiant. The term "*rope-a-dope*" was coined by Muhammad Ali to describe his strategy for defeating George Frazier in their famed world heavyweight championship bout (Andrevski, 2020). His strategy was to lean on the ropes and allow Frazier to plummet him with punches while he covered himself and blocked most of the punches. The result was that Frazier tired to the point that Ali could mount an offense that took Frazier out. The term is metaphorically applied here to describe how parents can withdraw from certain situations with their children. Parental withdrawal is confusing because parents, in essence, are seemingly giving over control to their child, creating the fear that their child will dominate them.

Controlling children's behavior and *nurturance*, being warm and affectionate, are the two major parenting behaviors that parents are assumed to possess and are the bedrock of most parent education models (Philips et al., 2014.) To suggest that effective parenting may require parents to vacate these sacred acts is counter-intuitive and illogical, yet paradoxically parents can have more control at times when they withdraw from the situation. Having power or *control* in a relationship has more to do with who guides the ever-evolving nature of the relationship, not who is most active (Haley, 1993). Creating confusion by withdrawing when active engagement is expected can create a novel learning experience and have transformational effects.

DOI: 10.4324/9781003381679-13

While withdrawing may not be appropriate for all parenting situations, there are some circumstances, particularly those that are intractable, where this technique can be valuable. Children who openly defy parental directions or whose modus operandi is to engage parents in power struggles are the most difficult for parents to manage. These children make up a large percentage of children who are patients in mental health treatment programs (Webster-Stratton & Reid, 2010). *Oppositional Defiant Disorder (ODD)* and *Conduct Disorder (CD)* are challenging behavioral disorders in that they have their roots in early childhood and persist throughout the lifespan. Mishandled power struggles between parents and children in early childhood and abusive and neglectful parenting are associated with ODD and CD in children and adolescents.

While no parent training technique exists for the confusion/rope-a-dope position, some parenting experts, such as Dreikurs (1964), advised parents to withdraw from a power struggle or to delay responding if they were angry. The rationale for delaying a response is based on the belief that the parent must be in control of their own emotions before they respond to the child's misbehavior. For example, if the toddler is refusing to take a bath and fighting the parents' efforts, the parent's rush of adrenaline to force the child to comply can come at the expense of the parent–child relationship. The parent is advised to not physically force the children to comply and leave it until the anger subsides. In Adlerian models, a power struggle leads to either parent or child winning and the other losing. The belief is that no one should win, and there are times when it is better for the parent to do nothing than do the wrong thing. *Communication models* of parenting as espoused by Faber and Mazlish (1980) would suggest that the parent stay positive and find verbal ways for resolving the issue.

The confusion/rope-a-dope technique differs from simply a parent removing themselves from the power struggle with the child. The rationale for using the technique is not based on a principle of the parent controlling their own anger by leaving the interaction with the child, but on the principle of providing a novel implicit parenting behavior that will have a profound effect on the child's neural responses.

The rationale for using confusion as a technique is its similarity to a systemic approach in changing families. Systemic family therapy, for example, posits that families get stuck in certain patterns and the homeostatic function prevents them from changing, resulting in a feeling of hopelessness (Haley, 1993). There is also a resistance to new thoughts or feelings. Breaking up this pattern is needed for real change to take place. The confusion technique could allow for novelty because underlying premises are changed by the new context. The caveat for using confusion in parenting is that it may be misinterpreted and lead to greater disconnect between parent and child.

The Relation of Confusion and Learning

In parent training models, confusion is not a popular or desirable technique to bring about change. Trainers are encouraged to do the very opposite of confusion—make skills and training modules clear and understandable so that a person of any education level can understand it. The case can be made, however, that persons are already in a state of confusion when they are participating in a group training or a therapy session. In fact, the child and parents are already experiencing a failure of synchronicity between their view of reality and their experiences, creating a confused state that is rigid and lacks options for change. While humor and other forms of implicit interventions have gained some status in changing rigid patterns, using confusion has not. Except for a few therapy models, such as Neurolinguistic Programing (NLP) (Charvet, 2019) and the experiential family therapy model popularized by Whitaker and Malone (1981), intentional use of confusion is frowned on. This fear of using confusion to bring about change can be alleviated by understanding the deeper meaning of confusion and how it is related to brain processes and learning.

Learning is accompanied by emotional responses due in part to the integration of new knowledge with old knowledge (Lodge et al., 2018). Thirty years ago, neuroscientists discovered the neural base in the role of emotion in learning new information (LeDoux, 1992). Anxiety and confusion have been generally associated with impeding the learning process in the classroom (Kennedy & Lodge, 2016). Only recently, emotions, such as confusion, have been studied in terms of their positive role in learning. Essentially, confusion causes cognitive incongruity and when the incongruity is resolved, deep learning can happen (Vogl et al., 2020). The current research regarding emotions related to learning beliefs, referred to as *epistemic emotions*, focuses on surprise, confusion, and curiosity.

Educators are becoming more aware that epistemic emotions can open students to greater learning by enhancing critical thinking and debate through dialectical thinking (Vogl et al., 2020). Belief systems are generally tied to closed or rigid thinking, while epistemic emotions of curiosity, surprise, and confusion are not tethered to belief systems and can engineer transformational change. Students have a greater ability to question and come to different solutions when they encounter situations that bring epistemic emotions to the fore.

One of the first researchers to address the role of confusion in learning was Mandler (1990) and the *discrepancy theory*. Discrepancy theory is based on the view that when new information conflicts with old information, an emotional response occurs and a shift in thinking to the discrepant information follows. If discrepancies cannot be resolved quickly when there is a mismatch of incoming information with existing information, cognitive disequilibrium occurs. D'Mello et al. (2014) found that when confusion is used strategically when learning difficult topics, participants learned more effectively than straightforward methods to induce memory.

D'Mello and associates (2014) studied the interaction between participants and computer-generated entities that acted as tutors in a series of discussions that contained both accurate and flawed information. The results of these discussions left participants confused when they were asked to determine the more effective and scientific arguments. Confused participants scored higher on a post-test and demonstrated greater problem-solving and critical thinking. The researchers concluded that confusion can be beneficial to learning when used appropriately. The best way to use confusion is to closely align the confusion to the content of the learning session, and the instructor provides guidance to resolving the discrepancy. Consequently, participants' confusion is eliminated over the session and deep learning takes place. The caveat is that struggling students may not be able to resolve the incongruity and, therefore, the confusion technique may hinder rather than help them (see Table 11.1).

Presenting information in a confused manner followed by a clarifying reframe has dramatic effects on both learning and behavior (Kardes et al., 2007). Confusion enhances learning because it increases attention and focus so that distractions are reduced. In addition, the study by Kardes et al. demonstrates that confusion followed by clarification can increase desired behavior; in this case, this technique increased purchases of a product. The researchers presented information about various products to participants and found that a confusing presentation of technical jargon did not increase interest in the products. What increased the interest and the desire to purchase products was cognitive closure which clarified the confusion. The researchers concluded that to increase interest and desired behavior, the best method might be to reduce resistance rather than emphasize persuasion.

The *impasse theory of learning* has much in common with the concept of confusion. When an impasse is experienced in learning, a person will feel confused, which will lead to efforts to resolve the confusion. In a confused state, the person must curtail activity, rethink the present circumstances, and engage in problem-solving (D'Mello et al., 2014). Consequently, relationship training, such as parent education, should challenge participants via confusion interventions to increase participants' processing of information through critical and dialectical thinking. Confusion should be viewed as the first step in a sequence and not as a single-step procedure. Confusion is considered the vehicle which sets in motion other processes that allow for *deep learning*. This deeper level of processing is associated with deep learning when there is a mechanism for resolving the confusion.

TABLE 11.1 Relation of Confusion and Learning

How Confusion Impacts Learning
Confusion is necessary for learning
Confusion increases attention and focus
Learning is the integration of new knowledge with old knowledge from a state of confusion
Confusion causes cognitive incongruity that is necessary for deep learning when resolved
Confusion is an epistemic emotion essential for dialectical thinking
Confusion followed by clarification can change behavior
Systemic therapists use confusion to induce change

Confusion and Transformational Change

Enhanced learning resulting from the resolution of confusion induces transformational change in actions and behaviors. This principle is well established in systemic psychotherapy (Haley, 1993; Minuchin & Fishman, 1981). For example, Haley (1993), the founder of strategic family therapy, believed that it is important in family therapy not to reduce anxiety or stress but to increase it. He believed that families who are in a state of equilibrium are not sufficiently motivated to change. In terms of a system like the family, the state of equilibrium keeps them rigidly holding on to the status quo rather than allowing for change when faced with challenges. The stability around the symptoms prevents the family from changing and acts as a type of resistance. The way to affect the resistance is to increase the level of discomfort in the family. The use of increasing the stress in this way is consistent with the idea of using confusion, because both would have the same outcome.

When parents enter parent education or when a counselor begins working on parenting issues with a family, the natural progression of this training will produce confusion. A word generally used to describe the state of confusion is *resistance*. Parents say they need help but seem to sabotage their own efforts by not following through or by not making desired progress. The trainer's expectation for transformational change is met with the parents' ingrained beliefs that make change difficult and slow. It is common to experience confusion, misunderstanding, and resistance when met with new information, although this is not considered a welcomed experience by trainers. Instead of trying to prevent the confusion, trainers would be better advised to *utilize* that confusion to enhance the learning and change process. The problem is that the old way of thinking and processing information must be changed, and the tension of trying to process the new information through the old way of thinking produces a state of anxiety and confusion.

Confusion that does not lead to positive outcomes occurs when the resolution is too complex to understand. Negative confusion can lead to disengagement and withdrawal from the learning environment (Lodge & Kennedy, 2016). There should always be a path to clarity and resolution. Confusion can be misinterpreted as lack of intellectual acuity, which inhibits confessing publicly that one is confused. Information presented quickly with various media may seem easily understood initially, but upon further inquiry may seem very confused.

Confusion is a signal that things are beginning to be questioned or changed. Dismantling the old beliefs and replacing them with new ones need not be rushed so that prepared training modules can be completed by the trainers. Confusion should be seen as a necessary step toward clarity and understanding. Perhaps the best strategy for dealing with the state of confusion in training is to sit with it, be comfortable with it, and not rush to resolve it, as is commonly practiced in meditative practices of Buddhism. Zen Buddhists understand reality (samsara) to be a persistent state of suffering and confusion; there is no controlling, dominating, or changing it. In embracing confusion, Zen Buddhists believe enlightenment comes.

In embracing confusion, a family can acknowledge that change is occurring, and deeper and more effective learning is taking place.

Another aspect of learning and behavior change is confidence in one's ability to learn. Research on confidence and overconfidence has yielded interesting results. For example, some researchers have concluded that *overconfidence* is much more detrimental for outcomes than doubt or confusion (Moore & Healy, 2008). Overconfidence is a cognitive bias that leads individuals to overestimate their abilities, knowledge, or judgment. While a certain level of confidence is essential for motivation and decision making, excessive overconfidence can have detrimental effects on the learning process. The effectiveness of learning can be hindered when individuals display overconfidence and can manifest in various forms, such as overestimating one's comprehension of a topic, underestimating the effort required for a task, or misjudging the accuracy of one's judgments.

Overconfidence can disrupt one's ability to monitor and regulate their own cognitive processes, including their judgments and learning strategies (Moore & Healy, 2008). First, overconfident individuals may fail to accurately assess their current knowledge or skills, leading to suboptimal study strategies and reduced engagement in productive learning activities. They may underestimate the need for additional learning efforts or overestimate their mastery of a subject, leading to poor planning and allocation of resources. Furthermore, overconfidence can impair individuals' ability to accurately gauge the difficulty of tasks or the likelihood of success. As a result, they may not adequately adjust their learning strategies in response to challenges, leading to reduced learning outcomes. Research has shown that accurate awareness of one's current functioning is essential for effective learning, and overconfidence can undermine this critical component of the learning process (Abdelrahmana, 2020).

Memory plays a central role in learning, as it involves the encoding, storage, and retrieval of information (Brem et al., 2013). Overconfidence can negatively impact memory in several ways. When individuals are overconfident in their understanding of a topic, they may not engage in sufficient rehearsal or elaboration of the material if they believe they have already mastered it. This can result in shallow encoding and poor retention of information. Moreover, overconfident individuals may neglect to revisit and review previously learned material, believing that they have already acquired it sufficiently. This leads to the decay of memories over time, further reducing the effectiveness of learning. Additionally, overconfidence can interfere with the accuracy of memory retrieval, as individuals may be more prone to recall incorrect information or distort memories to align with their overconfident beliefs.

As discussed in systemic theories, *feedback* is a vital component of the learning process, providing individuals with information about their performance and guiding their future actions (Smith & Karam, 2018). However, overconfidence can hinder effective feedback processing. Overconfident learners may dismiss negative feedback as irrelevant or inaccurate, believing that they are already proficient in a particular skill or subject. Conversely, they may selectively attend to positive feedback that confirms their overconfident beliefs while ignoring constructive criticism. This biased feedback processing can result in a stagnation of learning, as individuals fail to make necessary adjustments and improvements based on feedback.

Learning is not a static process but one that requires adaptability to changing circumstances and evolving knowledge. Overconfidence can impede adaptability by fostering a rigid mindset. Overconfident individuals may resist new information or perspectives that challenge their existing beliefs, leading to a lack of intellectual humility and openness to learning. In addition, when overconfident individuals encounter failure or setbacks, they may attribute them to external factors rather than their own limitations. This defensive attribution can prevent them from recognizing and addressing their weaknesses, inhibiting personal growth and learning.

In sum, confusion can enhance learning and behavioral change while overconfidence impedes both learning and behavior and change. Confusion aids learning because it helps people detect an inconsistency between cognitions, beliefs, and behaviors referred to in the literature as *cognitive dissonance*. Cognitive dissonance theory (CDT) is based on the writings of Festinger (1957). When there is an inconsistency in information or cognitions, confusion and distress occur until there is a resolution which depends to a large degree on the extent of the confusion. According to Festinger, alteration in onc's cognitions, adding innovative cognitions, or altering one's appraisal of the cognition are ways in which one can resolve the inconsistency (see Table 11.2).

TABLE 11.2 Three Primary Ways the Confusion/Rope-a-Dope Technique Can Be Implemented

How to Use Confusion as a Technique	
1. In kids with Oppositional Defiant Disorder (ODD) and Conduct Disorder (CD)	• Mishandled power struggles between parents and children in early childhood, and abusive and neglectful parenting are associated with ODD and CD in children and adolescents • The rationale for using the technique is based on the principle of providing a novel implicit parenting behavior that will have a profound effect on the child's neural responses • Systemic family therapy posits that families get stuck in certain patterns, and the homeostatic function prevents them from changing, resulting in a feeling of hopelessness • There is also a resistance to new thoughts or feelings. Breaking up this pattern is needed for real change to take place • The confusion technique could allow for novelty because underlying premises are changed by the new context

(Continued)

TABLE 11.2 (Continued)

How to Use Confusion as a Technique	
2. To challenge old, outdated belief systems	• A word generally used to describe the state of confusion is *resistance* • Parents say they need help but seem to sabotage their own efforts by not following through or by not making desired progress • The trainer's expectation for transformational change is met with the parents' ingrained beliefs that makes change difficult and slow • It is common to experience confusion, misunderstanding, and resistance when met with new information; however, this is not considered a welcomed experience by trainers • The problem is that the old way of thinking and processing information must be changed, and the tension of trying to process the new information through the old way of thinking produces a state of anxiety and confusion • Confusion is a signal that things are beginning to be questioned or changed • Perhaps the best strategy for dealing with the state of confusion in training is to sit with it, be comfortable with it, and not rush to resolve it. Embracing confusion is acknowledging that change is occurring, and deeper and more effective learning is taking place
3. To mitigate cognitive dissonance	• While a certain level of confidence is essential for motivation and decision making, excessive overconfidence can have detrimental effects on the learning process • The effectiveness of learning can be hindered when individuals display overconfidence and can manifest in various forms, such as overestimating one's comprehension of a topic, underestimating the effort required for a task, or misjudging the accuracy of one's judgments • Overconfidence can interfere with the accuracy of memory retrieval, as individuals may be more prone to recall incorrect information or distort memories to align with their overconfident beliefs • Confusion can enhance learning and behavioral change while overconfidence impedes both learning and behavior and change • Confusion aides learning because it helps people detect an inconsistency between cognitions, beliefs, and behaviors

The Neuroscience of Confusion

The brain networks activated by confusion reveal a complex interplay of cognitive processes when individuals confront conflicting information or ambiguous situations. Understanding the neural basis of confusion provides insights into how the brain adapts, learns, and ultimately resolves cognitive dissonance. The experience of confusion, though often challenging, is a fundamental aspect of cognitive growth and adaptation.

The neural region associated with processing and managing confusion includes the prefrontal cortex, a brain region responsible for higher order cognitive functions. When individuals encounter conflicting information, this region becomes highly active as it engages in critical thinking, problem-solving, and decision making processes. In addition, the *anterior cingulate cortex (ACC)* is involved in detecting cognitive conflicts, or situations that cause confusion. ACC monitors inconsistencies in information and signals the need for resolution. Increased activity in the ACC is associated with the emotional discomfort often linked to confusion. Another brain region, the *hippocampus,* crucial for memory and learning, is engaged when individuals attempt to reconcile their existing knowledge with new, contradictory information. It helps form new associations and integrate conflicting data into existing cognitive frameworks.

The research on brain activity and confused states is underdeveloped and researchers have noted the difficulty in identifying the existence of a confused state. Most research on the state of confusion used facial cues or feedback as the basis for determining confusion (Arguel et al., 2017). Consequently, the procedures for determining the state of confusion require further development since neither facial expression nor feedback are adequate determinants of confusion. Several recent studies have focused on reducing this deficiency by using EEG technology to identify and describe when participants were experiencing confusion (Liang et al., 2018). Liang et al. (2018) aimed at exploring brain activity when students were in a confused state when they were presented with conflicting or incomplete information. The study consisted of two situations: First, students were presented with an explicit situation in a math-solving scenario that contained only partial information; the second situation involved an implicit procedure where the content was concealed in the problem. The implicit problem where the lack of information is in the problem itself is difficult to consciously solve since it presents itself subliminally.

To induce confusion in the explicit experiment, Liang et al. (2018) used math calculations as the way to create confusion in problem-solving. Participants were asked to complete calculations where some numbers were replaced with symbols. In the implicit experiment, participants had to use inductive reasoning to determine the sequence patterns of numbers to solve the equation. The results indicated that more cognitive effort was needed during both explicit and implicit confusion states. The prefrontal region of the brain was more active when processing unfamiliar information, while the parietal and temporal areas showed more activity during periods of insufficient information.

Other studies have found similar results to the above study using EEG technology. For example, Xu et al. (2023) used an interdisciplinary approach to investigate confusion while reasoning. The findings confirmed the variances in the power of different brain waves in confused and non-confused states, and a higher cognitive effort when participants were confused. The researchers concluded that confused states can be detected from non-confused states during learning and can provide useful information for monitoring confusion and recognition when confusion has been resolved.

Another avenue in understanding the neuroscience of confusion/rope-a-dope technique is via research on novelty and surprise. The confusion/rope-a-dope technique can be considered a novelty because it cannot be predicted from present circumstances. The technique unique, spontaneous, and out-of-the-box behaviors that do not lend themselves to cognitive explanations. Neuroscience research reveals that working memory is involved in processing novelty (Nikolić, 2019). The working memory utilizes mechanisms for making sense of the integration of new and old information in resolving contradictions and seemingly disparate elements. Furthermore, researchers have found that the reward network responds more to the unexpectedness of input rather than to the gratifying properties (Berns et al., 2001). This means that the brain finds unexpected input more rewarding than expected input. The brain network involved in the reward system is the nucleus accumbens.

Researchers have found that surprise activates the body's *orienting system* resulting in increased nervous system stimulation, increased heart rate, and greater attention to new input (Asplund et al., 2010). Furthermore, it stunts the attention to other subsequent events to the surprise event, which means that a surprise event garners most of the attention capacity.

In addition to the research on surprise, research on novelty shows similar interesting results on brain activity. For example, animal studies show that new experiences reduce the strength of existing representations in the hippocampus and prefrontal cortex, which improves learning of new strategies (Park et al., 2021). For new experiences to be recalled, the process of *long-term potentiation*, or continuous strengthening of neural connections must occur while simultaneously remaining flexible to accommodate new information. The implication of this research is that novelty decreases the synaptic network between the ventral hippocampus and the frontal cortex, which makes it possible for new learning to occur.

A recent research study using animal subjects found an interesting association between the memory system and periods of remembering and learning (Gómez-Ocádiz et al., 2022). A major finding was that neural indicators from the hippocampus allow the brain to change from remembering to learning approaches. Various life happenings and events require that the brain recalls stored memories to deal with them. This process of memory recall works well for familiar events, but not so well when the brain experiences novelty or surprises when learning new responses are needed. The researchers concluded that at the precise moment that novelty was introduced to the animal subjects, a signal was sent from the hippocampus that resulted in a change from memory orientation to learning.

According to Montgomery et al. (2021), when there is new input, there is less focus on what already is familiar. The input can then be analyzed and thoroughly investigated. It is vital that a quick determination is made of the input to determine if it is new and novel or familiar. Once the new stimulus is understood and becomes familiar, less attention would be paid to it. In fact, Woloszyn and Sheinberg (2012), in their study of visual input in monkeys, believe that the brain constantly attempts to change its response to novelty by altering its original response of confusion to a recognition that the input is old and familiar. Focusing on the two major types of cells in the brain, *excitatory* and *inhibitory*, Woloszyn and Sheinberg found that they respond differently contingent on visual input. When viewing preferred, familiar input, the excitatory neurons were stimulated, while inhibitory neurons were more active when novel input was introduced. For example, seeing a familiar object such as a banana increases the response of excitatory neurons and activates a behavioral response. On the other hand, seeing a novel or unfamiliar object allows for the inhibitory neurons to signal a learning situation.

Researchers have found that experiencing new and novel situations can improve emotional and mental functioning (Heller et al., 2020). People have more positive emotions when their daily routines include novel experiences. Corresponding neural activity shows that the hippocampus and the striatum, the brain regions associated with processing novelty and reward, are active. Heller et al. (2020) concluded that novelty is related to emotional well-being.

Power Struggles

Many different parenting situations require parents to consider various interventions to stop or alter the behavior. One of the most difficult child behaviors for parents to curtail is a conflict that leads to a power struggle. Simply put, a power struggle between children and parents is when they have different agendas; they are not on the same page; and there is a battle over identity, values, or needs (Gray & Chapel, 2021). Engaging in power struggles is a natural occurrence for toddlers who are establishing themselves as a separate entity and for parents who view parenting as a need to control unwanted child behaviors. To maintain control, parents have rules and boundaries that they impose on children. Consequently, parent–child power struggles are a natural part of the parent–child relationship and often represent the child's growing independence and autonomy. These struggles manifest as disagreements, resistance, and confrontations in which both children and parents vie for dominance or influence. While power struggles can occur at any age, they tend to be most pronounced during specific developmental periods.

Power struggles in early childhood often revolve around issues related to physical autonomy, such as toileting, dressing, eating, and bedtime (Morin, 2021). Young children are striving to establish their independence, while parents are attempting to set boundaries and ensure safety. The child's limited language and impulse control may contribute to confrontations. The burden is on parents to appropriately handle the power struggle. The most common strategies for managing power struggles at this stage include offering choices within acceptable limits, maintaining consistency, and using positive reinforcement.

Part of the difficulty parents have with toddlers is the mistaken belief that toddlers are misbehaving, and that misbehavior is on purpose (Lerner, 2021). Parents who engage in power struggles with their child lack developmental knowledge of appropriate toddler behavior. This misguided view is implicated in their responses to the child's reluctance in following parental imperatives. Just like their parents, toddlers are not being manipulative when they refuse to comply, they are being strategic to get their needs met.

Temperament, which refers to the innate characteristics of the child, is a major aspect of toddler behavior and plays a role in their engagement in power struggles (Kopala-Sibley et al., 2018). Toddlers are known for their curious and exploratory nature, often leading to power struggles with parents as they navigate the complex task of developing autonomy while still relying on adults for support and guidance. Temperament encompasses a range of characteristics, such as activity level, adaptability, intensity of reactions, mood, and attention span, among others. These traits are relatively stable throughout the life course and can influence how a person interacts with their environment.

Toddlers with high reactivity may be more prone to emotional outbursts and intense reactions when they encounter obstacles (Miller, 2023). These emotional responses can lead to power struggles if parents are unable to effectively manage the child's emotional state. Toddlers with low adaptability may have difficulty transitioning from one activity to another or accepting changes in routine. These challenges can lead to power struggles when caregivers need to redirect the child's behavior. Toddlers who are highly sensitive to sensory input may experience discomfort or irritation more easily. This discomfort can lead to power struggles if caregivers are unaware of these sensitivities or do not take them into account. Short attention spans can make it challenging for toddlers to focus on tasks or follow instructions, potentially leading to power struggles when caregivers need the child's attention.

Middle school is a transitional period during which children begin to assert their independence and question authority. Consequently, power struggles between parents and middle school-age children often emerge (Figure 11.1). These struggles can lead to increased conflict and tension within the family (Hill & Tyson, 2009). During middle childhood, power struggles shift to areas like homework, chores, and social activities. Children's increasing cognitive development enables them to assert their preferences and question rules. Parents may find themselves negotiating with their children more frequently. Encouraging open communication, setting

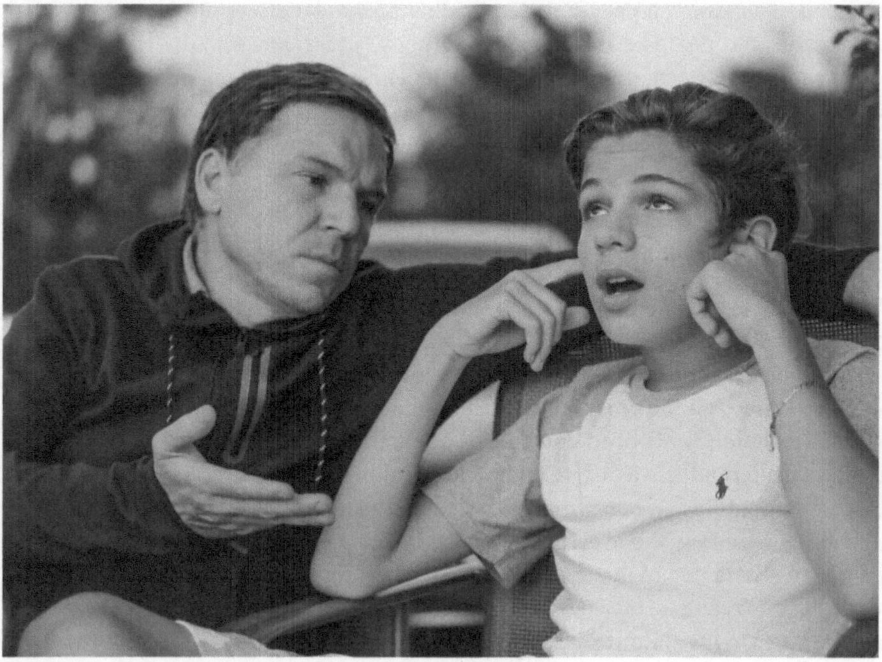

FIGURE 11.1 Power struggles between parent and teenager often result from poor communication. (Photo by Kindel Media from Pexels)

clear expectations, and involving children in rulemaking can help mitigate power struggles during this stage.

Middle school-age children are in the process of developing their identities and seeking greater emotional autonomy. They may challenge parental authority as they test their own boundaries and make independent decisions (Hill & Tyson, 2009). Peer influence becomes more significant during the middle school years. Parents may find themselves in power struggles when their children start to prioritize peer opinions and values over those of their family. Miscommunication or a lack of effective communication between parents and their middle school-age children can lead to power struggles. Differences in perspectives and failure to understand one another's needs can escalate conflicts.

The adolescent stage, a developmental stage characterized by significant physical, emotional, and social changes, is particularly conducive to power struggles. Adolescents are exploring their identity and seeking greater autonomy, often pushing against parental authority. Power struggles may revolve around curfews, choice of friends, academic decisions, and lifestyle choices. These conflicts, if not managed effectively, can impact family dynamics and the well-being of all individuals involved. By gaining a deeper understanding of the dynamics at play, parents and adolescents can navigate this challenging phase more constructively. Parents are often caught between granting more independence and maintaining necessary boundaries. Parents generally deal with power struggles in adolescence by maintaining open communication, negotiating differences in expectations, and respecting the teenager's perspective.

The Confusion/Rope-a-Dope Technique for Power Struggles

Power struggles with children is one of the major parenting issues that affect parent–child relations during the formative years. Parents typically use first order parenting to deal with them, which tend to be of the explicit, or verbal style. Second order parenting, on the other hand, uses implicit techniques. The suggestion to use implicit techniques is not to conclude that explicit techniques are ineffective, but to offer an alternative way of parental intervention that is based on sound neuroscience underpinnings. When parents use the confusion/rope-a-dope technique, they essentially withdraw themselves from the conflict. While withdrawal can be a confusing technique due to the unexpected and surprising characteristics, there are no studies that investigate the success of removing oneself from a negative interaction and thus proving withdrawal's effectiveness.

One of the most useful parental techniques in power struggles with their children is withdrawing or seemingly giving up power. It may also be one of the most difficult for parents to do. The difficulty in using this technique is that withdrawing from the conflict gives the impression that the child wins and this feels counterintuitive for parents. It goes against what they believe is necessary to be an adequate parent.

Nurturance and control are considered the basic parenting responsibilities and much of parenting is a balancing act between providing love and emotional support versus setting limits and imposing consequences. While both are necessary and need to be engaged in, too much or too little of either can spell issues with children. For example, systemic therapists point out that parents who overindulge their children, intrude into their children's lives, and fail to maintain boundaries because of a need to be emotionally connected to their child will produce dependent children who lack a strong sense of self (Bowen, 2015). Additionally, parents who are fixated on their child's behavior to guide or regulate the behavior will impede the natural progression of the child learning to self-regulate and will produce children who are emotionally immature and impulsive. The fear that children will be out of control unless parents actively stop the behavior is very real for some parents. The overuse of control by parents to prevent children from winning in a conflict can increase children's sense of alienation from parents and contribute to further poor relationships.

An analysis of power dynamics in the family on the definition of power reveals lack of clarity and mislabeling. For example, on the surface, the loudest or most physically engaged family member in a conflict may be considered to have the most power but, in fact, may have the least power in terms of controlling the outcome. According to Haley (1993), the family member who defines the interactional patterns within the family has the most power in the family. By controlling who can speak and what they can speak about, a member can control the flow and, therefore, functions as a type of executor of the family. Consequently, a reserved member may weld more power than a loud member.

Having power and expressing it is a human need that both parents and children desire. The need to control aspects of one's life and self-regulate emotional content is necessary for humans at all stages, but first presents itself as vital in small children. *Self-efficacy* is rooted in a sense of power and control. Children's sense of power is rooted in their need to have control over themselves rather than control over parents (Faull, 2023). What seems powerful to children may differ from what seems powerful to adults. The imposing physical difference between parents and children creates for children a sense of powerlessness in that parents can force their will by physical means. As children age, their view of power changes. Parents make decisions, control resources, such as money, and can set limits on children's outside activities. This change is most prominent in adolescents when they become aware of the larger social network.

Second Order Parenting and the Confusion/Rope-a-Dope Technique

The above discussion on power in the parent–child relationship sets the stage for understanding the nuances of how parents can increase their repertoire of interventions. As previously stated, parents have available to them many first order techniques and skill development procedures for changing unwanted child behavior. These interventions are referred to as first order because the goal is to apply overt, verbal, and specific interventions for specific problems. This interest in focusing on eliminating specific child behaviors is shared by parents and parenting experts. The problem of defining behavior problems is an issue that affects the type of intervention used by the parent (Corelli, 2023). The implication here is that when defiant behavior is labeled and interventions are enacted to change the behavior, that behavior may change but will pop out again in another round of unwanted behavior. While many of these parenting techniques are successful, they fail to provide a complete contextual understanding of the problem. They also limit interventions to conscious interventions without understanding the unconscious processes involved. Interventions that are outside of conscious awareness are generally neglected.

Second order parenting, on the other hand, believes that unconscious processes drive transformational change, and that conscious cognitive understanding of the change process is not necessary. This is why an intervention utilizing the confusion/rope-a-dope technique could be used to address some difficult parenting issues. For example, when the parent does something unexpected or confusing, it results in a conscious and unconscious attempt to resolve the situation. Most of this mental activity occurs unconsciously. The following story helps to illustrate how the parent using confusion can change child behavior (see Table 11.3).

James and Mary had their first child later than most parents. They married when James was 34 and Mary was 30. They both had been reared in stable families where the mother was the primary caregiver and their fathers were career-oriented and worked to support the family financially. James and Mary were breaking the mold in that both had careers and wanted to advance in their careers. They wanted to establish themselves in their careers and enjoy their relationship before introducing children. They had been married five years when their first child, Dylan, was born. Dylan received much attention from both parents, who had rearranged their work schedules so that one of them would be always home with him. Dylan was developing normally, and James and Mary felt good about their parenting until Dylan became 2 years old. While they were familiar with temper tantrums as an issue in parenting toddlers, they were not prepared for dealing with them.

When the tantrums first started, they reacted by giving in. Dylan had favorite toys that he would use to bang on furniture or throw against other fixtures in the house and reacted violently if the toy was taken from him. He would throw himself on the floor kicking and screaming. This behavior was so disturbing to James and Mary that they wanted to stop it immediately, and they would give the toy back. Their response was ineffective and contributed to increased temper tantrums. They talked about consulting with a parenting expert and made an appointment with a therapist that specialized in toddler issues. Before they could keep the appointment, a spontaneous and unrehearsed interaction occurred between James and Dylan. As James was watching TV while Dyaln played on the floor, Dylan began banging on the furniture with a toy. James immediately responded by taking the toy and first attempting to redirect Dylan with a different toy. Dylan reacted by throwing himself on the floor headfirst, kicking and screaming at the top of his lungs. While James had thought this behavior somewhat amusing before, he had always resisted

TABLE 11.3 Second Order Parenting and the Confusion/Rope-a-Dope Intervention

The Unconscious Processes of Second Order Parenting and Confusion
Second order parenting is driven by unconscious processes that produce transformational change
Conscious cognitive understanding of the change process is not necessary
Confusion interventions are effective with difficult misbehavior in children
The confusion/rope-a-dope intervention is unexpected and novel
Confusion causes the hippocampus to signal the prefrontal cortex that the brain should shift from excitatory to inhibitory response
Resolution from the confused state is accomplished unconsciously leading to different behavior

laughing. It struck him particularly funny that taking the toy away could produce such an outburst of emotion in Dylan. James was overcome with laughter and laughed hysterically for what seemed like minutes and then left the room with the toy. When he returned to the room, Dylan was playing peacefully at his play table.

Another example of parents using the confusion technique and withdrawal from conflict is during the teenage years when parents and adolescents have frequent conflicts. Megan is a 16-year-old high school junior who excels in academics and in sports. She is a star player on the girl's school soccer and lacrosse teams in addition to being on the academic honor roll with a straight A average. She recently began her first romantic relationship with 19-year-old former student, T. J., at her high school who is now a college freshman at a nearby college. He was the star quarterback on the football team and has an athletic college scholarship. She had a crush on him in high school but because he was several grades ahead of her, they had little contact. They met at a summer bonfire party on the beach and soon began dating. He was known in high school for being a ladies' man who loved to party and who had many girlfriends. When Megan's parents found out that she was dating T. J. when she claimed to be going out to a movie with her girlfriend, they were upset and confronted her. The confrontation did not go well. Megan accused them of spying on her and overreacting. She defended T. J.'s reputation, claiming that he cared about her and had changed. She threatened to move out of the home if they refused to let her see him. Equally upsetting to her parents was the decline in Megan's grades and poor performances on her sports teams.

Megan became so angry during the discussion that she took the position that they had no authority over her. At 16 years old, she believed that she could make her own decisions and would do so if they continued to restrict her. At that point, her parents, who had remained calm throughout the talk, stood up and quietly left the room. Without saying anything more, they simply withdrew from the conflict. They did not remove themselves for an effect, but out of love for their daughter to give her some space. What occurred next was not anticipated by her parents. In the morning, Megan apologized for her outburst and threatening to leave home. She said she was glad that they knew about her relationship with T. J. and wanted to talk more to work out an agreement with them.

Although these examples seem simplistic on the surface, they illustrate well the underlying dynamics of how confusion/rope-a-dope interventions could be effective in changing child behavior. First, the intervention of the parents is unexpected and confusing. The child does not expect parents to withdraw from the conflict, or not to take it seriously. It is novel and not familiar to the child, resulting in a signal from the hippocampus to the prefrontal cortex that the brain response should shift from excitatory to inhibitory response and initiate a learning process. The parents withdrawing from the conflict is new information which is at odds with past behavior. The child's inhibitory system is activated which reduces the strength of the existing representations in the hippocampus. Resolution from the confused state is accomplished more unconsciously, leading to the child behaving differently. The new behavioral response occurs because of the greater attention to new input.

References

Abdelrahmana, R. M. (2020). Metacognitive awareness and academic motivation and their impact on academic achievement of Ajman University students. *Heliyon, 6*(9), e04192. https://doi.org/10.1016/j.heliyon.2020.e04192; Published online 2020 September 2.

Andrevski, G. (2020). When a rope-a-dope strategy makes sense. *Smith Business Insight*. Retrieved November 1, 2023, from https://smith.queensu.ca/insight/content/when-a-rope-a-dope-strategy-makes-sense.php

Arguel, A., Lockyer, L., Lipp, O. V., Lodge, J. M., & Kennedy, G. (2017). Inside out: Detecting learners' confusion to improve interactive digital learning environments. *Journal of Educational Computing Research, 55*(4), 526–551.

Asplund, C. L., Todd, J., Snyder, A. P., & Marois, R. (2010). A central role for the lateral prefrontal cortex in goal-directed and stimulus-driven attention. *Nature Neuroscience, 13*(4), 507–512. https://doi.org/10.1038/nn.2509

Berns, G. S., McClure, S. M., Pagnoni, G., & Montague, P. R. (2001). Predictability modulates human brain response to reward. *Journal of Neuroscience, 21,* 2793–2798. https://doi.org/https://doi.org/10.1523/JNEUROSCI.21-08-02793.2001

Bowen, M. (2015). *The origin of family therapy: The NIMH family study project*. Rowman and Littlefield.

Brem, A., Ran, K., & Pascual-Leone, A. (2013). Learning and memory. *Handbook of Clinical Neurology, 116,* 693–737. https://doi.org/10.1016/B978-0-444-53497-2.00055

Charvet, S. R. (2019). *Words that change minds* (3rd ed.). Bloomanity.

Corelli, T. (2023). *Why most parenting advise is wrong*. Retrieved October 25, 2023, from https://www.linkedin.com/pulse/why-most-parenting-advice-wrong-todd-corelli?trk=article-ssr-frontend-pulse_more-articles_related-content-card

D'Mello, S., Lehman, B., Pekrun, R., & Graesser, A. (2014). Confusion can be beneficial for learning. *Learning and Instruction, 29,* 153–170. https://doi.org/10.1016/j.learninstruc.2012.05.003

Dreikurs, R. (1964). *Children the challenge*. Dutton.

Faber, A., & Mazlish, E. (1980). *How to talk so kids will listen and listen so kids will talk*. Avon.

Faull, J. (2023). Unplugging power struggles. *PEPS*. Retrieved October 25, 2023, from https://www.peps.org/ParentResources/by-topic/development/unplugging-power-struggles

Festinger, L. (1957). *The theory of cognitive dissonance*. Stanford University Press.

Gómez-Ocádiz, R., Trippa, M., Zhang, C., Posani, L., Cocco, S., Monasson, R., & Schmidt-Hieber, C. (2022, July). A synaptic signal for novelty processing in the hippocampus. *Nature Communications, 13*(1), 4122. https://doi.org/10.1038/s41467-022-31775-6

Gray, J., & Chapel, L. (2021). *Power struggles in relationships*. Retrieved October 10, 2023, from https://study.com/learn/lesson/power-struggle-relationships-overview-examples.html

Haley, J. (1993). *Uncommon therapy: The psychiatric techniques of Milton H. Erickson, M. D.* W. W. Norton.

Heller, A. S., Shi, T. C., Ezie, C. E. C., Reneau, T. R., Baez, L. M., Gibbons, C. J., & Hartley, C. A. (2020). Association between real-world experiential diversity and positive affect relates to hippocampal–striatal functional connectivity. *Nature Neuroscience, 28,* 800–804. https://doi.org/10.1038/s41593-020-0636-4

Hill, N. E., & Tyson, D. F. (2009). A meta-analytic assessment of the strategies that promote achievement. *Developmental Psychology, 45*(3), 740–763. https://doi.org/10.1037/a001536

Kardes, F. R., Fennis, B. M., Hirt, E. R., Tormala, Z. L., & Bullington, B. (2007). The role of the need for cognitive closure in the effectiveness of the disrupt-then-reframe influence technique. *Journal of Consumer Research, 34*(3), 377–385. https://doi.org/10.1086/518541

Kennedy, G., & Lodge, J. M. (2016). All roads lead to Rome: Tracking students' affect as they overcome misconceptions. In S. Barker, S. Dawson, A. Pardo, & C. Colvin (Eds.), *Show me the learning. Proceedings ASCILITE* (pp. 318–328). https://2016conference.ascilite.org/wp-content/uploads/ascilite2016_kennedy_full.pdf

Kopala-Sibley, D. C., Olino, T., Durbin, E., Dyson, M. W., & Klein, D. N. (2018). The stability of temperament from early childhood to early adolescence: A multi-method, multi-informant examination. *European Journal of Personality, 32*(2), 128–145. https://doi.org/10.1002/per.2151

LeDoux, J. E. (1992). Brain mechanisms of emotion and emotional learning. *Current Opinions in Neurobiology, 2,* 191–197. https://doi.org/10.1016/0959-4388(92)90011-9

Lerner, C. (2021). *Why is my child in charge? A roadmap to end power struggles, increase cooperation, and find joy in parenting young children.* Rowman and Littlefield.

Liang, Y., Liu, X., Qiu, L., & Zhang, S. (2018). An EEG study of a confusing state induced by information insufficiency during mathematical problem-solving and reasoning. *Computational Intelligence and Neuroscience, 2018,* 1943565. https://doi.org/10.1155/2018/1943565

Lodge, J., & Kennedy, G. (2016, September 13). Confused? Don't worry because that can be a good thing. *The Conversation*. Retrieved September 8, 2023, from https://theconversation.com/confused-dont-worry-because-that-can-be-a-good-thing-64421

Lodge, J., Kennedy, G., Lockyer, L., Amael, A., & Pachman, M. (2018, June 28). Understanding difficulties and resulting confusion in learning: An integrative review. *Frontiers in Education, 3*. https://doi.org/10.3389/feduc.2018.00049

Mandler, G. (1990). Interruption (discrepancy) theory: Review and extension. In S. Fisher & C. L. Cooper (Eds.), *On the move: The psychology of change and transitions* (pp. 13–32). Wiley.

Miller, C. (2023). DMDD: Extreme tantrums and irritability. *Child Mind Institute*. Retrieved October 13, 2023, from https://childmind.org/article/dmdd-extreme-tantrums-irritability/

Minuchin, S., & Fishman, H. C. (1981). *Family therapy techniques*. Harvard University Press.

Montgomery, D. P., Hayden, D. J., Chaloner, F. A., Cooke, S. F., & Bear, M. F. (2021). Stimulus-selective response plasticity in primary visual cortex: Progress and puzzles. *Frontiers of Neural Circuits, 15*. https://doi.org/10.3389/fncir.2021.815554815554

Moore, D. A., & Healy, P. J. (2008). The trouble with overconfidence. *Psychological Review, 115*(2), 502–517. https://doi.org/10.1037/0033-295X.115.2.502

Morin, A. (2021). How to avoid power struggles with children. *Verywell Family*. Retrieved October 10, 2023, from https://www.verywellfamily.com/how-to-avoid-power-struggles-with-children-1094751

Nikolić, J. (2019, December 2). How does the brain deal with novelty? *Sapien Labs*. Retrieved October 27, 2023, from https://sapienlabs.org/lab-talk/how-does-the-brain-deal-with-novelty/

Park, A. J., Harris, A. Z., Martyniuk, K. M., Chang, C.-Y., Abbas, A. I., Lowes, D. C., Kellendonk, C., Gogos, J. A., & Gordon, J. A. (2021). Reset of hippocampal–prefrontal circuitry facilitates learning. *Nature, 591*(7851), 615–619. https://doi.org/10.1038/s41586-021-03272-1

Philips, N., Sioen, I., Michels, N., Sleddens, E. F. C., & De Henauw, S. (2014). The influence of parenting style on health-related behavior of children: Findings from the ChiBS study. *International Journal of Behavioral Nutrition and Physical Activity, 11*(1), 95. https://doi.org/10.1186/s12966-014-0095-y

Smith, M., & Karam, E. (2018). Positive feedback in family systems theory. In J. Lebow, A. Chambers, & D. Breunlin (Eds.), *Encyclopedia of couple and family therapy*. Springer. https://doi.org/10.1007/978-3-319-15877-8_301-1

Vogl, E., Pekrun, R., Murayama, K., & Loderer, K. (2020). Surprised-curious-confused: Epistemic emotions and knowledge exploration. *Emotion, 20*(4), 625–641. https://doi.org/10.1037/emo0000578

Webster-Stratton, C. H., & Reid, M. J. (2010). The incredible years program for children from infancy to pre-adolescence: Prevention and treatment of behavior problems. In R. C. Murrihy, A. D. Kidman, & T. H. Ollendick (Eds.), *Clinical handbook of assessing and treating conduct problems in youth* (pp. 117–138). Springer Science. https://doi.org/10.1007/978-1-4419-6297-3_5

Whitaker, C., & Malone, T. (1981). *The roots of psychotherapy*. Brunner/Mazel.

Woloszyn, L., & Sheinberg, D. L. (2012). Effects of long-term visual experience on responses of distinct classes of single units in inferior temporal cortex. *Neuron, 74*(1), 193–205. https://doi.org/10.1016/j.neuron.2012.01.032

Xu, T., Wang, J., Zhang, G., Zhang, L., & Zhou, Y. (2023). Confused or not: Decoding brain activity and recognizing confusion in reasoning learning using EEG. *Journal Neural Engineering, 20*(2). https://doi.org/10.1088/1741-2552/acbfe0; PMID: 36854180

12

PARADOX

The Insight of Contradiction

In literature, a *paradox* is a literary device that, on the surface, seems contradictory but on further scrutiny conveys undeniable truth. In general, a paradox is a premise that appears to be logical and rational, yet contains contradictory elements that defy common sense (Oxford Wordpower Dictionary, 1993). While the definition of paradox alters slightly depending on the context, the impact of the paradox on understanding, thinking, and behavioral change is profound. Paradoxical statements present ideas that demand one take note to determine the meaning behind the statement. Breaking down the word paradox into its root meanings offers insight into its deeper meaning (Craiker, 2021). For example, *para* means "beyond" and *dox* comes from a Greek word that means "to think." A paradox requires that one *thinks beyond*, outside the box, or outside the normal way of thinking. A statement such as, "hurry up and slow down," seems contradictory, but if one's goal is to slow down, one may be in a rush to reach that goal. Some paradoxical statements may be logically impossible to resolve but they create significant mental gymnastics. For example, the paradoxical question, *which came first, the chicken or the egg?*, is contradictory and without an obvious answer (Figure 12.1). A more contemporary logical paradox is the argument made by modern-day *postmodern thinkers* who claim that there is no objective truth, and, therefore, all truth is relative. To say "all things are relative" is itself an objective truth, contradictory to postmodernists' value in relativity. Paradoxical thinking has been widely used in therapy, and a discussion of how paradox has been used to change families will be reviewed later.

DOI: 10.4324/9781003381679-14

Family Therapy and Paradoxical Interventions

Paradoxical thinking has been documented in various scholarly fields, including psychology (Sutton, 2022), religion (Kosloff & Solomon, 2020), and hard sciences such as physics (Matthews, 2022). The importance of paradox to change behavior has been demonstrated in the field of psychotherapy. Systemic family therapists such as Whitaker and Malone (1981) and Haley (1993) used paradox to influence the family. For Haley, this technique was used for clients who seemed to be stuck in a destructive cycle or who were resistant to therapy. For example, a writer with writer's block and paralyzed by fear of making mistakes might be given the suggestion to write something that was obviously poorly constructed. The therapist states that the purpose for the suggestion is to help the writer learn how to handle making mistakes, which additionally serves to reframe the writer's fear, overcoming poor writing. The reframe changes the focus from avoiding writing to recovering from poor writing. The implication is that the fear of writing is now manageable due to the change in how the writer sees the problem.

Another way to use paradox in therapy is when the therapist encounters a family that claims they need to change but refuses to follow through on any interventions

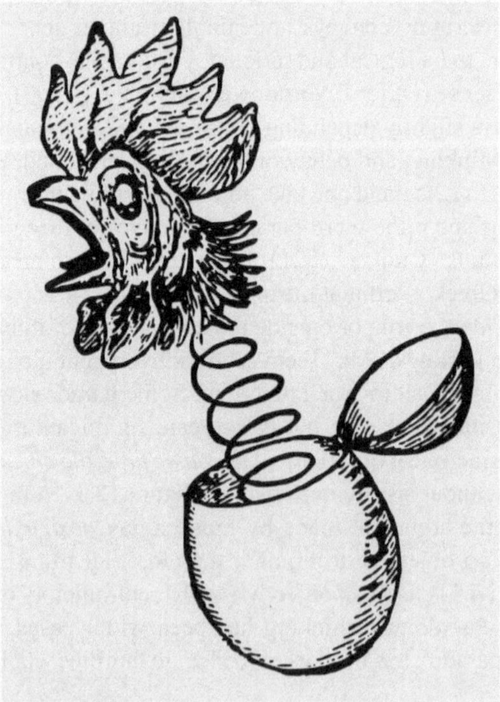

FIGURE 12.1 Paradoxical thinking can allow for unique perspectives and thinking outside the box.

(Haley, 1993). The *"go slow" intervention* is used to put the family in a therapeutic double-bind where whatever the family does will have positive outcomes. For example, if the therapist says the family may not be ready for the chaos that the change would bring and they should stay the course for now, either way the family responds would result in a positive outcome. If they do as the therapist suggests and stay the course, then they show greater cooperation, and if they move forward with changes then they will begin to reduce symptoms. While this technique may seem magical, it works because it fits with a systems view of how families function, especially in maintaining symptomatic behavior. Using paradox outside of this context may be misapplied and inappropriate.

Systemic therapists use paradox in therapy to change the pattern of communication from maintaining the symptoms to creating a new pattern that promotes growth and health (Haley, 1993). Consequently, according to Haley, therapy is meant to be brief not to uncover the underlying cause of the problem, since paradoxical thinkers do not believe that understanding the cause of the problem will change it. Many of the paradoxical interventions used appear counterintuitive but can have dramatic effects. For example, for a child who refuses to eat a nutritious meal and instead insists on eating nothing but potato chips so that mealtimes are stressful and irritating to parents, a systemic therapist might suggest that instead of forcing their child to eat a balanced meal, allow them to eat all the potato chips they want. The rationale behind this intervention is the child will, in time, learn the negative consequences of eating nothing but potato chips and will self-regulate to a more balanced meal.

Such interventions as this appear are logically contradictory to the goal of the child eating a balanced meal. It is based on the supposition that cognitive awareness and insight is not necessary for change and that change takes place implicitly through unconscious processes. Furthermore, it is postulated that the change that takes place is transformational or second order. The structure and maintaining mechanism of the symptoms are altered. When clients engage in these interventions, their resistance to change works toward enacting change so that by being resistant to the intervention, they change.

In the process whereby paradoxes cause second order change, the therapist *prescribes the symptom* by instructing the client to enact the problem behavior they want to avoid. This maneuver allows the client to have a greater understanding of the control they have over the behavior. If the client can consciously create the problem behavior, they are able to change it as well. The therapist maintains a neutral attitude toward the problem behavior which allows for the client to learn from the intervention (see Table 12.1).

Hameiri et al. (2014) applied paradoxical thinking to changing the most intractable positions held in opposition to each other. The idea of applying paradoxical thinking to intractable social or political ideologies, which are shared by like-minded individuals, is a new paradigm for resolving conflicts. Social and political conflicts are the most difficult to peacefully resolve because they reflect

TABLE 12.1 How Paradox Works to Change Behavior

Paradox and Second Order Change
Paradoxical thinking is useful in various scholarly fields, particularly psychotherapy
A paradox is effective in reducing resistance to change
A paradox can induce a double-bind circumstance
Communication patterns change from maintaining the symptoms to changing their behavior
Paradox facilitates second order parenting because the structure of the problem is altered
Paradoxical change occurs because the unconscious mind processes the metaphoric meaning

ideological identities that are firmly implanted. Such conflicts have long histories, carry over into perpetuity, and are characterized as rigid where information that does not reinforce the prevailing beliefs are defended against and quickly disregarded. A successful intervention should unfreeze the previously held contradictions and alter the view of conflict and of the opponent.

According to Hameiri et al. (2014), the typical way to create second order change is to use interventions that reduce or block the entrenched beliefs or to allow for a context that permits new ideas to arise. These approaches are conscious, explicit cognitive interventions where the new information counters the old rigid beliefs systems. Furthermore, these interventions are based on *consistency theory*. For example, when new information is inconsistent with one's belief system, resulting in cognitive dissonance, this encourages one to shift from the established belief system to a more functional belief system. The underlying weakness in consistency theory is the reliance on the strength of the inconsistency caused by the challenge to held beliefs.

Hameiri et al. (2014) believed that a new paradigm was needed to adequately create the change that is needed for intractable belief systems. They believed that paradoxical thinking was a novel approach that had the promise to be successful in changing belief systems because it did not offer new information to cause inconsistency. In addition, they believed that paradoxical thinking would not lead to a defensive reaction, would be easily applied, would have validity, and could be used broadly by professionals.

Hameiri et al. (2014) were influenced to use paradox from reviewing clinical literature that suggested that when persons are provided with an exaggeration that is consistent with their held beliefs, they are prone to change those beliefs regardless of how entrenched they are. For example, instead of resisting the thing they fear, clients were encouraged by the approach and accepted the fear. The caveat to this approach is that if clients are not motivated to change as many people with rigid belief systems generally are not, the outcome may not be as productive.

Assumptions about Using Paradox

An underlying assumption about paradoxical interventions is that persons can be understood only from the relationships in which they are involved. Consequently, to think of them as *independent entities* is a misconception. The position that persons can only be understood through their relationships has been criticized because it raises an ethical question. For example, Haley (1976) has been criticized for saying that it is acceptable to lie to families if it will facilitate change (labeled "*beneficial lie*"), because it undermines the individual's right to be evaluated based on their individual behavior (MacIntyre, 1987). Ethical concerns could be raised about interventions that may have long-term psychological effects (Peluso & Freund, 2023). The concern about ethics in therapy centers on the *informed consent right* of the client who has a right to know the treatment and procedures used by the therapist. The assumption that the client makes when they enter the therapeutic relationship is that the therapist is honest and has a *fiduciary relationship* with the client. The use of deceit by the therapist can be seen as a violation of the fiduciary commitment to the client. The client must be able to believe that the therapist is trustworthy, transparent, and is acting to improve their well-being.

Resistance and intractable problems have been the impetus for using paradoxical interventions (Peluso & Freund, 2023). Resistance to therapy may present itself when the client fails to complete homework assignments or follow through on other aspects of the treatment. The scenario plays out with the therapist pursuing more compliance with the interventions and the client becoming even more resistant. The consequence of this stand-off is that the client will deteriorate more, and therapy will be declared a failure. The therapist must stay loyal to treating the client and use any means that would improve the well-being of the client. Since, from the therapist's perspective, termination of therapy can take place only if the client sufficiently improves, the client would then either transfer to another therapist or request to terminate therapy. From the standpoint of the therapist who uses paradox, the loyalty principle means that if the therapist can intuit that paradox would be effective in reducing the symptoms and in improving the client's emotional and mental functioning, then not using a paradoxical intervention would be unethical. Browning and Hull (2021) argue that many of the concerns over ethics in using paradox are unjustified due to a lack of nuanced reasoning. While some paradoxical interventions may be dishonest and manipulative, other interventions are direct, honest, and balanced. Browning and Hull point out the different types of paradox and tie them to sociological and historical contexts.

Other criticisms of paradoxical interventions are based on the lack of rigorous research methods, and consequently have not been acknowledged as an integral part of psychotherapy (Ascher & Turner, 1979). According to Ascher and Turner, most research presents case studies using clinical subjects. Furthermore, most of the reports of change come from therapists and not from clients and are, therefore, unreliable. Others have made clear arguments that paradoxical interventions are effective.

The first prominent psychotherapist to use paradoxical interventions was Afred Adler (1925/2011). He believed that dialectics form the basis of therapy, and that paradox was a form of dialectics. Adler believed that the patient takes an uncooperative stance with the therapist and a paradoxical intervention swings the patient toward cooperation. By not challenging the patient and accepting the resistance, the therapist is able to forge a therapeutic alliance with the patient. Adler's use of paradox includes giving the patient permission to have their symptoms, predicting that symptoms will return, reframing symptoms as positive, and prescribing the continuation of the symptoms. The use of the Adlerian model of paradoxical interventions was continued by Dreikurs (1968) for parenting misbehaving children.

The name most associated with paradoxical approaches and the effectiveness of the approach is Milton Erickson (1980). While it is the case that rigorous research may be lacking in paradoxical interventions in therapy, it should not be concluded that the approach is ineffective. The work of Milton Erickson, which gave birth to a whole school of systemic therapies, provides ample evidence of the effectiveness of this approach. His contribution to psychotherapy was profound and based on the *power of suggestion* of language. He used a novel approach to induce hypnotic states that were paradoxical in nature which were intended to change clients by facilitating change, not by directing the outcome. He believed that once the change process began, it would create its own outcome. Believing that all persons are different, Erickson did not have a standard set of interventions. Rather, his interventions were created individually for each client, which has been described variously as a *utilization approach*, using what the client offers about themselves or their problems (Gorton, 2005). He wanted to fully understand his clients and developed a style of relating where he could facilitate small changes in their behavior that would start and cause an avalanche of changes. He relied on his unconscious perceptions which he viewed as the source of creative wisdom. His novel approach attempted to connect to the client's unconscious which contained the storehouse of resources for change. While he used hypnosis at times, his approach was not the common method of inducing hypnosis.

Erickson (1980) deviated from common practice in psychotherapy. He did not believe that understanding the past was necessary for change; what *was* necessary for change was doing something different. The change need not be large because any change, regardless of how small, will have cascading effects and usher in larger change. The change was always initiated by the client and not by Erickson and in this sense, he was considered *nondirective*. He believed that showing genuine empathy was necessary for change to occur. Unless the therapist had genuine empathy, the client would feel manipulated, and that the therapist was phony. Having real concern for the client and using what the client brought to therapy (e.g., the client's own story, expressions, and language) established rapport. At the same time, the therapist must be comfortable with themselves and trust their intuitive perceptions. When thoughts and perceptions emerge into consciousness that may not rationally seem to connect to what is being said, Erickson believed that this was important and necessary to share with the client. Erickson was against rigid alliance to a particular type of psychotherapy and only used interventions that were genuine and comfortable for both the therapist and the client. Even when the client demonstrated little hope for change, Erickson maintained his empathic responses and genuine care for the client.

In addition to using paradoxical interventions, Erickson told stories, used extensive metaphors, and anecdotes, many of which were from his own life and experiences (Short, 2017). Erickson believed that one should enjoy the process of living more than attempting to reach a particular goal. Becoming and growing and even waiting were underlying suggestions to help start the change process. Erickson would infuse words and phrases into the dialogue that would go beyond the verbal conscious understanding so that the wisdom of the unconscious would be activated and affect the client's understanding.

One of the most unique perceptions that come from reading Erikson is that each client is unique, and the approach is unique to that client (Short, 2017). One size does not fit all and there is no repeatable formula for doing psychotherapy. This means that the therapist should not have a predetermined therapy model for all clients. Rather, his paradoxical interventions were spontaneous and fit the context of the client and the direction in therapy was determined by the unique history and interactional patterns that characterized the social environment of the client. Consequently, interventions must be geared to the situation at hand. Erickson viewed problems as opportunities for problem-solving. Problems provide the impetus to marshal efforts to overcome and reach a new level of well-being. Dreading and attempting to avoid problems only add to the despair that accompanies failed efforts.

Erickson's view of the unconscious differed from Freud and other psychoanalysts in that his view gave more credence to the *positive power of the unconscious* (Short, 2017). Erickson believed that the unconscious operated on metaphors, stories, and imagination and he used them to facilitate the change process. He believed that the unconscious mind could process the meaning of stories, metaphors, or paradoxes while the conscious mind could not. His view of hypnosis used casual conversational language instead of the common practice of inducing trance and was also viewed as an unconscious process that the conscious mind could not comprehend. Erikson's perception of the unconscious aligns with recent neuroscience research that demonstrates the significance of the unconscious processes in decision making and problem-solving (Newell & Shanks, 2014). While decision making has been thought of as a rational process engaging the neocortex, recent research has shown that the unconscious makes the decision and transfers this information to the conscious mind. Likewise, problem-solving takes place unconsciously and when a solution is made, the unconscious informs the conscious mind. A trick in perception then happens as the person perceives that the problem was solved by the rational processes of consciousness rather than worked out by the unconscious.

Erickson believed that persons tend to stay stuck in their problems because change is uncomfortable (Short, 2017). Paradox, confusion, and surprise all worked to destabilize this comfortable stuck position. This means that in any type of learning experience, persons must be destabilized to learn new behaviors. This perspective is important for parent education training, which may need to expand the types of training modules to include exercises that activate the unconscious implicit processes. The phrase "no pain, no gain" emphasizes the need to allow for some level of confusion, discomfort, and uncertainty in the training model for positive change to occur.

Erickson's model was based on experiences and full sensory activation instead of a structured model of academic and logical processes (Short, 2017). Change was based on movement away from the rigid automatic responses and insightful understanding of one's behaviors. The underlying premise is that putting one's past under the microscope provides little help in changing behavior. The change is unconscious and, therefore, does not need conscious awareness.

On parenting, Erickson focused on the importance of all behavior, and not narrowly on eliminating bad behavior. The implication is that bad behavior is useful and can be mobilized to produce second order change. For example, parents can be too narrowly focused on eliminating bad behavior of their children and their own perceived weaknesses in parenting by adding new skills.

Erickson's view of psychotherapy differed from his contemporaries in the goal or outcome of therapy (Short, 2017). For example, most outcomes in therapy are thought of as resulting from specific cause-and-effect action. When a particular intervention is applied to a particular problem, the outcome is expected to be a desired outcome. For Erickson, this was not the case. Therapy outcomes were not conceptualized as linear, but instead took a nonlinear path. He recognized that patients often regressed and reverted to past unproductive behavior. More than that, his paradoxical process of therapy, which is counterintuitive by design, gave directions to continue unwanted behavior. Conscious understanding by the patient was not needed for the change to occur and the attempt to make it conscious would inhibit the desired change.

Erickson's approach downplayed using skill-building techniques and instead built a deep and personal relationship with the client (Short, 2017). The first principle was that therapy was a joint project between the therapist and the client. Therapy was not something done to the client, rather it was done together with the client's collaboration. If the deep personal relationship is missing, the therapy interventions would be ineffective.

According to Erickson, the important first step is observation (Short, 2017). Observing strengths instead of weaknesses and hidden resources in the client and using them as the basis for interventions is primary from an Ericksonian perspective. Observation includes how the client uses language, expresses emotions, displays nonverbal gestures, and engages in recurring behavioral patterns. The therapist should pay close attention to what the client avoids saying, which can be referred to as *listening with the third ear*. Observation is extremely important for understanding the client's problem development. Observation sometimes leads to the need for interpretation, but Erickson believed that the therapist should refrain from interpreting because it can lead to the client feeling judged. The therapist should show acceptance and support for all positions stated by the client. It is only in showing complete acceptance that the client will divulge significant thoughts and feelings.

Trusting the client and accepting what they bring to therapy is rooted in the belief that clients possess an inner tendency to grow and develop toward health and well-being. The process of therapy allows the client to lead in the change process (Short, 2017). Therapy from a growth perspective includes the possibility for growth in both the therapist and the client. Because the therapist does not have a blueprint for how therapy will develop, there is no need for targeted interventions designed to change particular behaviors in the client. If the answers lie within the person as Erickson believed, answers that come from outside, as from the therapist, will have little impact on the outcome. Erickson believed that the unconscious contained the creative answers that the client may be asking the therapist for. Change facilitated in this way may happen outside the client's awareness where they recognize a change but cannot verbalize how it happened.

Paradoxical interventions are associated with facilitating transformational or second order change by embracing the principle of inescapability, or not being able to avoid or ignore change (Short, 2017). When the therapist asks the client to perform the behaviors that are inescapable, the underlying repetitive resistance to change occurs. In complying to the therapist's directives, the client must acknowledge the inescapability of the behavior and not focus on resisting the change that is simultaneously occurring. The client changes whether they follow the directive or do not follow the directive.

An important aspect of Erickson's views about therapy is that it should be experiential; that is, therapy should involve action rather than merely providing didactic or intellectual input (Short, 2017). Experiential activities provide a way for the client to uncover insights and solutions that seemed unsolvable. The therapist is a facilitator, not an expert on what the client will discover from the experience. The nature of the experience was not the deciding factor for the benefits to the client. Rather, any experience could lead to a change in perspective, mood, or understanding of their problem.

Neuroscience and Paradox

Most of the research on the neuroscience of thinking has been on deductive and inductive reasoning (Belekou et al., 2022). The ability to think logically and critically is an important aspect of the human brain, which is understood as the process of deductive thinking. In *deductive reasoning*, a valid argument with irrefutable properties can provide conclusive evidence that the outcome is true. If the principles are sound and valid in an argument through the deductive process, the outcome cannot be questioned. Researchers have postulated several theories for how the brain processes deductive reasoning. One theory is the *mental model theory* which views deductive reasoning as a visuospatial procedure grounded in rule-based processes where a spatial depiction of the symptomatic problem is made (Brunetti et al., 2014). The brain region that would be expected to be active if deductive reasoning is processed in the parieto-occipital region of the right hemisphere. An opposing view, *formal rule approach*, posits that deduction is a linguistic process activated in the left hemisphere governed by a set of linguistic rules (Rodriguez-Moreno & Hirsch, 2009). A third model for understanding the brain process during deductive reasoning is *dual process reasoning*, which assumes integration of the two brain systems that cooperate in processing deductive reasoning. The first brain region is the quick automatic activation of the frontotemporal region that is associated with making judgments about what is true, and the second region is a slower network that activates the parieto-occipital and working memory.

While the neurobiological substrates of deductive or logical reasoning have been outlined, a paucity of research exists for paradoxical thinking. One study that investigated if logical deductive reasoning and paradoxical statements activate the same brain regions was conducted by Papageorgiou et al. (2016). The findings of that study concluded that logical deductive reasoning activated the parietal–occipital region and paradox activated the fronto-orbitofrontal region.

To rectify the paucity of research of paradoxical reasoning, Belekou et al. (2022) investigated the brain activation of rational deductive reasoning and nonrational or paradoxical statements. Using fMRI imaging techniques, the researchers observed subjects making decisions on the correctness of logical and paradoxical statements. Results indicated that different brain regions are active for deductive reasoning and paradoxical reasoning. The study concluded that two different brain networks are activated by deductive and paradoxical reasoning. Paradoxical thinking activates the frontotemporal network, while deductive reasoning activates the frontoparietal network. The *frontotemporal network* is an essential element in the understanding of paradoxes and other nonliteral forms of language, such as metaphors (Figure 12.2). According to Belekou et al. (2022), the activation of the frontotemporal network is due to a process of revision in which two propositions are in conflict. The subject must then choose the proposition that carries the least cost. This study, which supports the earlier study by Papageorgiou et al., suggests that logical reasoning and paradoxical reasoning engage different brain networks and, therefore, have different outcomes.

Second Order Parenting and Paradoxical Interventions

While paradoxical interventions have been grounded in family therapy, the application for parenting is enormous. Paradoxical interventions are second order because the goal is to facilitate transformational change via implicit, unconscious

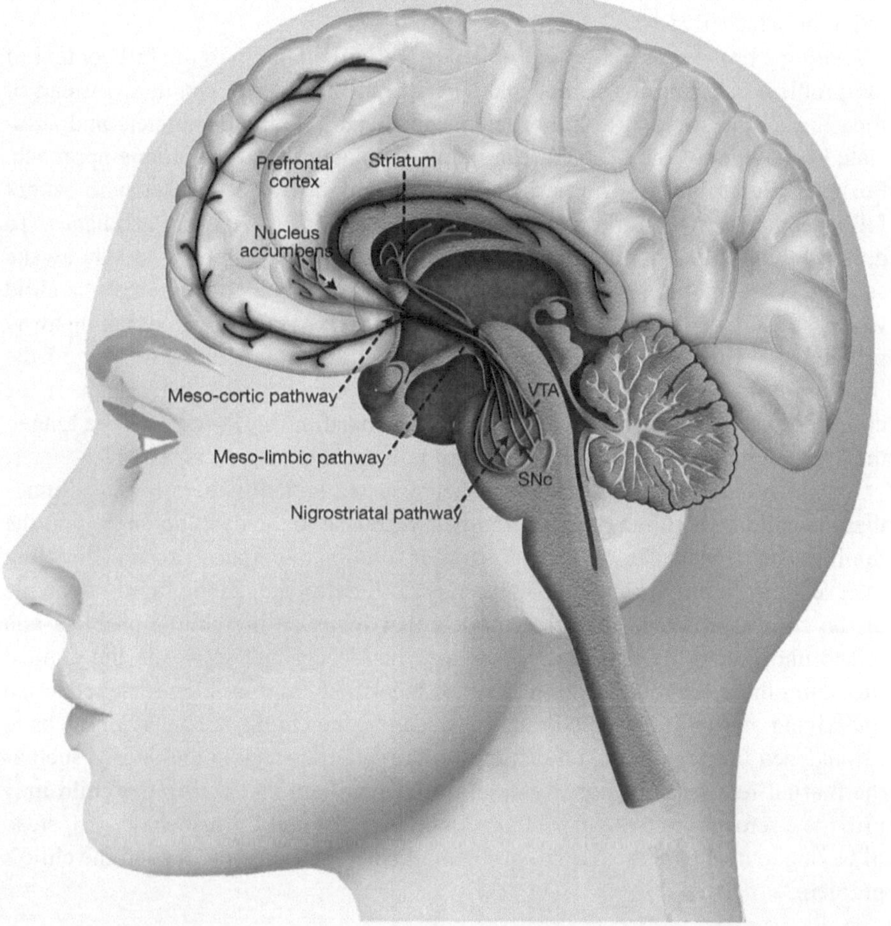

FIGURE 12.2 Paradoxical thinking activates the frontotemporal network, which is an essential brain network in understanding nonliteral language, such as metaphors, and in interpreting truth. (Arias-Carrión et al., 2010, CC BY-SA 4.0)

processes. These interventions do not require insight or knowledge of how they cause change. Brain processes provide an explanation for the ensuing change and provide a heuristic understanding of the change process. Second order change is enhanced by paradoxical interventions because the basis is to try something different. Parents persist in doing the same things repeated even if they do not work. Something different and unexpected by the parent can have enormous effects on the child's behavior. This can be true because brain processes are activated in the child. To do something different, the parent may need to alter how they view the problem. If the problem is long-standing, the parent may need to reassess from a different perspective.

Getting a broader view of the problem by careful attention to the full context of the problem can help the parent make small but meaningful changes. Instead of focusing on the solution to the problem, understanding the parameters and associated behaviors of the problem can help formulate a new and unique approach. For example, a mother who is disturbed every night by her toddler who cannot fall asleep after story time punishes her daughter by taking away privileges. To do something different could be to tell her daughter that it is okay to stay awake as long as the light in her room is turned off. The outcome could be that the child would be more compliant with following this directive than the parent taking away privileges. Telling the child to stay awake but with the imperative to shut off the light prescribes the symptom while at the same time slightly changing it. If the child falls asleep faster, the outcome is better, and if the child stays awake longer, they have followed the suggestion and are in control of staying awake.

Second order change is a primary focus of systemic family therapy and assumes that the child's identified problem can be a response to the dysfunction within the family system (Madanes, 1980). A first order solution of emphasizing and directing interventions to only change the child may do little to change the family dynamic or the child's problem. Parenting models that focus on the child's problem and fail to understand the family dynamic may be largely ineffective. In the clinical literature, there are many examples of an identified child problem that reflect an underlying marital issue. According to Madanes, the child's misbehavior needs to be analyzed for its protective function of other relationships in the family, such as the marital relationship. For example, a noncompliant and acting out child may provide a refocus from the marital dysfunction to the child's misbehaving. Instead of having to deal with the marital problem, the parents can unite around the child's problem.

Other Paradoxical Interventions with Children

According to Haley (1984/2011), the goal of therapy is for the client to spontaneously act differently, not because of being told how to act by the therapist. The role of the therapist is to inspire change, not direct it. In parenting strategies, paradoxical interventions can penetrate the child's resistance and disarm their fear and anger networks. Power struggles between parents and children can be neutralized by using paradoxical interventions. The basic premise of paradoxical interventions is to ask the child to continue doing the disruptive behavior. The paradox means that if the child persists in troubling behavior, the parent wins because of the imperative to continue the bad behavior; on the other hand, if the child defies the parent and changes, the parent still wins because the problem behavior has been removed. The child is placed in a *therapeutic double-bind*, because regardless of the behavior engaged in, improvement in the child's well-being will occur. On the other hand, if the parent confronted the child's negative behavior directly and engaged in a power struggle, the child's resistance to the parent would be expected to increase. The underlying belief is that for the child to change, the parent must be in control of the process covertly. The parent being in control of the process, however, does not mean that the parent is coercive, but is providing an opportunity for the child to evaluate choices and make better decisions. That is, the goal is for the child to exert adaptive internal control, not controlled externally by the parent. The parent's love and support for the child is unabated by the child's bad decisions.

As mentioned earlier, parents use a double-bind to set a scenario where the parent can congratulate the child on their behavior regardless of what they do. With any parenting intervention, parents are encouraged to be in control of their emotions, and not show anger or sarcasm. One of the most common problems with children, especially with pre-teens and teens is a messy room. Eating in their room and leaving dirty dishes around and having dirty clothes strewn about the floor is a common annoyance to parents and can become a source of ongoing strife and conflict. A paradoxical intervention might be something like this:

> I know you don't like to put your dirty dishes in the dishwasher and get upset with me and yell that I should leave you alone, so do you want to yell now and get it over with or wait until I remind you about the dirty dishes?

This frame of the problem puts the child in a therapeutic double-bind and provides an opportunity for the child to make a different decision on how to act. The double-bind is not prescriptive, and the child is free to make a bad choice. Parents cannot react in anger at a bad choice because they have given the green light for how the child chooses to respond. The double-bind also disarms the child who is trying to upset parents. When the parent asks the child to persist in their negative behavior, the parent is controlling the process because in the child's resistance, the parent makes the requested behavior positive (Hage, 2023).

Another paradoxical intervention used by systemic therapists is encouraging the client to set aside specific times to engage their symptomatic behavior because they are not spending enough time with their problems. For example, with a child who is doing poorly in school because they are spending too much time on Facebook, the parent might suggest that the child set aside specific times for Facebook so that their study would not take away too much time from Facebook. This illustrates the idea that clients need to do something to change, not simply think about it. Change takes place because of action and not insight.

From a systemic therapy model, a goal of paradoxical parenting is to sufficiently challenge the client or child rather than make them comfortable (Haley, 1984/2011). The more comfortable the client becomes, the less therapeutic change will occur. Once there is a bond between the therapist and client, the client will then accept the therapist's interventions, which should make the client uncomfortable with their own behavior that facilitates problems. This means that the therapist must push for a behavior that the client has not been able to do for themselves. If the therapist makes the client uncomfortable enough in the session, change outside of the session is more likely to occur. For example, an out-of-control teenager who frequently becomes irate with parents is asked by the therapist to become irate with him and scream profanities at him that he screams at his parents. The results might be that the teen will stop screaming at his parents to avoid having to do so in front of the therapist. While these paradoxical interventions can appear to some to be anti-therapeutic, harsh, and even unprofessional, the rationale rests on the belief that real change depends on challenging the client/child in the short term.

Not only does the therapist exaggerate the symptoms by prescribing a continuation of them, but also asks the client to refrain from change. Suggesting that the client refrain from changing aligns the therapist with resistance, leaving the client to align with change and will likely escalate change. Problematic child behaviors that concern parents include resistance to healthy foods and regular mealtimes, noncompliance when asked to complete their assigned chores, lying to parents, stealing, and spending time on social media, among an assortment of other complaints. Although commonplace and not as disruptive and stressful or confrontational as noncompliance, lying to parents can be a difficult behavior for parents to resolve. This is true because parents are unable to control the situation and must either accept the child's explanation or challenge it (Hage, 2023). Challenging what the parent perceives to be a lie may present more problems because the child may feel less trust in the relationship and, consequently, be prone to lie more. A paradoxical intervention may be more effective because it does not directly challenge the child. For example, predicting when the child will lie and granting acceptance can sidestep the animosity of a confrontation. The parent could say, "When you and Ashley go to a movie at the mall, I want you to come up with a lie. I will be disappointed if it's not a good lie." This strategy will take the child by surprise. The parent is abrogating the control function and turning the interaction with the child into a humorous exchange. It can be assumed that the child's automatic response to lie will be interrupted and the decision to lie will be a more conscious choice. By being paradoxical, the parent has changed the rules of engagement from an adversarial position to one that can be more cooperative. Other paradoxical interventions could be used in a lighthearted and humorous way, such as in games in which one must decide if they will lie or tell the truth. If the child tells the truth, the parent can reward good behavior so that long-term behavior change can take place.

Stealing can be a particularly disturbing behavior from a child and can have legal consequences depending on the context. A paradoxical intervention introduced by the parent in a playful mood can have powerful effects on the child continuing to steal (Hage, 2023). For example, while the child is at school, the parent could hide items around the house and, when the child comes home, he/she could be given the imperative to "steal" the items without being caught. If the child is caught, the parent engages the child through chasing, arresting, and putting in jail. The goal in the intervention is to place the focus on getting caught and simultaneously giving no consideration to being successful in stealing. The fun part of the game is getting caught and, therefore, will garner more attention than being successful in stealing. The paradoxical intervention means that stealing will become more evident and the hidden and disguised behavior will decrease. As stealing is more overt and recognized, it will come under the child's self-control.

One of the most difficult age groups to effectively change their behaviors is adolescents. Normal adolescent period is bereft with problems, but severe mental health issues in the form of oppositional defiant disorder (ODD) or conduct disorder (CD) present special challenges. It can be assumed that the resistance of adolescents in being compliant represents a positive relation to the degree of rebelliousness they exhibit (Sheras & Jackson, 1978). Likewise, the more resistant an adolescent is to change, the greater the effectiveness of the paradoxical intervention. Using paradoxical directives to intervene with adolescents having severe mental health issues is believed to be the first step toward breaking the inescapable hold of the resistance to change.

Sheras and Jackson (1978), in a classic study using paradoxical interventions for an adolescent residential treatment program, provided ample evidence for the effectiveness of paradox to treat adolescent problems. The advantage to using paradoxical interventions is reducing resistance by advising the client to continue with the symptom. The process of change begins with the adolescent noticing that change, which will be more functional than past behavior, is possible. All the subjects in the study by Sheras and Jackson had been removed from regular schools because of their extremely disruptive behavior and mental illness diagnoses. The paradoxical interventions were used for behaviors such as fighting, withdrawing, showing disrespect to clinicians, and passive aggression.

One case Sheras and Jackson (1978) discussed was with a 15-year-old bully, Willie, whose favorite target for both verbal and physical assaults was a much smaller 14-year-old boy, Richie. The staff was concerned that the smaller boy could be severely injured. The bullying behavior violated the school rule of no verbal or physical violence. The staff devised a paradoxical two-week intervention plan that consisted of both boys showing no friendly gesture of communication to each other for the two-week period when they would be allowed to encounter each other verbally and physically, which would take place in the presence of the staff. This directive was presented to both boys in a contract that each signed. They were assured of receiving some tangible rewards if they complied with the contract. The results indicated that the bullying behavior decreased, but was not eliminated, while friendly behavior increased. A caveat is needed in this type of intervention because it is possible that harm could come to Richie that would appear to be directed by the staff. This intervention aligns with the ethical concerns regarding paradoxical interventions and should only be used by experienced clinicians who can control the setting for the intervention.

As mentioned earlier, ODD and CD are two serious behavior problems with children and generally require professional help. Parents lose patience and resort to overcontrol when children are oppositional and, thus, negative patterns persist. The strength of paradoxical interventions with these disorders is a more relaxed and non-confrontational approach. When parents use surprise and novel interventions, children may respond positively and are more likely to change their behavior.

Paradoxical interventions with an ODD teenager can be illustrated by the following case. Josh is a 13-year-old boy who has exhibited increasing defiant behavior at home and at school. He is a frequent rule-breaker at school and has also been aggressive with peers, resulting in suspension from school on several occasions. Using a behavior economy approach and rewarding good behavior did not help, and the parents are frustrated and angry. The parents decide to have a different approach. As usual, they sit down with Josh after one of his noncompliant behaviors, but this time do something other than talk about the consequences and imposed restrictions on his behavior. They use a paradoxical intervention and suggest that he continue his behavior but in a way that is less attractive for him. In the conversation, his father admits that his behavior is beyond their control, and he is encouraged to continue with his noncompliant behavior for the next week, but he should write down the behavior and why he did it. They decide to meet again in a week and discuss it. At the follow-up, Josh was asked if he made notes of his noncompliant behavior and he replied that it did not feel right to break rules on purpose, so he refrained from doing so. The negative interaction pattern was disrupted and Josh's behavior overall improved.

An alternative intervention could have been to give Josh the responsibility for making the rules for them for one week. The purpose of doing this intervention is to break the negative pattern, and to support Josh in analyzing his choices and being more responsible for how his behavior affects his parents. Follow-up could have addressed how Josh felt about making the decisions for everyone, or addressing if he did not make any rules, why not? The outcome of this intervention could open the door to more productive discussion of rules and rule violations in the home which could lead to more cooperation and negotiations.

The Feasibility of Paradox as a Parenting and Parent Training Intervention

As discussed earlier, paradoxical interventions developed from its application to therapy, which was primarily from the work of Milton Erickson. The therapy background included work with families and children, focusing on parenting that improves the emotional well-being of children. The paradoxical interventions differ from common practices in parenting because the parent is not overtly attempting to stop negative behavior. It is non-confrontational and introduces humor and lightheartedness into the exchange.

The overuse of any parenting intervention loses its effectiveness, and the same is true with paradox. Many parents use grounding, spanking, or lecturing as punishments for misbehaving. When paradoxical interventions are effective, they are used sparingly and there is no risk of harm to the child.

Despite the criticisms of manipulation and ethical concerns in paradoxical interventions, there is evidence that paradox can be effective in changing negative resistive patterns (Peluso & Freund, 2023). While most of the research on the effectiveness of paradoxical interventions has been with adult subjects, it seems plausible to assume that children who are resistant to parents' directives and noncompliant to other authority figures tend to respond favorably to paradoxical interventions. The use of paradoxical interventions is novel and surprising to children. As a result, the rules of engagement are altered so that automatic negative patterns are disrupted. A disruption in the negative patterns can lead to a transformational change in the child's behavior.

The brain network involved in responding to paradoxes is the frontotemporal network that is activated by nonliteral messages, which allows for coordination of competing messages. The conscious or rational networks of the brain are not activated by paradoxical interventions. Instead, it is a nonlinear process that is resolved implicitly by the unconscious brain.

References

Adler, A. (2011). *The practice and theory of individual psychology*. Martino Fine Books/Amazon Publishing Group. (Original work published 1925)

Arias-Carrión, O., Caraza-Santiago, X., Salgado-Licona, S., Salama, M., Machado, S., Egidio Nardi, A., Menéndez-González, M., & Murillo-Rodríguez, E. (2010). Orquestic regulation of neurotransmitters on reward-seeking behavior. *International Archives of Medicine, 7*, 29. https://doi.org/10.1186/1755-7682-7-29

Ascher, L. M., & Turner, R. M. (1979). Paradoxical intention and insomnia: An experimental investigation. *Behavior Research and Therapy, 17*(4), 408–411. https://doi.org/10.1016/0005-7967(79)90015-9

Belekou, A., Papageorgiou, C., Karavasilis, E., Tsaltas, E., Kelekis, N., Klein, C., & Smyrnis, N. (2022). Paradoxical reasoning: An fMRI study. *Frontiers in Psychology, 13*. https://doi.org/10.3389/fpsyg.2022.850491

Browning, S., & Hull, R. (2021). Reframing paradox. *Professional Psychology: Research and Practice, 52*(4), 360–367. https://doi.org/10.1037/pro0000384

Brunetti, M., Perrucci, M. G., Di Naccio, M. R., Ferretti, A., Del Gratta, C., Casadio, C., & Romani, G. (2014). Framing deductive reasoning with emotional content: An fMRI study. *Brain Cognition, 87*, 153–160. https://doi.org/10.1016/j.bandc.2014.03.017

Craiker, K. N. (2021). What is paradox? Definition and examples. *ProWritingAid*. Retrieved November 5, 2023, from https://prowritingaid.com/paradox-definition

Dreikurs, R. (1968). *Children: The challenge*. Meredith.

Erickson, M. H. (1980). *The collected papers of Milton H. Erickson on hypnosis* (Vols. 1–4, E. L. Rossi, Ed.). Irvington. https://doi.org/10.1176/appi.ajp.162.7.1255

Gorton, G. E. (2005). Milton Hyland Erickson 1901–1980. *American Journal of Psychiatry, 162*(7), 1255.

Hage, D. (2023). *Paradoxical techniques (resisting resistance increases resistance)*. Retrieved November 13, 2023, from https://deborahhage.com/paradoxical-techniques/

Haley, J. (1976). *Problem-solving therapy*. Jossey-Bass.
Haley, J. (1993). *Uncommon therapy: The psychiatric techniques of Milton H. Erickson, M. D*. W. W. Norton.
Haley, J. (2011). *Ordeal therapy: Unusual ways to change behavior*. Crown House Classics. (Original work published 1984)
Hameiri, B., Porat, R., Bar-Tal, D., Bieler, A., & Halperin, E. (2014). Paradoxical thinking as a new avenue of intervention to promote peace. *Proceedings of the National Academy of Sciences, 111*(30), 10996–11001. https://doi.org/10.1073/pnas.1407055111
Kosloff, S., & Solomon, S. (2020). The paradox of faith: How existential concerns motivate both prosocial and antisocial religious behaviors. In K. Vail, III & C. Routledge (Eds.), *Science of religion, spirituality, and existentialism* (pp. 435–454). Academic Press.
MacIntyre, A. (1987). *A short history of ethics*. Routledge.
Madanes, C. (1980). Protection, paradox, pretending. *Family Therapy Process, 19,* 73–85.
Matthews, R. S. (2022). *The paradoxical meeting of depth psychology and physics*. Routledge.
Newell, B. R., & Shanks, D. R. (2014). Unconscious influences on decision making: A critical review. *Behavioral and Brain Sciences, 37*(1), 1–18. https://doi.org/10.1017/S0140525X12003214
Oxford Wordpower Dictionary. (1993). Oxford University Press.
Papageorgiou, C., Stachtea, X., Papageorgiou, P., Alexandridis, T., Tsaltas, E., & Angelopoulos, E. (2016). Aristotle meets Zeno: Psychophysiological evidence. *PLoS One*, *11*, e0168017–e0168067. https://doi.org/10.1371/journal.pone.0168067
Peluso, P. R., & Freund, R. (2023). Paradoxical interventions: A meta-analysis. *Psychotherapy (Chic), 60*(3), 283–294. https://doi.org/10.1037/pst0000481; Epub 2023 March 16; PMID: 36931813
Rodriguez-Moreno, D., & Hirsch, J. (2009). The dynamics of deductive reasoning: An fMRI investigation. *Neuropsychologia, 47,* 949–961. https://doi.org/10.1016/j.neuropsychologia.2008.08.030
Sheras, P. L., & Jackson, S. B. (1978, August). *Paradox as an intervention strategy with emotionally disturbed adolescents*. Paper presented at the Annual Convention of the American Psychological Association, Toronto, ON.
Short, D. (Ed.). (2017). *Principle and core competencies for Ericksonian therapy, 2017 edition*. The Milton H. Erickson Foundation. Retrieved November 20, 2023, from https://www.iamdrshort.com/PDF/Papers/Core%20Competencies%20Manual.pdf
Sutton, J. (2022). How does paradoxical intention really work in therapy? *Positive Psychology*. Retrieved November 6, 2023, from https://positivepsychology.com/paradoxical-intent/
Whitaker, C., & Malone, T. (1981). *The roots of psychotherapy*. Brunner/Mazel.

13
POSTSCRIPT

Transformational Change via Unconscious and Implicit Methods

The purpose of this book was twofold—first, it was designed to make a case for the role of the unconscious in parent education training; and second, to highlight some interventions in which change occurs implicitly outside of conscious awareness. It requires thinking outside the box to improve the effectiveness of parent education models and parenting in general. The purpose does not include replacing parent education models or parenting practices in general, but to add consideration for the unconscious, and for implicit methods in parent education and parenting. This approach is bolstered by recent findings in neuroscience for learning, decision making, solving problems, and processing information. All these areas of research are relevant in improving the effectiveness of parent education. This chapter summarizes the major thesis of the book to bring together how indirect and implicit parenting can be used by parents and parent educators. While it may seem redundant, the purpose is to leave the reader with a clear understanding of how the unconscious is essential in transformational change.

A corollary to the two major purposes is the emphasis on parenting that results in transformational change, labeled second order parenting (Maier, 2008). Much of the parenting literature focuses on first order change, or on direct instructions intent on changing the behavior of the child. Second order parenting incorporates the whole interactive system of the child for change. The change is viewed as transformational because it is discontinuous with the past, and the change process may or may not be conscious depending on the intervention.

Transformational change is based on new neuroscience research highlighted in earlier chapters of this book that have rewritten how the unconscious influences consciousness. Once viewed as a deep caldron of hidden motives that can only be exposed by long and painful psychotherapy, the unconscious is now known to

DOI: 10.4324/9781003381679-15

be active in consciousness and jointly working together with consciousness (Carruthers, 2017). In fact, it is the unconscious that is most active in solving problems even while one is distracted from the problem or sleeping (Kahneman, 2011). The solution appears to be worked out in the unconscious that invades the conscious with a decision either as an "aha experience" or as an apparent conscious reflection of a solution to the problem (Solms & Friston, 2018). As we are unaware of unconscious processing, the conscious mind then tricks itself into believing that the solution was gained through conscious awareness (Figure 13.1).

Implications from research on the conscious and unconscious in problem-solving and decision making for parent education are enormous. For example, attention should be placed on training modules that assess the emotional activity of participants. How they feel about what they are learning should be emphasized. As discussed in this book, neuroscience research demonstrates that emotions are essential for learning. This means that instead of limiting emotional responses, parent trainers should develop interventions that promote emotional experiences.

In the same way that solving problems is the main activity of the unconscious, rational thinking also has been found to take place in the emotional center of the brain and not the neocortex. Decision making does not appear to be based on a logical process of weighing pros and cons to take the right approach. Rather, decisions are made based on how one feels about them. This suggests that paying more attention to emotions in decision making could improve the way decisions are made. It also suggests that parents should be more in tune with their emotions and the emotions of their children in disciplining misbehavior. For parent education, trainers should be cognizant of how parents are emotionally processing the material in

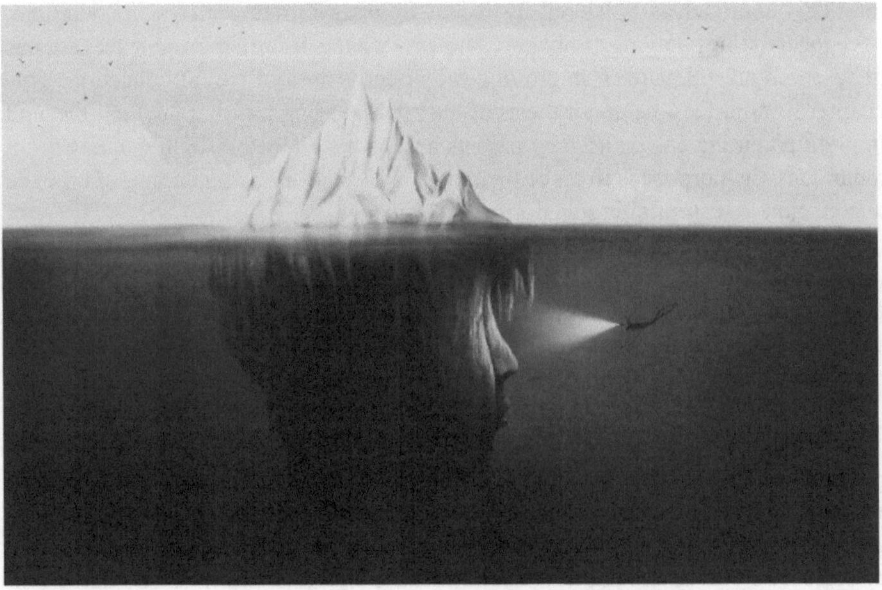

FIGURE 13.1 Most of the brain functions outside of our conscious awareness.

the training modules. For example, evaluation of the effectiveness of the program from parent feedback should include their emotional assessment, and not only their rational assessment, of the training program.

The theoretical frame for transformational change evolved from systems theory, which has been applied to improving family relationships for many decades in the form of psychotherapy. While therapy with children and families has been reviewed throughout the book, the systems/dialectical approach in this book is not a therapy model. Rather, it is a heuristic model for understanding the nuances of parent–child relationships and how the interactions between parents and children change over time. Dialectical thinking allows for flexibility in parenting due to the recognition of the ongoing relationship between parent and child that must change in reference to new input.

Throughout this book, the writings of Milton Erickson (1980) have been underscored because of his outside the box thinking in working with his clients. While his writings were done before recent advances in brain research allowed for definitive examination of brain activation in processing information, modern neuroscience confirms that his views of the positive intent and creative responses in decision making and change evolved from the unconscious rather than the conscious mind. His therapeutic focus was to address the unconscious and, as such, conscious resistance was bypassed. Erickson's approach in this book is stressed to illustrate that the change process is unconscious and happens outside of conscious awareness through interventions such as modeling and observation, storytelling, reframing, humor, confusion, and paradox.

Suggestions for unconscious and implicit interventions are not prescriptive but meant to illustrate how they can be used to facilitate change. Families with child problems are each uniquely different and require diligent exploration and understanding of the family interactional patterns (Erickson, 1980). Contrary to contemporary beliefs of what are important skills to be taught in parent education based on research of desired parental behaviors, the position taken in this book is to address the uniqueness of each family. This means that rather than applying a predetermined skills program it is more effective to address what each family needs to change. Following the lead of Erickson, the family oversees change, and the parent trainer is the conduit.

Unconscious and implicit interventions are underdeveloped in the parent education because learning is considered a conscious cognitive process. As more research accumulates that reveals a definite unconscious link to learning and behavior, more focus will be placed on implicit intervention methods. New interventions in parent education could discover how the conscious and the unconscious work together and to engage the unconscious to facilitate problem-solving and transformational change. The view that changing the unconscious is done through repeated conscious means should be replaced with the view that the unconscious mind, when presented with a problem, does not need practice to change. Instead, change is brought about by allowing the unconscious time to form a creative answer and inform the conscious brain of its conclusion.

The book suggests six distinct implicit interventions that activate unconscious processes—modeling and observation, storytelling, reframing, humor, confusion, and paradox. These interventions tend to be unconscious and may not provide immediate insight into how change occurred. Recent research has debunked the commonly held view that observation alone is insufficient to learn something new and required practice. In a seminal study, Cross et al. (2009), concluded that the same brain areas were active regardless of whether the subject was participating in the activity or was merely observing. This study is important for parenting because it reveals how children learn from observing and not solely through behavioral practice. In addition, this study provides ample support for the view that children learn many ways of reacting from observing parents without conscious acknowledgment on their part or the part of the parent that learning has taken place. Infant imitation studies have demonstrated that infants can learn and recall memories that were formed from observation before language development (Meltzoff & Williamson, 2013).

Storytelling is an implicit intervention that impacts children's behavior unconsciously. It increases oxytocin levels and prosocial behavior (Suzuki et al., 2020), engages multiple brain networks, and allows for integrative processes. Young children are especially influenced by stories because their brains respond to the narrative in visual and representative ways rather than in logical or rational thinking. Storytelling is a natural communicative tool that is used in every cultural group and is one of the primary ways that cultures continue to influence those within the culture.

The use of storytelling to discipline children has not been fully developed. The most common form of storytelling to directly influence children's behavior in Western societies is called discipline stories, which tend to be print stories about specific struggles or transitions the child may need help with. Responding to the child's misbehavior through spontaneous and original stories created by the parent, however, has not been developed except by psychotherapists in counseling. To aid parents and use storytelling to change unwanted behavior, guidelines for parents have been developed. The guidelines are not meant to prescribe exactly how parents should tell stories, but to provide a flexible roadmap that can be adapted to the specific circumstance with their child. The story should be well disguised but relevant to the problem the child is having. Like other implicit interventions with children, storytelling reduces negative exchanges with the child and aids in creating a collaborative relationship. It is a natural way to communicate and influences children indirectly. Because the intervention is implicit, the child's response is not predetermined and may vary.

Reframing has long been an intervention to facilitate change in psychotherapy. It has powerful implications for the use in parent education and parenting. Reframing changes the understanding of the problem which allows for new solutions to be tried (Haley, 1997). In parenting recurrent problems, parents get stuck in "doing more of the same," which exacerbates the problem. Reframing the problems seems like a minor adjustment, but if the conception of the problems changes, the result is a different problem that brings with it the hope of a solution.

Recent neuroscience research implies that the brain has a negative bias, which means that even minor stressors and problems can be labeled in very negative terms (Moser et al., 2014). Efforts to change negative thoughts and behaviors into positive ones are difficult and mainly ineffective. A negative cycle can dominate the brain and the processing of information since the reward system in the brain can be activated by both negative and positive thoughts. Research has not provided a definitive answer for how to change negative thoughts into positive ones, but it is clear that telling someone to think positively does little to change the negative cycle.

Reframing is an intervention that goes beyond attempting to change negative thoughts into positive thoughts. This is because reframing is about process and not outcome. Reframing is not concerned with the history of the negative cycle or fixing it in the present. Rather, it is about how the problem is manifested and maintained in the present (Haley, 1997). Reframing is based on the view that implicit processes are paramount in creating transformational change. When a parent reframes the problem with the child, the whole context of the problem changes, including the history, maintenance, and solution to the problem. Viewing the problem differently changes the neuropathways and behaviors that maintain it. Consequently, new solutions can begin to emerge that will provide solutions that have not been attempted before.

Humor is an important communication tool that is present in all human interactions. In some interactions, humor is underdeveloped such as in disciplining a child. No doubt, the emphasis on explicitly controlling the child's misbehavior results in the reticence in using humor. Humor is typically spontaneous and introduces novelty and the unexpected into an exchange between parent and child (Cohen, 2002). Although no single succinct definition of humor captures the whole meaning, there is research evidence that demonstrates the profound effect of humor on reducing stress, increasing the immune system, bonding, and improving emotional well-being (Brockington et al., 2021). Lack of humor or reduced expression of humor is common in mental and emotional disorders.

Humor improves learning and emotional regulation because it activates the frontal brain network that is involved in emotion regulation, bonding and attachment, and in resolving discrepancies in processing information (Rutter, 1990). The reward system of the brain is also activated by humor. When unexpected elements are introduced into conversation, the brain releases dopamine which is the pleasure chemical associated with many of the positive effects of humor. Furthermore, researchers reveal that humor reduces the preoccupation with pain for children with cancer and improves the efficacy of dealing with small failures and disappointments. Not all humor results in positive outcomes due to lack of its appropriateness to the current circumstances.

Although humor was shunned as a common intervention in psychotherapy until recently, some therapists, such as Carl Whitaker and other marriage and family therapists, promoted the use of humor with families. Humor that is genuine, spontaneous, and bonding changes the way the family views the problem and enhances transformational change. In taking oneself less seriously, clients improve self-direction, allow the unconscious to act in providing answers through an "aha experience," and change the perception that one is deficient and needing help. These benefits may not be acknowledged by the clients because they happen outside of conscious awareness.

Parents naturally use humor with their children but need to be aware of the child's developmental level because what children find humorous changes as they age (McGhee, 1999). Young children find flatulence noises funny but not always as they age. Older children respond to more cognitively complex humor where there is a discrepancy in perceptions. To be effective in humor discipline, as in other forms of discipline, parents must understand the developmental level of the child. When parents use humor, there is an increase in endorphins that deactivates activity in the amygdala, part of the emotional center of the brain, which implicitly reduces negative emotions. Humor activates a complex network of brain regions that work to reduce anxiety and increase dopamine, the pleasure chemical in the brain (American Physiological Society, 2008). While the child may experience the chemical change in their brain when the parent reacts to them with humor, they are not conscious of how this occurred.

The confusion/rope-a-dope intervention is similar to the Adlerian model in which parents are encouraged not to engage in a power struggle with the child but, in its place, to withdraw from the situation at hand (Dreikurs, 1964). The rationale for using the confusion intervention is not based on the parent not engaging in a power struggle, but based on the belief that confusion is grounded in how learning and changing behavior occurs. Confusion can help change entrenched destructive interactional patterns and change the neural brain patterns in the child.

Until recently, confusion and emotions were viewed as impeding the learning process. Research on the neural underpinnings of learning in recent years, however, has rewritten the effects of confusion and emotion in learning (Lodge et al., 2018). Cognitive incongruity caused by confusion is not viewed as necessary for deep learning to take place. Discrepancy theory developed out of the belief that new input conflicts with old information, activating the epistemic emotions and resulting in discrepancies to resolve. Generally, researchers have found that learning that occurs from this confused state is more effective than learning that occurs from explicit and straightforward methods.

Emotions such as surprise, confusion, and curiosity, labeled "epistemic emotions," are viewed as necessary for learning (Vogl et al., 2020). Epistemic emotions are effective in learning because they are not rooted in ideology or belief systems. Instead, they allow the brain to incorporate new input that bypasses rigid belief systems and enhance transformational or second order learning.

Researchers have found that epistemic emotions facilitate critical and dialectical thinking (Vogl et al., 2020). In a recent study on the effects of confusion on learning, confused subjects compared to nonconfused subjects scored higher on post-test and showed more ability to think critically and solve problems more efficiently. This finding demonstrated that when confusion is aligned with the content and when the instructor offers appropriate guidelines for resolving the confusion, learning is enhanced.

Parent education and parenting interventions by parents could be improved by understanding the relation between learning and confusion. Introducing confusion into the training will enhance learning when it is followed by clear and understandable resolutions. On the other hand, when learning material is presented with too much attention to explicit conscious learning modules, learning outcomes are not as productive or efficient.

Finally, paradox is also generally minimized or avoided altogether in parent training and by parents because of the fear that a paradox will increase confusion and therefore lead to poor learning outcomes. Paradox is counter to the typical way that change is facilitated, in which intervention trainers or therapists attempt to remove entrenched rigid beliefs by consciously introducing new information that contradicts the belief system (Hameiri et al., 2014). This mode of thinking is based on consistency theory, which postulates that the lack of consistency between the new information and the belief systems will enable one to shift their beliefs toward the more functional new information.

Instead of the typical way of thinking about change, Hameiri et al. (2014) believed that change is enhanced by paradoxical thinking. For example, when one is placed in a paradoxical situation where they are met with input that is consistent but is an exaggeration of their belief system, this tends to change even their rigid belief system. Change may be small and seemingly inconsequential initially but can mushroom into enormous change (Erickson, 1980). Paradoxical thinking is more concerned with how change occurs than the outcome of the change. The change that takes place is due to action and not due to the developing of insight.

There is little neuroscience research on paradox, but what exists shows that paradoxes activate the orbitofrontal region of the brain, the area associated with emotion, and the reward network (Roll et al., 2020). Papageorgiou et al. (2016) found that logical deductive reasoning activates the parietal–occipital region, while paradox activates the orbitofrontal region.

Second Order Parenting

This book is intended to disrupt long-held beliefs about parenting and parent education by expanding interventions to include implicit and unconscious interventions. As discussed previously, when parents enter parent education training, they bring with them well-established attitudes and beliefs about parenting. To a large degree, these attitudes will determine if the training was successful. When these attitudes change because of training and parents change their parenting behaviors, second order parenting occurs (Figure 13.2). Ordinary or usual methods of facilitating change, that are direct and explicit, may need to be supplemented with implicit and unconscious methods of facilitating change. One of the most popular criticisms of utilizing the indirect methods discussed in this book is that they can be understood to be manipulative. However, this book presents that indirect methods are no more manipulative than direct methods, since the goal in both is to change behavior. While one is done explicitly through the conscious mind, the other is done implicitly through the conscious mind. Furthermore, there is mounting evidence that the bedrock of transformational, second order change is dialectical and paradoxical thinking, which are facilitated by implicit and indirect methods.

While skill-building exercises use didactic presentations, video, role-play, and group discussion, second order parenting is accomplished by using indirect, implicit, and unconscious methods using dialectical and paradoxical interventions. The use of paradoxical and dialectical interventions apart from psychotherapy, philosophy, and religion has been minimal until several decades ago where paradox was applied to mathematics, the hard sciences, and logic (Kainz, 1988). One area of research that has produced much interest applying paradox is organizational

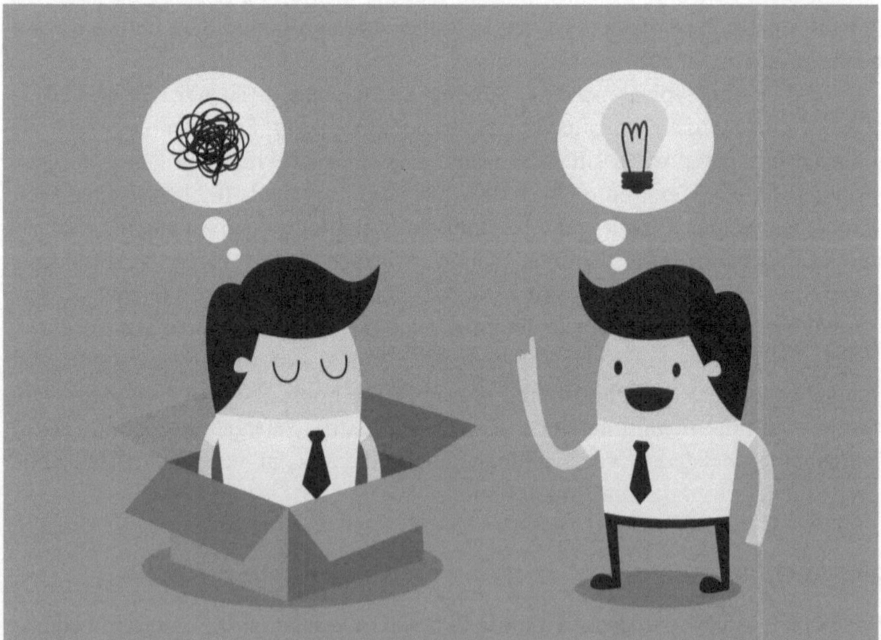

FIGURE 13.2 Second order parenting techniques encourage out-of-the-box thinking, which provides opportunities for creative and innovative outcomes; a space for the unconscious to experience aha moments; and the potential for transformational change.

management (McGuire et al., 2006). In some studies, the distinction between paradox and dialectics are vague and not clearly defined, but it is helpful to see the similarities and differences in the two concepts.

Both dialectics and paradox are about contradictions, or two elements in opposition with each other. A paradox is composed of two contradictory, logically interconnected elements that are illogical when paired together (Lewis, 2000, cited in Hargrave & Van de Ven, 2017). In a paradox, one element undermines or forestalls the opposing element in an either/or manner. Paradoxes promote creativity in that the tension between these two elements facilitate new behaviors and thinking outside the box. On the other hand, a dialectic is comprised of two opposite elements that interact to produce a synthesis, which will have an opposite, and the process repeats. A dialectic is characterized by both/and, meaning both positions are tenable and with recognition that no position is permanent. Studies in organizational management have focused on the interplay between paradox and dialectics for understanding the structure and daily operation of organizations. While little research exists on the relation of paradoxical and dialectical thinking, a review of that literature can analyze the nuances of applying paradoxical and dialectical thinking to parenting.

The writings of Erika Christakis (2016) are helpful as a starting point in understanding how paradoxical and dialectical thinking are similar and how they can work together to produce transformational change. Her book on preschoolers opens a new door in understanding how parents can interact with their young children. For Christakis, parenting is a paradoxical situation in that the young child's brain is hardwired to learn quickly and effortlessly, but learning is a challenge. The parent's approach to learning differs from a child's natural inclinations for learning, creating a paradoxical relationship between parent and child. According to Christakis, a basic paradox is that parents are viewing the child from the adult position while children just want the freedom to be themselves. The fatal assumption that parents make is in the belief that they know what children think and feel because they were once a child. Unfortunately, parents are unable to grasp how their children think and must alter this assumption before they can adequately move forward with interacting with their children. In today's world, children are spending considerably less time outdoors in imaginative play and more time inside looking at a screen. Parents must get inside the mind of their child and allow them free play without parental structure. Christakis offers five tips that help parents resolve this paradoxical situation with the child: (1) calibration—the parent's interventions with their child should be developmentally appropriate; (2) coaching—the parents' role is as facilitator for the child in cascading up the learning ladder; (3) communication—the best thing parents can do for their child is to be a good listener; (4) creativity—allow for spontaneous self-expression; and (5) connection—validating the child's efforts.

Like paradox, dialectics refers to opposing positions that define the nature of reality, and the nature of this opposition is to create a synthesis—instead of being a compromise between the positions, a synthesis is something new, unpredicted, and novel (Hargrave & Van de Ven, 2017). This means that the synthesis is a resolution to the conflict of the positions. In power systems, this means that each side of the dialectic must have enough power to oppose the other. If power is one-sided, no resolution of the conflict can occur. The dialectical position requires that both sides interact according to the rules of engagement for dialogue with the opposing view. This conflict differs substantially from the paradoxical view which is attempting to manage, but not resolve, the conflict.

As noted earlier, in parent–child relationships, dialectical and paradoxical interventions are effective with many issues affecting the relationship, but more so when there is a high degree of resistance and/or conflict. Bradley et al. (2017) applied a dialectical model to four parenting interactions that are relevant for the child's development: "supportive presence, respect for autonomy, stimulation, and hostility" (p. 3214). The use of paradox and dialectical interactions are implicit ways of communicating. The danger with direct interaction with children is that the opposite effects from what the parent wants can happen. Researchers have found that when parents interject themselves into the child's activities, even though the child does not need parental input and is fully engaged in their activity, the child is more likely to lack regulating emotional reactions and have more difficulty with delaying gratification (Obradović et al., 2021). Overinvolvement of parents into their children's lives may have similar negative outcomes to underinvolvement.

The above research underscores that when parents become too vigilant in their parenting, the natural flow and spontaneous interchanges between parents and children take on a rigid character that stifles creative and emotional deep communication. Not only do children recognize when parents have an agenda in communicating with them, they resist and are less compliant. It follows that a danger in parents' focusing too much on parenting, and perhaps overevaluating their parenting skills, can result in undesirable outcomes.

Parental Determinism and Intensive Parenting

In recent years, there has developed global attention to the role parents play in child well-being, which has morphed into improving parents' skills in all their interactions with their children (Yerkes et al., 2021). The terms *parental determinism* and *intensive parenting* have been used to describe this obsession with parenting behaviors. The phrase parental determinism, used more in the academic literature, refers to the view that parents determine how their child develops. The phrase intensive parenting is used more in blogs and media writings to describe parental overinvolvement with their children, such as "helicopter parenting" (Figure 13.3). While these terms differ in their use in the literature, both definitions point to overinvolvement in parenting and making parents responsible for child outcomes. No one can deny the importance of parents' influence on their child; what is at hand, however, is the rush by governmental agencies, educators, and childcare agencies to train all parents in parenting skills so that children will develop optimally.

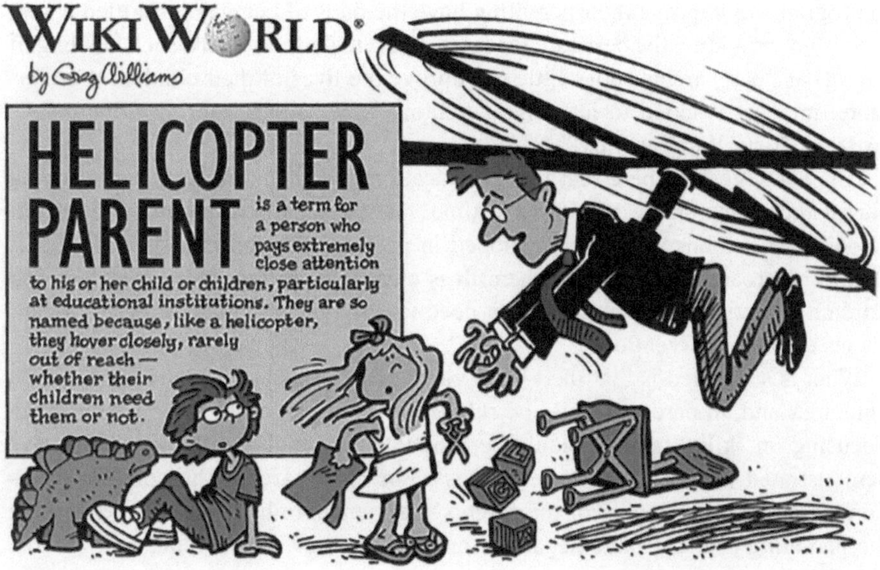

FIGURE 13.3 Overinvolved parents produce children who lack the ability to make their own decisions, robbing them of taking responsibility for themselves (Williams, 2007, CC BY-SA 3.0).

An underlying motif in this book is that the focus on making parents responsible for child outcomes and remediating poor parenting by teaching parents skills undermines the natural flow of parenting and may be more detrimental to children than doing nothing. The current focus on parents being both the cause of child problems and the cure pushes parents into a more intensive relationship with their children. In terms of physical health, there is research that intensive parenting may reap some benefits (Yerkes et al., 2021). On the other hand, there is little support for the presumption that intensive parenting will increase psychological well-being. Yerkes et al. (2021) cites research that indicates children of intensive parents have greater emotional difficulties and, during adolescence, have greater issues with establishing autonomous behavior.

Parental determinism is a theoretical framework that has been forced on parents globally with negative effects on parents (Fargion, 2023). The most vocal critics of parental determinism reside in England specifically and Europe generally, although many countries, including the United States, have programs aimed at parents to improve parenting skills. Public policies about parenting have coalesced around improving the well-being of children by focusing on how parents interact with their children. Some writers have criticized the evidence-based claim of these programs because comparing children of extreme trauma or neglect to children raised without trauma or neglect has little relevance to most children and their parents (Lee, 2011). While most parenting policies are optional, parents who do not participate in programs to improve their parenting have the onus of being an unskilled parent who is not providing the best care for their children. Unfortunately, such labeling of parents as "bad parents" does little to improve the lives of their children. Furthermore, mothers respond to intensive parenting expectations with negative results (Adams, 2020; Widding, 2018).

It is not suggested here that parent education does not work and that teaching parents parenting skills is a waste of time. As stated earlier, implicit and unconscious interventions are underdeveloped in parent education models and models should be broadened to include them. It is clear that children learn from parents' implicit behaviors and parents do not need to only telegraph parenting from conscious explicit interventions.

What is suggested is that the global view that parents are responsible for child outcomes and all parents should be subject to improving their skills is contested. Focusing on skills training should be limited to the high-risk parents who have demonstrated lack of parenting readiness. For most parents, the constant attention on the child's behavior or the parents' assessment of how they are performing the parenting role can have negative consequences for both parents and children (Li, 2024).

Some basic parenting knowledge would benefit all parents, such as knowledge of child development and developmentally appropriate expectations. Providing free playtime, encouraging outdoor experiences, and supporting the child's interest are simple things that any parent can do regardless of the social status, family form, or income level. Simply acknowledging that children learn from what parents do before language develops can enhance child outcomes. Parenting need not be overwhelming but should be relaxed, supportive, and flexible, building on parents' strengths and their knowledge of relationship skills.

References

Adams, E. A. (2020). Intensive parenting ideologies and risks for recidivism among justice-involved mothers. *Women & Criminal Justice, 30*(5), 316–335. https://doi.org/10.1080/08974454.2020.1741487

American Physiological Society. (2008, April 10). Anticipating a laugh reduces our stress hormones, study shows. *ScienceDaily*. Retrieved September 5, 2023, from www.sciencedaily.com/releases/2008/04/080407114617.htm

Bradley, R. H., Iida, M., Pennar, A., Owen, M. T., & Vandell, D. L. (2017). The dialectics of parenting: Changes in the interplay of maternal: Behaviors during early and middle childhood. *Journal of Child and Family Studies, 26,* 3214–3225. https://doi.org/10.1007/s10826-017-0805-6

Brockington, G., Moreira, A. P. G., Buso, M. S., da Silva, S. G., Altszyler, E., & Fischer, R., & Mollh, J. (2021). Storytelling increases oxytocin and positive emotions and decreases cortisol and pain in hospitalized children. *Proceedings of the National Academy of Science USA, 118*(22), e2018409118. https://doi.org/10.1073/pnas.2018409118. Published online 2021 May 24.

Carruthers, P. (2017). The illusion of conscious thought. *Journal of Consciousness Studies, 24*(910), 228–252.

Christakis, E. (2016). *The importance of being little: What preschoolers really need from grownups*. Viking.
Cohen, L. J. (2002). *Playful parenting: An exciting new approach to raising children that will help you nurture close connections, solve behavior problems, and encourage confidence paperback*. Ballantine.
Cross, E. S., Kraemer, D. J. M., Hamilton, A. F., Kelley, W. M., & Grafton, S. T. (2009). Sensitivity of the action observation network to physical and observational learning. *Cerebral Cortex, 19*(2), 315–326. https://doi.org/10.1093/cercor/bhn083
Dreikurs, R. (1964). *Children the challenge*. Hawthorne.
Erickson, M. H. (1980). *The collected papers of Milton H. Erickson on hypnosis* (Vols. 1–4, E. L. Rossi, Ed.). Irvington. https://doi.org/10.1176/appi.ajp.162.7.1255
Fargion, S. (2023). Representations of parenting and the neo-liberal discourse: Parents' and professionals' views on child-rearing practices in Italy. *Journal of Family Studies, 29*(3), 188–204. https://doi.org/10.1080/13229400.2021.1905049
Haley, J. (1997). *Leaving home: The therapy of disturbed young people*. Brunner/Mazel.
Hameiri, B., Porat, R., Bar-Tal, D., Bieler, A., & Halperin, E. (2014). Paradoxical thinking as a new avenue of intervention to promote peace. *Proceedings of the National Academy of Sciences*, *111*(30), 10996–11001. https://doi.org/10.1073/pnas.1407055111
Hargrave, A. H., & Van de Ven, A. H. (2017). Integrating dialectical and paradox perspectives on managing contradictions in organizations. *Organization Studies*, *38*(3–4), 319–339. https://doi.org/10.1177/0170840616640843
Kahneman, D. (2011). *Thinking, fast and slow*. Farrar, Straus, and Giroux.
Kainz, H. (1988). *Paradox, dialectic, and system: A contemporary reconstruction of the Hegelian problematic*. The Pennsylvania State University Press.
Lee, E. (2011, August). The tyranny of parental determinism. *Spiked*. Retrieved February 2, 2024, from www.spiked-online.com/2011/08/24/the-tyranny-of-parental-determinism/
Li, P. (2024, January 13). Intensive parenting: Effects & 7 tips on how to quit. *Parenting for Brain*. Retrieved February 2, 2024, from https://www.parentingforbrain.com/intensive-parenting/
Lodge, J., Kennedy, G., Lockyer, L., Amael, A., & Pachman, M. (2018, June 28). Understanding difficulties and resulting confusion in learning: An integrative review. *Frontiers in Education, 3*. https://doi.org/10.3389/feduc.2018.00049
Maier, H. (2008). First and second order change: Powerful concepts in preparing child-care practitioners. *Journal of Children in Contemporary Society*. https://doi.org/10.1300/J274v17n03_04
McGhee, P. E. (1999). *Health, healing and the amuse system: Humor as survival training*. Kendall/Hunt.
McGuire, T., Dougherty, D. S., & Atkinson, J. (2006). "Paradoxing the dialectic:" The impact of patients' sexual harassment in the discursive construction of nurses' caregiving roles. *Management Communication Quarterly, 19*(3), 416–450. https://doi.org/10.1177/0893318905280879
Meltzoff, A. N., & Williamson, R. A. (2013). Imitation: Social, cognitive, and theoretical perspectives. In P. D. Zelazo (Ed.), *The Oxford handbook of developmental psychology (Vol. 1): Body and mind* (pp. 651–682). Oxford University Press.
Moser, J. S., Hartwig, R., Moran, T. P., Jendrusina, A. A., & Kross, E. (2014). Neural markers of positive reappraisal and their associations with trait reappraisal and worry. *Journal of Abnormal Psychology, 123*(1), 91–105.
Obradović, J., Sulik, M. J., & Shaffer, A. (2021). Learning to let go: Parental over-engagement predicts poorer self-regulation in kindergartners. *Journal of Family Psychology, 35*(8), 1160–1170. https://doi.org/10.1037/fam0000838
Papageorgiou, C., Stachtea, X., Papageorgiou, P., Alexandridis, T., Tsaltas, E., & Angelopoulos, E. (2016). Aristotle meets Zeno: Psychophysiological evidence. *PLoS One*, *11*, e0168017–e0168067. https://doi.org/10.1371/journal.pone.0168067

Roll, E. T., Cheng, W., & Feng, J. (2020). The orbitofrontal cortex: Reward, emotion, and depression. *Brain Communication, 16*(2), 196. https://doi.org/10.1093/braincomms/fcaa196; PMID: 33364600; PMCID: PMC7749795

Rutter, M. (1990). *Helping troubled children*. Plenum.

Solms, M., & Friston, K. (2018). How and why co nsciousness arises: Some considerations from physics and physiology. *Journal of Consciousness Studies, 25*(5–6), 202–238.

Suzuki, S., Fujisawa, T. X., Sakakibara, N., Fujioka, T., Takiguchi, S., & Tomoda, A. (2020). Development of social attention and oxytocin levels in maltreated children. *Scientific Reports, 10*(1), 7407. https://doi.org/10.1038/s41598-020-64297-6

Vogl, E., Pekrun, R., Murayama, K., & Loderer, K. (2020). Surprised-curious-confused: Epistemic emotions and knowledge exploration. *Emotion, 20*(4), 625–641. https://doi.org/10.1037/emo0000578

Widding, U. (2018). Parental determinism in the Swedish strategy for parenting. *Social Policy, & Society, 17*(3), 481–490. https://doi.org/10.1017/S1474746417000513

Williams, G. (2007). Helicopter parents. *Flickr*. https://www.flickr.com/photos/wikiworld comic/1236894043

Yerkes, M. A., Hopman, M., Stok, F. M., & De Wit, J. (2021). In the best interests of children? The paradox of intensive parenting and children's health. *Critical Public Health, 31*(3), 349–360. https://doi.org/10.1080/09581596.2019.1690632

GLOSSARY

Acculturation Individuals and families immigrating to a new culture go through a process of acculturation; stories aid in retaining the heritage and shared values of a subculture's original homeland.

Adaptability Ability to change when circumstances demand it.

Add-on Change A change that is not part of the essence of a thing.

Adlerian Model Nonpunitive approach to parenting based on the child learning to take responsibility for his/her actions.

Adolescence A period of child development marked by identity issues, ranging from teenage years to early 20s.

Adrenaline The excitement hormone.

Affiliative Humor Humor that is shared and creates bonding.

Aggressive Humor Aggressive humor, including sarcasm and certain forms of teasing and jokes, is used to enhance oneself at the expense of others' feelings. It is a way to feel superior and has an overall negative effect on prosocial behavior in that it results in hostility, depression, lower self-esteem, and lack of social support. *See* **Sarcasm.**

Aha Experience Describes a moment when the lack of insight quickly becomes this amazing new insight regarding the problem at hand, accompanied by newfound confidence and understanding.

Ambivalence Can be a frequent state in the parent–child relationship due to parental inconsistent verbal and modeling behavior.

Amygdala The part of the brain that is responsible for processing emotions like fear and stress.

Anterior Cingulate Cortex (ACC) Involved in detecting cognitive conflicts, or situations that cause confusion.

Antithesis Georg Hegel believed that the process of competing phenomena (i.e., thesis) and its opposite (i.e., antithesis) leads to a synthesis, which describes how change in humans and society take place. *See* **Synthesis** *and* **Thesis.**

Approach System The first parental system is the approach system. The brain secretes bonding hormones, such as oxytocin, that make it rewarding for parents to provide caregiving behaviors to their young child.

At-Risk Families Families below the poverty line with an inequity of resources available to them.

Attachment A bond between child and caregiver (usually the mother), which results from the quality of the caregiving.

Attachment Theory is Reductionistic Suggests that mental health issues prevalent in adulthood result from early childhood experiences.

Attachment Trauma Results from the caregiver not creating an optimum environment for attunement and persists because the caregiver does not repair the mis-attunement.

Attunement Thoughts and feelings of one individual that reflect similar thoughts and feelings of another individual.

Authoritarian Parenting Seeks to maintain control by closed and rigid communication patterns. Authoritarian parenting leads to children who lack initiative and have more problems at home and in a school setting.

Authoritative Parenting The most functional family style. Authoritative parenting is the most effective because it fosters trust; bidirectional, open communication patterns; and emotional attunement.

Autonomy The process of identity development. Power struggles in early childhood often revolve around issues related to physical autonomy, such as toileting, dressing, eating, and bedtime. Middle school-age children are in the process of developing their identities and seeking greater emotional autonomy. *See* **Power Struggles.**

Behavior Activation System The brain's activation system is roughly the reward system of the brain that is stimulated when positive emotions are numerous, and is referred to as the "dopaminergic reward circuit," which includes the nucleus accumbens, the ventral striatum, and the ventral tegmental area.

Behavioral Model A model that posits that children learn how to behave in social situations through others' positive or negative reinforcement.

Beneficial Lie Haley (1976) has been criticized for saying that it is acceptable to lie to families if it will facilitate change because it undermines the individual's right to be evaluated based on their individual behavior.

Bidirectionality Reciprocal interaction patterns that mutually affect each other.

Bidirectional Relationship Refers to a relationship that includes interrelated interactions and behaviors.

Bobo Doll Experiment To demonstrate that children learn from interaction patterns, Bandura initiated research that confirmed that when children witness violent actions by an adult, they are more prone to commit violent actions.

Borderline Personality Disorder A mental illness characterized by a general lack of consistent self-identity.

Boundary Alignment When rules of engagement align between persons.

Boundaries Barriers or rules between individual parts of a system, which determine the system's function, composition, and interaction among parts.

Brain-Based Parenting A term for applying neuroscience to parenting. It assumes that applying neuroscience research to specific parenting behaviors will result in better outcomes for children. *See* **Neuroparenting.**

Brain Plasticity Typically refers to the ability of the neural pathway connections in the brain, particularly those related to emotion and thought, to be altered by interactions with the environment or through implicit psychobiological processes. Psychotherapy grounded in nonverbal and implicit methods demonstrate that some level of brain plasticity continues throughout life and can amend earlier neural connections.

"Breaking the Will" "Breaking the will" of a child, or, breaking the will without breaking the spirit so that the child submits to parental authority, is associated with using harsh punishment. *See* **Harsh Parental Behavior.**

Bucharest Early Intervention Project (BEIP) This was a landmark study that began in 2001 and it demonstrated that experiences affect the development of the brain.

Change When Baxter and Montgomery (1998) use the word "change," they mean that things are always in flux. Change is not a value term and can be positive or negative depending on the circumstances.

Change without Change *See* **First Order Change.**

Character Perhaps the greatest effect in learning from storytelling is the use of characters since they allow for a human face to be put on facts or problems. *See* **Storytelling.**

Child Neglect and Abuse Parenting that does not meet the child's need or is harsh and physically punishing. *See* **Harsh Parental Behavior** *and* **Corporal Punishment.**

Circular Causality This is the belief that there is no linear progression of cause and effect due to the complex interactional patterns that characterize human nonlinear communication.

Cognition Rational thinking and perceptions. Referred to as "the way" by Berkman (2018).

Cognitive Dissonance Inconsistency between cognitions, beliefs, and behaviors.

Communication Models Categorize common communication patterns.

Conduct Disorder (CD) A challenging behavioral disorder that has its roots in early childhood and persists throughout the lifespan. *See* **Oppositional Defiant Disorder.**

Conference on the Welfare of the Child A conference under President Theodore Roosevelt addressing the responsibility of determining future pathways for children who resided outside their parents' homes.

Conflict Resolution The process of negotiating outcomes in a conflict.

Conscious Competency Ladder This model, which was developed six decades ago, is a good description of a generic approach to skill development.

Conscious Control Conscious control of thoughts is one of the developmental accomplishments that comes with aging.

Consciously Skilled Consciously skilled is the third stage of the conscious competency ladder and the beginning of learning new skills to replace automatic responses. *See* **Conscious Competency Ladder.**

Consciously Unskilled Becoming aware that a person's skills arc underdeveloped. For example, at this stage there is a realization that communication skills are poor, and the level of empathy is low amid other poor skills. *See* **Conscious Competency Ladder.**

Consistency Theory The typical way to create second order change is to use interventions that reduce or block the entrenched beliefs, or to allow for a context that permits new ideas to arise.

Continuity over Time Because temperament has a genetic component, it is reasonable to assume that research conducted in one time frame would apply to later research, but this assumption is somewhat nebulous and may change over time due to interactions with the parent.

Constitutive Change Part of the nature of a thing, in contrast to add-on change. *See* **Add-On Change.**

Contradiction Refers to the acknowledgment that any given point of view, belief, perspective, assumption, and the like have opposing positions that are equally valid.

Control Having power or control in a relationship has more to do with who guides the ever-evolving nature of the relationship, not who is most active. *See* **Power Struggles.**

Convergent Thinking Analyzing options to solve a particular problem and settling on one option considered to be the best.

Coping Humor A type of adolescent humor, which aids in adjusting to stressful events. For example, looking unkempt in a social setting is something that would otherwise cause embarrassment, but can be seen humorously to play off the embarrassment.

Corporal Punishment Physical punishment of the child, such as spanking.

Cortisol The stress hormone.

Creativity Spontaneous and unique actions or thoughts.

Critical Thinking Critical thinking is the ability to think rationally by weighting alternative positions and ideas and determining the most appropriate and useful position. It requires an unbiased mind.

Culture A system of patterned behavior where children grow and develop, and that is shared by their parents and community. This is a social background that consists of values and customs which bind together large groups in society.

Declarative Memory Declarative memory is conscious memory of past events and can be recalled from conscious awareness. This type of memory is not present during the first years of life when the infant is forming attachment relationships.

Deductive Reasoning Reasoning that occurs in a stepwise manner to a final premise.

Deep Learning When there is a mechanism for resolving the confusion.

Default Mode Network This is activated when an emotional response to artistic expression occurs.

Deferred Imitation Occurs when infants can recall preverbal memories of past events.

Deficit Approach This assumes that all participants have similar deficits and need the training that is either general or individualized for participants.

Democratic Families Democratic families allow for mutual respect and freedom, which gives the child a framework for learning that choices can have consequences.

Dialectical Thinking Dialectical thinking shares the concept of wholeness with systems theory and describes a process for change through contradiction, conflict, and oppositions.

Differentiation The balance between fusion and disengagement is labeled differentiation, the ability to emotionally separate while maintaining closeness.

Difficult Temperament Defined as the child having poor adaptability, a negative mood pattern, being withdrawn, and slowness in being calmed.

Diffuse Parenting A family with a diffuse boundary would allow anything in.

Direct Intervention First order change occurs due to direct interventions that are rational and understood by the participants.

Discipline Stories These address common concerns and challenges of children and are generally print stories. Discipline stories are different from fairy tales because the purpose of discipline stories is to change behavior in the present moment.

Discrepancy Theory Based on the view that when new information conflicts with old information, an emotional response occurs and a shift in thinking to the discrepant information follows. If discrepancies cannot be resolved quickly when there is a mismatch of incoming information with existing information, cognitive disequilibrium (or cognitive dissonance) occurs. *See* **Cognitive Dissonance.**

Disengaged Families with too little closeness are described as disengaged, which is characterized by lack of intimacy and emotional support.

Disinhibition Behaviors that are more likely to occur from observation.

Disparaging Humor A style of humor that is related to developmental issues for adolescents, and is associated with aggressive media.

Divergent Thinking Divergent thinking entails an open mindset and a recognition that beliefs, thoughts, or arguments can be seen from multiple points of view, generating multiple options.

Dopamine The pleasure hormone related to the reward system.

Dual Process Reasoning A model for understanding the brain process during deductive reasoning is dual process reasoning, which assumes integration of the two brain systems that cooperate in processing deductive reasoning. The first brain region is the quick automatic activation of the frontotemporal region that is associated with making judgments about what is true, and the second region is a slower network that activates the parieto-occipital and working memory.

Dunning–Kruger Effect A research study by Dunning and Kruger (1999), referred to as the Dunning–Kruger effect, illustrates that people are unaware of and inflate their perceived skill level. They showed that the lowest skill-level person rated themselves as being highly competent.

Dysregulation of Emotional Development Neuroscience research has demonstrated that dysregulation of emotional development occurs due to attachment trauma, or attachment disorder.

Easy Temperament Characterized as being adaptable, having a positive mood pattern, and easily soothed.

Ecological Learning This refers to how learning takes place within a nested system of influence from the child to the family, to the community, and to the culture.

Emotional Self-Regulation Central to the early relationship with the caregiver/mother, emotional self-regulation is the ability to monitor and control one's own emotional responses. The caregiver facilitates emotional regulation for the infant by responding with emotional attunement through gaze, facial expression, body posture, and tone of voice. As the child matures, emotion regulation moves from external control (the mother) to internal or self-regulation.

Emotional Thought Emotional thought is the platform where reasoning, emotion, and bodily states come together and where creativity emerges.

Emotionally Fused Families that are too close are described as emotionally fused, where members do not develop functional self-awareness or go through the process of individuation. *See* **Differentiation.**

Epigenesis The investigation of how genes interact with environmental factors.

Epinephrine Hormone related to the reward system.

Epistemic Emotions Emotions related to learning beliefs, such as surprise, confusion, and curiosity.

Equifinality Equifinality is a principle of systems theory based on the knowledge that a particular starting point can produce many outcomes, or vice versa that many starting points can produce a single outcome. Applied to parenting, the principle of equifinality suggests that inflexible parenting, which expects certain outcomes in their children, may be harmful to children in the long run.

Evidence-Based Research A study that builds on prior research to add significant contribution.

Excitatory Neurons One of the major types of cells in the brain. When viewing preferred, familiar input, the excitatory neurons were stimulated. *See* **Inhibitory Neurons.**

Expectations-Behavior Anticipation of future happenings.

Expected Behavior The life course includes behaviors that generally happen to all people within a culture.

Experiential Therapy An important aspect of Erickson's views about therapy is that it should be experiential, that is, therapy should involve action rather than merely providing didactic or intellectual input.

Explicit Conscious Process What one is aware of.

Extended Families The kinship network beyond the nuclear family.

Fairy Tales Within the folklore genre, fairy tales typically feature magic and mythical creatures.

Feedback As discussed in systemic theories, feedback is a vital component of the learning process, providing individuals with information about their performance and guiding their future actions. *See* **Feedback Loops.**

Feedback Loops Feedback loops between the system and the environment provide both new input from the environment and the system's response to the new input.

Felt Moments The process of change occurs in the here and now, through implicit and nonverbal communication.

Fiduciary Relationship The assumption that the client makes when they enter the therapeutic relationship is that the therapist is honest and has a fiduciary relationship with the client. *See* **Informed Consent Right.**

Fight or Flight Response The fight or flight response is meant to protect us when there is perceived danger.

First Order Change Change brought about by direct, conscious efforts to change the family dynamic.

First Order Parenting (FOP) First order parenting occurs due to first order change. *See* **First Order Change.**

Formal Operations A concept of Piaget where the child begins to reason in a more complex manner.

Formal Rule Approach Posits that deduction is a linguistic process activated in the left hemisphere governed by a set of linguistic rules.

Formalized Skill-Building Exercises Predetermined and packaged modules that can be done online.

Frontotemporal Network The frontotemporal network is an essential element in the understanding of paradoxes and other nonliteral forms of language, such as metaphors.

Gelotology The study of laughter.

Genes Heritable DNA.

Global Attachment Emerging research on attachment is labeled global attachment, which characterizes the way a person generally relates to important people in his/her life.

"Go Slow" Intervention The "go slow" intervention is used to put the family in a therapeutic double-bind where whatever the family does will have positive outcomes.

Goals Outcomes that would not have happened unless an intervention occurred.

Good Parenting Good parenting comes from parents who have developed skills from expert training. It is related to positive outcomes in children, which prepares them to function effectively within their sphere of influence of family and friends.

Goodness of Fit In the parent–child relationship, goodness of fit refers to how well the child's temperament fits with the temperament of the parent.

Gray Matter Important for processing information from the connections in the brain. Gray matter seems especially important early in development. *See* **White Matter.**

Harsh Parental Behavior Harsh parental behavior, such as hitting, yelling, and constant anger at a child, results in smaller brains in adolescence and derailed social and emotional development. *See* **Child Neglect and Abuse** *and* **Corporal Punishment.**

Head Start The UK program Sure Start and the US program Head Start were aimed at poor, uneducated parents. *See* **Sure Start.**

Herbaika Cards Created to increase cognitive development.

Hierarchy Hierarchy is a principle of systems theory that demonstrates the organizational structure of a system; that is, a system is organized from the least to the most complex.

Hippocampus A brain region that is crucial for memory and learning, and is engaged when individuals attempt to reconcile their existing knowledge with new, contradictory information.

Homeostasis Homeostasis, or equilibrium, defines the desire and attempt on the part of a system to maintain a steady state.

Human Growth Hormone Hormones related to increasing genetic material.

Humor An experience that is pleasant, metaphoric, and paradoxical.

Humor Styles Questionnaire A questionnaire that categorizes types of humor.

Hypothalamic Pituitary Axis Regulates stress in the body.

Imitation Children learn from observing parents and others in their sphere of influence, imitating the observed behaviors.

Impasse Theory of Learning When an impasse is experienced in learning, a person will feel confused, which will lead to efforts to resolve the confusion. In a confused state, the person must curtail activity, rethink the present circumstances, and engage in problem-solving.

Implicit Unconscious Process Actions and thoughts that are outside of awareness.

Incongruity Resolution Theory Incongruity resolution theory is a theory of humor based on the process involved in resolving an inconsistent experience. When the joke is understood, the resolution brings a feeling of satisfaction, like solving a problem.

Incredible Years Program This is an evidence-based parenting education program that offers individual programs for parents with infants (0–1), toddlers (1–3), preschoolers (3–6), and school-age children (6–12).

Incremental Change A change that progresses over time with the goal to create an outcome that does not alter the system.

Independent Entities No interaction among entities.

Indirect Parenting Techniques Interventions by the parent that are hidden and that alter behaviors without conscious focus.

Infant Sociability Infant sociability refers to the degree to which infants respond to their parents.

Informed Consent Right The concern about ethics in therapy centers on the informed consent right of the client who has a right to know the treatment and procedures used by the therapist. *See* **Fiduciary Relationship.**

Inhibition Refers to behaviors that are less likely to be mimicked.

Inhibitory Neurons One of the major types of cells in the brain. Inhibitory neurons are more active when novel input is introduced. *See* **Excitatory Neurons.**

Insecure Attachment Children with insecure attachment tend to have parents who have not dealt with their upbringings and who often make the same mistakes that their parents made with them. *See* **Life Narrative.**

Instructional Humor Processing Theory (IHPT) Posits that students must first cognitively process and judge the appropriateness of the humor and determine if the humor enhances the recall of information.

Internalization A child internalizes what is observed from those who are in close contact; these internalized observations become the source for the child's memory and automatic behaviors.

Inuits Native inhabitants of Anarchical.

Joining Joining the family system means that the therapist must adopt their language and style and be able to play a role in the family.

Jokes A type of humor, typically told verbally, that includes a story with a funny punchline.

Learning Learning is accompanied by emotional responses due in part to the integration of new knowledge with old knowledge.

Less of the Same Change in behavior so that a person behaves differently than the regularly expected behavior.

Life Narrative If a person can tell their life story, showing both positive and negative events and connecting them to their later development, they tend to develop a secure attachment style. *See* **Insecure Attachment** *and* **Secure Attachment.**

Limbic System Emotional and memory center of brain.

Listening with the Third Ear In therapy, the therapist should pay close attention to what the client *avoids* saying, which can be referred to as "listening with the third ear."

Logical Consequences Logical consequences do not follow directly from the children's behavior like a natural consequence, but describe the relationship between statements and action, acting as a true consequence of the behavior. *See* **Natural Consequences.**

Long-Term Potentiation For new experiences to be recalled, the process of long-term potentiation (or the continuous, strengthening of neural connections) must occur while simultaneously remaining flexible to accommodate new information.

Memory Memory plays a central role in learning, as it involves the encoding, storage, and retrieval of information. *See* **Hippocampus.**

Memory Reconsolidation The process of replacing old memory that affects current functioning.

Mental Model Theory A theory for how the brain processes deductive reasoning, which views deductive reasoning as a visuospatial procedure grounded in rule-based processes where a spatial depiction of the symptomatic problem is made. *See* **Deductive Reasoning.**

Metaphor A figure of speech that is applied to an object or action that cannot be taken literally. Metaphors are symbolic language that relates ideas and powerful influential messages indirectly.

Mindfulness The art of being present in the moment.

Mind-Wandering The state of the mind when it is at rest or unfocused.

Mirror Neurons Mirror neurons, discovered over 20 years ago in studies with macaques, are activated both by doing an activity and by observing an activity, while other motor neurons are activated only by motor action or observation.

Misbehavior Defined by the parent when the child knowingly refuses to comply with parental wishes. *See* **Resistance.**

More of the Same Repeating an action and being reluctant to change it.

Morphogenesis Morphogenesis depicts change within the system and is the opposite of homeostasis. *See* **Homeostasis.**

Motivation Referred to as "the will" by Berkman (2018).

Moynihan Report A report that discussed the vulnerability of at-risk Black families in the 1960s. *See* **At-Risk Families.**

Narrative Brain The aspect of the brain that is active when one is engaged in literary activities.

Natural Consequences Actions occurring in response to the child's behavior without parental involvement, which are imposed by nature, society, or another person. *See* **Logical Consequences.**

Near-Infrared Spectroscopy (NIRS) A common practice for studying the brains of young children.

Negative Brain Bias The brain is geared toward forming memories from bad experiences that are then influential in directing behavior.

Negative Emotionality Negative emotionality refers to the infant having predominantly fear, anger, and distrust in the relationship with the parent. *See* **Positive Emotionality.**

Neuroparenting Neuroparenting is defined as child-rearing practices that are based on neuroscience research. *See* **Brain-Based Parenting.**

No-Lose Approach A principle in PET that considers both the parents' and the child's position. *See* **Parent Effectiveness Training (PET).**

Nondeclarative Memory Nondeclarative memory is present from birth and is characterized as learning that takes place outside of conscious awareness.

Nondirective A change that is initiated by the client and not by the therapist.

Nonlinear and Holistic *See* **Second Order Change** *and* **Ecological Learning.**

Nonlinear Interactional Pattern A pattern of interaction in which parents do not express anger toward children, which can be effective in creating a healthy and functional system.

Nonnormative Change Unexpected change, such as caused by accidents, illness, or economic status changes.

Normative Change Expected developmental change.

Novelty Unexpected change.

Nuclear Family Parents and child(ren) united by partnership and parenthood.

Nurturance Being warm and affectionate, one of the major parenting behaviors.

Nurturing Fathers' Program A program that consists of 2.5-hour sessions for 13 weeks. Fathers are exposed to nurturing interventions which can enhance their ability to communicate more effectively and be a more involved family member.

Observation Observation is the key to learning for young children. Parent education models typically do not emphasize observation as an intervention. Observation includes how the client uses language, expresses emotions, displays nonverbal gestures, and engages in recurring behavioral patterns.

Oppositional Defiant Disorder (ODD) A challenging behavioral disorder that has its roots in early childhood and persists throughout the lifespan. *See* **Conduct Disorder.**

Oral Storytelling Verbal stories passed down through the generations.

Orienting System Surprise activates the body's orienting system, resulting in increased nervous system stimulation, increased heart rate, and greater attention to new input.

Overconfidence A cognitive bias that leads individuals to overestimate their abilities, knowledge, or judgment.

Oxytocin A hormone and neuropeptide.

Paradigm Shifts When an accepted paradigm is challenged by new ideas that give better answers than the old ideas, a shift takes place.

Paradox Something that appears obviously false or contradictory on one level, but, when investigated, turns out to be true on another level. It may appear illogical and irrational since it contradicts one's expectation, but the paradoxical situation, person, or thing changes behavior in a positive direction.

Parent Education Education that trains parents to better understand parenting behaviors.

Parent Effectiveness Training (PET) Emphasizes communication between the child and parent.

Parental Determinism The belief that parents are both the cause and cure for the child's problems.

Parental Executive System This is based on the belief that parents can make conscious efforts to control negative and emotional responses.

Parental Meaning-Making Domain According to Hughes and Baylin (2012), if parents lack maturity and self-awareness, they will inevitably negatively affect their children.

Parental Reading System How adequately the parent can understand verbal and nonverbal communication.

Parental Resistance Parental resistance includes both (1) parents who model bad behavior and refuse to see the connection of their behavior and the problems with their child, and (2) parents who mean well, but are limited in their efforts to change.

Parental Reward System The parental reward system is activated by the release of oxytocin which stimulates the production of dopamine and the orbitofrontal cortex and the nucleus accumbens.

Parental Values The involvement of parents to hold the outcomes of their children in high regard.

Parenting Experts Anyone who portrays themselves as having professional knowledge of parenting.

Parenting Schema A parenting schema is a framework for behaviors toward children, which includes nurturing and disciplining behavior.

Permissive Parenting In permissive parenting style, parents allow for open communication but do not exert control over the child's behavior. The downside is that children of permissive parenting have issues with authority figures and may refuse to take responsibility for their actions.

Perry Preschool Project A longitudinal study that followed participants into their 20s, providing an intensive preschool educational program for poverty-level children.

Personality Personality is the term that is most often used for temperament as the child matures. It refers to the internal characteristics of a person, including his/her psychological makeup, moods, and disposition.

Person-Centered Identifying the elements of the child's temperament, and matching or not matching with parental practices. *See* **Goodness of Fit** *and* **Variable-Centered Method.**

Picture Book Stories Children's story books with descriptive pictures.

Positive Discipline Interventions Interventions that are nonpunitive.

Positive Emotionality Refers to the infant's ability to interact with the parent and the environment free of apprehension and fear. *See* **Negative Emotionality.**

Positive Parenting Program Referred to as the "Triple P," this model is a skills training integrative parenting approach that pulls from cognitive behavioral theory, social learning theory, and developmental components.

Positive Power of the Unconscious Unlike the conscious mind, Erickson believed that the unconscious operated on metaphors, stories, and imagination and he used them to facilitate the change process.

Positive Thinking An attitude of general optimism that one develops from a focus on thoughts that are conducive to healthy outcomes in mind and body.

Postmodern Thinkers Modern-day postmodern thinkers claim that there is no objective truth, and, therefore, all truth is relative. The claim that "all truth is relative" is itself an objective truth. This is a paradox. *See* **Paradox.**

Poverty Describes families who are below a certain monetary measure for minimal standard of living.

Power of Suggestion Milton Erickson used a novel approach to induce hypnotic states that were paradoxical in nature, which were intended to change clients by facilitating change, not by directing the outcome.

Power Struggles When persons test their status in the relationship by opposing rather than cooperating with each other. A power struggle between children and parents is when they have different agendas; they are not on the same page; and there is a battle over identity, values, or needs.

Predictive Mind Theory A recent development in neuroscience, labeled "predictive mind," is based on evidence that the brain is geared toward predicting future personal and social outcomes. The predictive mind theory embraces the ideas that (1) the primary brain orientation is about future social and personal outcomes, which occurs automatically, and (2) consciousness is only activated when predication fails.

Prefrontal Cortex The prefrontal cortex, known for cognitive functions, is the most affected brain region from sleep loss.

Prescribing the Symptom In the process whereby paradoxes cause second order change, the therapist prescribes the symptom by instructing the client to enact the problem behavior they want to avoid. *See* **Paradox** *and* **Second Order Change.**

Pretend Play Defined as play occurring in a narrative or story in which various objects represent other things. In pretend play, a child uses divergent thinking within a story narrative to create a fantasy where an object can symbolize other objects or characters. *See* **Divergent Thinking.**

Preventative Ounce Temperament Program This is a skills-based program that evaluates both the parents' and the child's temperament.

Priming The presentation of information that is not consciously perceived by the subject.

Process of the Problem What maintains the problem.

Prosocial Behavior Behavior of positive outcomes toward others.

Protective Function of the Child's Symptoms The child's misbehavior is an attempt to keep the focus on the child, rather than have the focus rest on a more serious problem between the parents.

Punitive Discipline Dysfunctional discipline methods, such as corporal punishment. *See* **Corporal Punishment.**

Qualitative, Irreversible Change Second order change is a qualitative, irreversible change in which there is a discontinuous process. *See* **Second Order Change.**

Quantitative Change Change that can be measured.

Reattachment The process of reattachment as an implicit and nonconscious process is not clearly articulated. Attachment and reattachment are not direct, rational processes.

Reframing Changing the context of a situation so that it also changes the meaning. Reframing is a frequent technique used by systemic therapists in the treatment of families and children.

Relative Openness A reflexive system.

Relational Dialectical Theory Refers to how contradictions and conflicts are structurally engrained in interpersonal interactions, especially in romantic and marital relationships.

Relief Theory A theory of humor which was first popularized by Spencer (1911) and based on the implicit meaning in the physiology of laughter, rather than the content of the joke. He concluded laughter was the release of pent-up emotions and subsequent increase of energy.

Redundancy Principle Repeatable patterns of interaction that occur without conscious awareness. *See* **Rules.**

Resistance While change in mind and behavior is the goal of parent education, change may not be welcomed by all participants. Resistance is what occurs when the changes are challenged.

Resilient Perseverance despite negative circumstances.

Responsible Fatherhood (RF) Program This is a federally funded program that works primarily with fathers who are currently incarcerated, or fathers reentering society who have been involved in the criminal justice system.

Reward Network The part of the brain that processes and secretes brain chemicals, such as dopamine.

Right Hemisphere The right hemisphere is associated with the formation of memory, and the development of implicit and nonconscious processes. It develops first and is associated with the development of attachment between infant and caregiver.

Right Lateralized Brain Beginning in childhood and continuing throughout the lifespan, the right lateralized brain components are integral in unconscious affective processes.

Roles In parenting, roles can be explicit or implicit, the same or complementary. Unacknowledged rules set the tone for roles. For instance, nurturing and disciplining behaviors tend to be complementary.

Rope-a-Dope The term "rope-a-dope" was coined by Muhammad Ali to describe his strategy for defeating George Frazier. The term is metaphorically applied in this book to describe how parents can withdraw from certain situations with their children. Parental withdrawal is confusing because parents, in essence, are seemingly giving over control to their child, creating the fear that their child will dominate them.

Rules Rules refer to repeatable patterns of interaction that occur without conscious awareness. *See* **Redundancy Principle.**

Salience Level A level of acceptance where important questions are answered.

Sarcasm One type of humor that adults engage in often is sarcasm, which is caustic and can increase the emotional pain a child is feeling about a certain circumstance.

Schemas Basic unconscious patterns for categorizing and understanding actions and behavior.

Schizophrenia A mental illness characterized by poor reasoning, hallucinations, and distorted perceptions.

Scientific Approach to Parenting This led to the belief that the children's behaviors could be understood from the application of scientific methods.

Seanchaí In Ireland, the itinerant seanchaí were storytellers who moved from one community to the next telling stories of honor and ageless knowledge. Telling stories of past heroes, such as kings, the seanchaí embellished historic myths and spawned national pride.

Second Order Change Second order change refers to changes that occur unconsciously or implicitly.

Second Order Parenting (SOP) Second order parenting occurs due to second order changes. *See* **Second Order Change.**

Secure Attachment Secure attachment in one's children, as it turns out, is highly correlated with how the parents positively dealt with and processed their own upbringing.

Self-Defeating Humor Humor that undermines one's goals and status.

Self-Efficacy Self-efficacy is rooted in a sense of power and control. Children's sense of power is rooted in their need to have control over themselves rather than control over parents. *See* **Power Struggles** *and* **Emotional Self-Regulation.**

Self-Enhancing Humor Promoting the self at the expense of others through humor.

Self-Help Approach Books and pamphlets that give advice on self-improvement.

Self-Image How one views oneself.

Self-Schooling Higher social class parents had more technical equipment and felt more confident in their role of self-schooling, and their children were engaged in more activities that were conducive to learning.

Skill-Building Teaches parents new behaviors that improve interactions with their child.

Smith–Lever Act In 1914, Congress passed the Smith–Lever Act, which established Cooperative Extension between land grant universities and the US Department of Agriculture for the creation and dissemination of resource materials.

Social Class It is well established from many research studies that social class is an important variable for outcomes with children.

Social Cognitive Model The social cognitive model of Albert Bandura (1977) is based on the belief that learning occurs when children observe and imitate their parents and others around them.

Social Contagion Humor has a social contagion factor; expressed in a group setting, humor has social effects that are not present in individual expressions. Humor promotes a feeling of well-being within the group and increases relaxation and acceptance among others. *See* **Humor.**

Social–Emotional Development The ability to form meaningful relationships with parents and others.

Socialization The process of socialization is fluid, continually changing, and adapts over the lifespan.

Sociocultural Theory This is another perspective on learning by observation, which was developed by Vygotsky (1978), who believed that children learn by social interactions that can be outside of conscious awareness. The interactions occur within a precise social and cultural setting.

Solutions Becoming the Problem Trying to solve problems with methods that do not work but nevertheless are continued.

Somatotopic Map The outer portion of the brain in which different areas of the body are reflected in specific areas of the brain.

STAR Parenting Program The underlying theoretical base of this program is cognitive behavioral theory, influenced heavily by the writings of Baumrind (1966) on authoritative parenting.

Story Drama The main idea behind the action and plots of a story.

Stranger Situation Paradigm The initial testing of Bowlby's attachment theory was done by Ainsworth et al. (1978). Several scenes occur where the mother is present with the infant and is replaced by a stranger and then returned to the room. Of primary concern in the stranger situation test was how the infant reacted when separated from and reunited with the mother.

Strengthening Families Program for Parents and Youth (10–14) The SFP 10–14 parenting education program is a seven-session parenting program based on combining two approaches that support healthy family development: (1) the biopsychosocial model and (2) the risk and prevention model.

Stress in Parenting When there is heightened stress, parents lack the ability to parent children without negative consequences.

Subjective Value The value a person places on thoughts and actions.

Subsystems Subsystems are created in the family to regulate emotional closeness and distance, which include the spousal subsystem, the sibling subsystem, and the parent–child subsystem. Each subsystem has different functions within the family unit and contributes to the overall quality of family relationships.

Superiority Theory A theory of humor that posits there is an element in humor that delights in making fun of others who are perceived to be different or inferior.

Sure Start The UK program Sure Start and the US program Head Start were aimed at poor, uneducated parents. *See* **Head Start.**

Synthesis The combination of thesis and antithesis. *See* **Thesis** *and* **Antithesis.**

System A unit consisting of interacting parts that make up a whole.

Systemic Approach Understanding human behavior as stemming from the interaction patterns within a group.

Systemic Therapy The application of general systems theory to individual and family problems.

Teasing Teasing is a type of humor discipline that acts as social control because it focuses on a desired social skill within groups.

Temperament Temperament is the contribution that children make to the interactions they have with parents, resulting in their own developmental trajectories. *See* **Personality.**

Theory of Mind What is produced by stories is a theory of mind, and the more that younger children are exposed to stories, the more developed their theory of mind is.

Therapeutic Double-Bind Placing a person in a catch-22 where any action on their part is an improvement. *See* Paradox.

Thesis The first statement or position. *See* **Antithesis** *and* **Synthesis.**

Threat Response The threat response occurs because humans desire the status quo and any change to the status quo causes a painful response.

Transformational Change A change that is noncontinuous with the past. *See* **Second Order Change.**

Unconscious Learning Term alluded to by Furedi; he stated that learning does not have to be taught. In fact, he did not believe that parents can learn how to parent from reading books or gleaning advice from experts. Children learn how to behave from the relationship with parents, and parents learn how to parent through their interactions with others.

Unconsciously Skilled The final stage in the Conscious Competency Ladder, which comes after much practice when the skills become natural and automatic. *See* **Conscious Competency Ladder.**

Unconsciously Unskilled The first step in the Conscious Competency Ladder, which states that, in general, persons are unskilled but do not have conscious awareness of it. *See* **Conscious Competency Ladder.**

Uninvolved Parenting In uninvolved parenting, children tend to be on their own because their parents offer no guidance. Children of uninvolved parents lack self-control and have more behavior problems than children raised by parents employing one of the other parenting styles.

Unity of Entities This term describes how things are bound together and cannot be separated into individual parts.

Utilization Approach Using what the client offers about themselves or their problems.

Variable-Centered Method A method used by researchers to test the goodness of fit. *See* **Goodness of Fit.**

White Matter White matter is necessary for forming connections across the brain. *See* **Gray Matter.**

Wholeness The concept of wholeness depicts the family as a unit of interactional parts that mutually affect each other.

Working Model This is an unconscious mental process that influences conscious actions in adulthood.

"Yes" Environment Creating a "yes" environment creates an entire atmosphere of emotional support, opening young, developing brains to receiving new experiences.

"Zero to Three" Movement Refers to the formative years for later development.

INDEX